Biomaterials

Innovation for world healthcare

Online at: https://doi.org/10.1088/978-0-7503-5187-4

IOP Series in Global Health and Radiation Oncology

Series editor

Wilfred Ngwa
Dana-Farber/Harvard Cancer Center, University of Massachusetts Lowell, Johns Hopkins University, USA

Editor biography

Wilfred Ngwa is the Director of the Global Health Catalyst, a cross-institutional collaboration initiative launched at Harvard to catalyse high impact collaborations in global health. He currently serves as Adjunct Professor at the University of Massachusetts, as Associate Professor of Radiation Oncology at Johns Hopkins University and as ICTU Distinguished Professor of Public Health. He is a chair of the Lancet Oncology Commission for Sub-Saharan Africa, has published three books on global health and serves on the editorial board of a number of journals, including ASCO's *Journal of Global Oncology, Ecancermedicalsciences*, and *Frontiers in Oncology*. He has won many awards from Harvard, the USA National Institutes of Health, and international professional organisations for his innovations and leading work in global health to address disparities in the USA and globally.

Aims and scope

This series includes books in the emerging area of global radiation oncology and its applications in global health. Building on the published book by the series editor entitled *Emerging Models for Global Health in Radiation Oncology*, it will further detail the work being done globally to promote cancer research and awareness, particularly in lower-income countries.

A full list of titles published in this series can be found here: https://iopscience.iop.org/bookListInfo/iop-series-in-cancer-research-for-global-radiation-oncology#series.

Biomaterials

Innovation for world healthcare

Mohan Edirisinghe
Department of Mechanical Engineering, University College London, London, UK

Merve Gultekinoglu
Department of Nanotechnology and Nanomedicine, Graduate School of Science and Engineering, Hacettepe University, Ankara, Turkey

Jubair Ahmed
Department of Mechanical Engineering, University College London, London, UK

IOP Publishing, Bristol, UK

ISBN 978-0-7503-5187-4 (ebook)
ISBN 978-0-7503-5185-0 (print)
ISBN 978-0-7503-5188-1 (myPrint)
ISBN 978-0-7503-5186-7 (mobi)

DOI 10.1088/978-0-7503-5187-4

Version: 20240201

IOP ebooks

British Library Cataloguing-in-Publication Data: A catalogue record for this book is available from the British Library.

Published by IOP Publishing, wholly owned by The Institute of Physics, London

IOP Publishing, No.2 The Distillery, Glassfields, Avon Street, Bristol, BS2 0GR, UK

US Office: IOP Publishing, Inc., 190 North Independence Mall West, Suite 601, Philadelphia, PA 19106, USA

To Taylor Alejandría Castilleja. The light of my life.

—Jubair Ahmed

Contents

Preface xi

Author biographies xii

1 The concept and manufacture of a new generation of biomaterials based on global healthcare needs 1-1

References 1-9

2 Microfluidic manufacturing 2-1

2.1 The principles of microfluidics 2-1

2.1.1 The history of microfluidics 2-1

2.1.2 Fluid dynamics in microfluidics 2-3

2.2 Materials used in microfluidic chip development 2-6

2.2.1 Inorganic materials 2-7

2.2.2 Organic materials 2-10

2.2.3 Hybrid materials 2-14

2.3 Microfluidic chip development technologies 2-15

2.3.1 Photolithography 2-16

2.3.2 Soft lithography 2-18

2.3.3 Three-dimensional printing 2-19

2.3.4 Milling 2-21

2.3.5 Hot embossing 2-23

2.3.6 Injection moulding 2-24

2.4 Microfluidic reactors 2-27

2.4.1 Mixing microfluidic reactors 2-27

2.4.2 Droplet-based microfluidic reactors 2-30

2.4.3 Multiple-field microfluidic reactors 2-34

2.5 Applications of microfluidic bio-fabrication 2-36

2.5.1 Microbubbles 2-36

2.5.2 Nanoparticles 2-51

2.6 Microfluidics for biological applications 2-65

2.6.1 Microfluidics for omics technologies 2-65

2.6.2 Microfluidics in gene therapy 2-67

2.6.3 Microfluidics in protein separation 2-70

2.7	Lab-on-a-chip diagnostic applications	2-73
	2.7.1 Paper-based microfluidic biosensors	2-74
	2.7.2 Microcirculation-based sensors	2-79
2.8	The future scope of microfluidic technology	2-83
	References and further reading	2-84
3	**Electrohydrodynamic manufacturing**	**3-1**
3.1	The principles of electrohydrodynamics	3-1
	3.1.1 Fluid dynamics in EHD	3-2
	3.1.2 Electric field in EHD systems	3-3
3.2	Material properties used in EHD	3-4
	3.2.1 Viscosity	3-4
	3.2.2 Dielectric properties	3-5
	3.2.3 Solvent evaporation kinetics	3-6
	3.2.4 Shear stress	3-6
3.3	Electrohydrodynamic fabrication techniques	3-9
	3.3.1 Electrohydrodynamic atomisation	3-9
	3.3.2 Direct writing	3-14
3.4	Electrohydrodynamic fabrication products	3-16
	3.4.1 Particles	3-17
	3.4.2 Fibres	3-19
3.5	Electrohydrodynamic technology-based biomedical engineering	3-23
	3.5.1 Tissue engineering	3-23
	3.5.2 Drug delivery	3-31
	3.5.3 Wound dressings	3-36
	3.5.4 Implant modification	3-42
	3.5.5 Surface patterning	3-45
3.6	Perspectives on the future development of electrohydrodynamic technology	3-47
	References	3-49
4	**Gyratory processes for manufacturing**	**4-1**
4.1	Centrifugal spinning	4-1
4.2	Pressurised gyration	4-3
	4.2.1 The principles of pressurised gyration	4-3
4.3	The operating parameters of pressurised gyration	4-6
	4.3.1 Rotational speed	4-6

	4.3.2 Gas pressure	4-7
	4.3.3 Collection setup	4-7
4.4	The physics behind pressurised gyration	4-9
	4.4.1 The effects of rotational speed without gas pressure	4-9
	4.4.2 The effects of gas pressure on fluid physics	4-10
4.5	The applications of pressurised gyration fibres	4-11
	4.5.1 Drug delivery	4-12
	4.5.2 Tissue engineering	4-31
	4.5.3 Filtration	4-50
4.6	Materials exploited by pressurised gyration	4-57
	4.6.1 Natural materials for wound healing	4-57
	4.6.2 Graphene	4-66
	4.6.3 Self-healing materials	4-76
	4.6.4 Composite materials	4-79
4.7	The morphologies produced using pressurised gyration	4-84
	4.7.1 The effect of the solvent on the morphology	4-84
	4.7.2 Beaded fibres	4-88
	4.7.3 The surface features of PG fibres	4-89
	4.7.4 Microbubbles for diagnostics	4-94
4.8	Variants of pressurised gyration	4-98
	4.8.1 Infusion gyration	4-98
	4.8.2 Melt-pressurised gyration	4-102
	4.8.3 Core–sheath pressurised gyration	4-106
	4.8.4 Nozzle pressurised gyration	4-113
4.9	The future scope of pressurised gyration	4-114
	References	4-115
5	**Future perspectives**	**5-1**
5.1	Biomaterials in healthcare	5-1
	5.1.1 Industrial scale-up	5-1
	5.1.2 Energy usage	5-2
	5.1.3 Environmental considerations	5-2
	5.1.4 Drug delivery	5-2
	5.1.5 Biosensors	5-3
	5.1.6 Regenerative medicine and tissue engineering	5-4
	5.1.7 Cell encapsulation	5-4
	5.1.8 Graphene and its derivatives	5-5

5.1.9 Artificial intelligence and machine learning 5-5
5.1.10 Soft robotics 5-6
5.2 The future of microfluidic technologies 5-6
5.3 The future of electrohydrodynamic technologies 5-7
5.4 The future of gyration-based manufacturing techniques 5-9

Preface

Materials Science & Engineering (MSE) has come a long way in the past decades and its development has contributed hugely to applications in the biomedical field. We as authors have a particular interest in these applications and as such, greatly believe that biomaterials are the future for a world where sustainability in terms of both environmental and from a materials standpoint can be achieved. The golden rule of MSE is that the composition leads to product forming which influences the microstructure. The microstructure of any material determines its properties and use cases. A more appropriate way to bind the relationship between material composition and properties, is through manufacture (scaled up production) alongside processing and forming.

This book is intended to introduce a few key methods of biomaterials manufacturing which takes into account our joint experience in the field. By reading this book, you will come to learn some of the key developments in the field of biomaterials science, biomedical engineering and other such intertwined disciplines which aim to leverage MSE to overcome many of the medical-related issues faced in everyday life. The book has a particular focus in the manufacturing of materials for healthcare applications; we have worked on this for decades and have realised the potential of microscale and nanoscale polymeric materials for a vast range of healthcare applications that range from tissue engineering and drug delivery to medical imaging and targeted gene therapy. Here we show the developments of such materials which include bubbles, particles and fibres.

We hope that by going through this work, you will have a better understanding of the current developments in what we term a new generation of biomaterials, being the morphologies of microbubbles, particles and fibres and make you ever more aware to the possibility of further developments, both in terms of manufacturing and the advancement in material choice and suitability while focusing on sustainability.

Author biographies

Mohan Edirisinghe

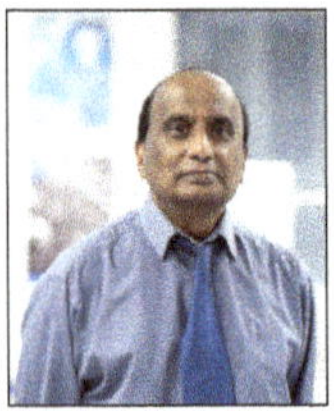

Mohan Edirisinghe, holds the Bonfield Chair of Biomaterials, within the Mechanical Engineering Department at University College London. He has published 600 journal papers (H-index of 72 with over 19 000 citations) and over a dozen key patents, given more than 125 invited/keynote lectures worldwide. He has supervised over 250 researchers including over 100 PhD graduations and he has been awarded grants to the value of £25 million, which have given him the opportunity to adventurously explore novel avenues of scaled-up forming of advanced materials for application in key areas such as healthcare. In 2015 was elected as a Fellow of the Royal Academy of Engineers in the UK. In 2020 he was elected a Fellow of the European Academy of Sciences and in 2021 he was appointed OBE (Order of the British Empire) for his services to Biomedical Engineering. He has won many awards for his research, in 2023 he was awarded two prizes: The RAEng Colin Campbell Mitchell Prize for his world-leading contribution to the industrial application of polymeric fibres by inventing novel fibre manufacturing vessels and processes, and The Royal Society Clifford Paterson Medal & Lecture Prize for his seminal research in engineering science of making small structures from soft matter in novel scalable ways, creating new frontiers in functional applications causing major advances in manufacturing and healthcare.

Merve Gultekinoglu

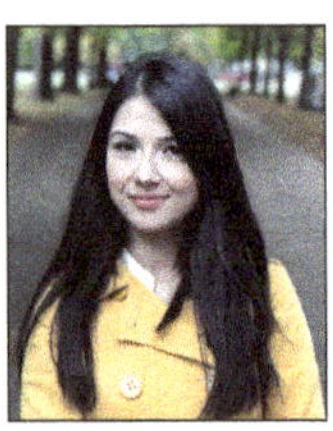

Merve Gultekinoglu, is an assistant professor at Hacettepe University in Ankara, Turkey, Department of Nanotechnology and Nanomedicine. Having studied BSc in Chemistry, she completed her MSc and PhD in the Department of Bioengineering at Hacettepe University. She completed her PhD in 2019 in the field of polymer synthesis and processing for fibre based-tissue scaffold manufacturing. Her research is in the field of biomaterials and tissue engineering with emphasis on polymer synthesis-modification, antibacterial systems, drug delivery systems, active targeting, tissue engineering and biofabrication techniques. In 2021, she won the Hacettepe University the Science Encouragement Award in the field of Medicine and Health. She is an active working group member of the European Union COST actions and focuses on new natural polymer classes and green synthesis methods in the fields of biomaterials and tissue engineering.

Jubair Ahmed

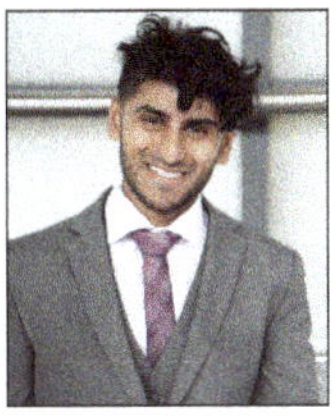

Jubair Ahmed, is a postdoctoral researcher at University College London. Having studied undergraduate Biochemistry at The University of Westminster, he went on to complete a MSc in Biomaterials & Tissue Engineering at University College London where he graduated top of his class, for which he was awarded the Armourers and Brasiers' Biomaterials Medal. Having completed his PhD in 2022, his research has focussed on the manufacturing of advanced into biomaterials which have various applications in biomedical engineering. To date, he has published 24 journal papers, with four journal front covers, a H-index of 11 and over 500 citations. His work has been published in leading journals such as in Biotechnology Advances and Langmuir. He believes that public engagement, especially via the use of non-conventional and modern mediums such as e-information sharing platforms and social media is the way forward in increasing public engagement in science.

Chapter 1

The concept and manufacture of a new generation of biomaterials based on global healthcare needs

Work on biomaterials has progressed for about six decades, and major developments have been made. Conventional biomaterials incorporating metals, ceramics, polymers, and their composites have ushered in new generations of biomaterials. However, the scale-up of laboratory innovations to the manufacturing stage is falling behind. This chapter elucidates some of these key developments *but then alerts the reader to the fact that this book is dedicated to a different new generation of biomaterials: small structures made from soft matter, mainly bubbles, particles, and fibres, and particularly their scalable manufacture for healthcare applications—innovative mass production manufacturing processes that work for the benefit of patients.*

History reveals that biomaterials are a type of functional material whose application in the human body is beneficial. Biomaterials have been investigated for about six decades and they are traditionally classified as biometals, bioceramics, biopolymers, and biocomposites. Titanium is a good example of a biometal, as it can be used in musculoskeletal applications. Hydroxyapatite is a well-known bioceramic which is also bioactive rather than simply being biocompatible. It is extensively used in orthopaedics, in which cellular entities such as osteoblasts are attracted by its presence; it therefore promotes a specific biological response at the surface of the material, thus actively encouraging the formation of a bond between body tissues and the material. The bioglass used in dental repair and toothpastes is another example. There are many polymers that are classified as biomaterials and even as biodegradable materials. Poly(lactic-*co*-glycolic) acid (PLGA) and polycaprolactone (PCL) are two such commonly used materials. As in many other materials engineering applications, these biometals, bioceramics, and biopolymers can be

doi:10.1088/978-0-7503-5187-4ch1

combined. HAPEX is a good commercial example; it is made by combining hydroxyapatite and high-density polyethylene to improve the mechanical properties of the former; it can be used to prepare eye and ear implants. For many decades, the science of biomaterials has been researched to invent new generations of biomaterials. Some notable examples are discussed below.

Some of these developments target specific applications that will significantly improve healthcare. New generations of resorbable copolymers for textile structures can be used to make haemostatic wound dressings which significantly shorten the clotting time of blood [1]. Biomaterial drug delivery vehicles, such as polymer micro- and nanoparticles and liposomes have been used to target dendritic cells in novel fields such as vaccination, a domain which increasingly needs to innovate at unprecedented rates. Dendritic cells, for example, which are specialised antigen-presenting cells that retain the ability to initiate and regulate immune responses, can now be utilised to develop vaccines at a rapid pace [2].

In the treatment of orthopaedics, various calcium phosphate materials have increasingly been applied for bone tissue replacement and augmentation. These calcium phosphate materials are of great benefit in bone tissue engineering applications due to their phase and chemical (ionic) composition (bioresistivity and bioresorption). Their microstructure also plays a crucial role, since chemical modification using biocompatible anions and cations allows for novel approaches in the newer generations of biomaterials [3].

The spotlight on biomaterials with antimicrobial action is of particular interest, and new bactericidal surfaces are being constructed primarily for their surface structures, which are superior to traditional chemistry-based approaches in terms of their long-lasting bactericidal effect. New developments in methods for modifying surface nanotopographies could represent a major advance in the manufacture of a new generation of biomaterials with antimicrobial capabilities. However, the question of whether this ideology can progress from laboratory to scaled-up manufacture is a crucial issue for success in terms of advancing global healthcare [4].

A new generation of biomaterials can also emerge as a result of prescribing design criteria for a specific application; a good example here is urinary hollow organ reconstruction, for which three aspects are identified: (i) to be able to mimic the nanofibrous collagen extracellular matrix, (ii) to facilitate a large number of cells on one side, and (iii) to simultaneously serve as a barrier on the opposite side, in order to achieve an asymmetric structure that can withstand the mechanical stresses that occur during tissue neogenesis [5].

The battle against dengue fever is another interesting challenge that can be addressed using biomaterials; for example, the cost-efficient production of highly specific nanoyeasts enables the accurate detection of the dengue virus (DENV) via immunoassays, producing high-avidity nanoyeast single-chain variable fragments (scFvs). This gives rise to the potential for large-population screening of DENV that can be scaled for use in developing economies. Recently, a highly efficient system for yeast display has been discovered that can express the DENV nonstructural protein1 scFvs on the yeast surface, providing a scFv-positive cell population of up to 64%. Accurate DENV antigen immunoassay performance (2.5% CV) has been achieved through the physical disruption of yeast cells in order to release the soluble scFvs. Through sonication, scFv-containing yeast fragments of about 90 nm can be achieved. This approach could be used to produce other highly specific biomaterials for diagnostic applications in environments where resources are limited [6].

Oral and dental applications can also define a generation of biomaterials. Biofabrication techniques that involve directly incorporating human oral mucosa tissue explants to create human bioengineered mouth and dental tissues have become a focal point in tissue engineering. Acellular fibrin–agarose scaffolds (AFASs), non-functionalized fibrin–agarose oral mucosa (n-FAOM) stroma substitutes, and novel functionalized fibrin-agarose oral mucosa stroma substitutes (F-FAOM) have been developed and analysed. After three weeks of *in vitro* development, histochemistry and immunohistochemistry were used to assess the extracelluar matrix components formed, and these were compared to native oral mucosa. The findings showed that the biomimetic characteristics of the biomaterials were improved in line with the functionalization of the material. The biomimetic capabilities of these materials reduced the time required for *in vitro* tissue development.

Other researchers have focused on specific biomaterials. A new type of polymeric material known as supermacroporous cryogel has been introduced. This been shown to possess significant potential in a range of bioengineering and biotechnological applications. Such cryogels have characteristic interconnected supermacropores which allow them to facilitate the unhindered diffusion of nearly all sizes of solute. These gels also allow for the mass transport of nano- and microparticles. The applications of these supermacroporous cryogels have been evaluated for a number of applications. Scaffolds made of these cryogels which were fabricated from agarose–gelatine were shown to have graded pore sizes and the mechanical strength to mimic cartilage. This approach can be used to design the next generation of cartilage tissue engineering scaffolds, which are not limited in the same way as other conventional approaches. These supermacroporous cryogel biomaterials have vast potential in a diverse range of biotechnology and bioengineering applications due to their inherent microstructures [7].

Another noteworthy biomaterial development has been the generation of porous-wall hollow glass microspheres, which have already demonstrated remarkable potential in drug delivery and regenerative medicine. For example, fluorescent nanocrystals and quantum dots can be used in assays and multispectral imaging systems that are able to detect fluorescence in aqueous phases. Qdot 605, for example, can be used to reliably assay the drug-eluting properties of a material. These nanocrystals can be used in the imaging and flow cytometry of head and neck surgery as well as other medical applications [8]. PLGA and PCL have come to the forefront of biodegradable polymers favoured for biomedical applications. Recently, a new generation of poly(lactide/ε-caprolactone) polymers (PLCLs) composed of ε-caprolactone (CL), l-lactide (l-LA) and d-lactide (d-LA) with an l-LA content of less than 72% have been synthesised using bismuth (III) subsalicylate as a catalyst. These novel polymers have the ability to remain uncrystallized or to show very little crystallisation during hydrolytic degradation, whilst also not producing resistant crystalline remnants. These properties are present because it is possible to control the average sequence lengths of d-LA and CL and because of their inability to form highly crystalline structures. The d-LA and CL units in terpolymers of l-LA/d-LA/CL disrupt the microstructural arrangement, preventing crystallisation; this has the effect of shortening their average block sequence. This creates a more disordered structure that has a lower glass transition temperature. These materials are therefore more elastomeric and less resistant to hydrolytic degradation. The degree to which d-LA replaces CL units can also be used to tune the glass transition temperature and to tailor the stress-related properties of l-LA/CL or racemic-LA/CL elastomeric copolymers at low glass transition temperatures (< 20°C) [9].

A study of polyphosphazenes, polymers that have an inorganic phosphorus and nitrogen backbone, has shown the potential of macromolecular substitution, which permits the facile attachment of different organic groups and drug molecules to the backbone polyphosphazene polymers. This can be leveraged in the development of a broad class of biomaterials. As a result, materials such as these may be more biocompatible than conventional biomaterials, and can be mixed with other clinically relevant polymers to develop new material approaches that exhibit unique erosion properties and more suitable near-neutral degradation products. As a biomaterial, polyphosphazene signifies a step into the next generation of biomaterials that provides the needed evolution of synthetic design. Polyphosphazenes have the potential to be used in regenerative bioengineering as well as in the delivery of active pharmaceutical ingredients [10].

One study which evaluated a novel biomaterial derived by decellularizing sturgeon chondral endoskeletal tissue made a notable contribution to cartilage tissue engineering. This study showed that decellularized sturgeon cartilage could be recellularized with human chondrocytes along with four other types of human mesenchymal stem cells (MSCs). *Ex vivo* and *in vivo* assessments were used to ascertain the suitability of the resulting materials as cartilage substitutes. The results of the *ex vivo* and *in vivo* studies showed that the scaffold had high biocompatibility and was able to sustain cell attachment, adhesion, proliferation, and differentiation. MSCs that were added to the cartilage-substitute scaffolds were biosynthetically active and could facilitate the remodelling of the extracellular matrix, where production of type II collagen and other relevant components was observed, especially when adipose-derived MSC tissue was used. These findings suggest that biomaterials obtained from decellularized cartilage could be suitable for generating tissue substitutes from a variety of different cell sources in the future [11].

Experimental characterisation advancement can also play a key role in the development of newer generations of biomaterials. For example, a study which characterised biomaterials using many different experimental procedures found that that differences in the microstructural patterns of the produced tissue substitutes correlated with their macroscopic mechanical properties. The study also showed that magnetic tissue substitutes could have their mechanical properties tuned by non-contact magnetic forces. Such an approach would be advantageous if it could be applied to other biomaterials and used to match the mechanical properties of the tissue substitutes to produce materials that are targeted for use in many different tissue engineering applications [12]. Another notable example of biomaterial processing has been the evolution of microscopical techniques, which has allowed material scientists to better characterise their materials. Polysulfones (PSFs) are a class of polymers with optical properties; they can perform second-harmonic generation (SHG), which is especially useful in advanced imaging. SHG imaging has been found to be capable of quantitatively revealing the mesostructure of PSF, which was seen to be polar and fibrilliform. With the availability of SHG-based endoscopy, PSF has become an attractive scaffolding material for implants and tissue engineering applications in which theragnostic nanoagents can be used; examples include disease detection and drug delivery [13].

Advances in chemistry will also help in the rapid development of the next generations of biomaterials. Organic bioelectronics are making a tremendous impact in the field of tissue engineering. These devices are not only biocompatible but also bifunctional, since they are conductive material platforms. In order to maximise their potential, it must be possible to integrate these materials into organic conductors, such as graphene or other biopolymers, in a targeted manner. This approach allows for the development of medical devices and tissue scaffolds that are capable of carrying many chemical, physical, and electrical stimuli [14].

Graphene and its derivatives are also beginning to make a striking impact. Over the last decade, research into graphene (as evidenced by the growing scientific literature) has shown the ability of graphene nanocomposites to tackle antimicrobial resistance by interacting with microorganisms. Graphene nanocomposites have been shown to have inherent antimicrobial mechanisms that have become apparent in *in vitro* and *in vivo* studies in which graphene nanocomposites have been used for antibacterial, antiviral, and antifungal applications [15]. Other advances in biomaterial synthesis have involved chemistry-led scenarios; an example is the structural and physicochemical characterisation of heparinised chitosan. This research stresses the need to develop new methodologies that align with sustainable trends in production. Specific chemical modification reactions and new assemblies can be applied to obtain new 'custom-made' chitosan biopolymers that provide a great deal of versatility for many different biomedical applications due to their structure and functionality [16]. New generations of biology-driven biomaterials are also just emerging. The importance of using the biological environments of materials to produce materials while studying the prevalent interactions with their natural environment and leveraging them to derive useful materials is the focus, and the key factor is the chemistry at the interface [17].

Scalable innovative manufacturing is a key aspect, and this is only considered in very few new generations of biomaterials introduced in the research literature. Adaptation by industry to manufacture these materials via mass production is a crucial issue if such materials are to be incorporated into global clinical practice for all-important patient care. This has only been discussed for very few scenarios. For example, hydroxyapatite (HA) nanoplates have been deposited on an AZ31 Mg alloy, with the result that the material had improved bioactivity and offered greater control over its biodegradability. Heat treatment at 60 °C following the anodization process also promoted nanoplate growth. Fouirer transform infra-red spectroscopy (FTIR) analysis of these materials corroborated the formation of HA on the surface of the AZ31B, which was found to be able to mimic the structure of natural bone and facilitate suitable cell proliferation and subsequent attachment. This study demonstrated a highly effective and novel method for modifying the surfaces of such alloys which also imparted vast potential for large-scale industrial production [18]. Hydrophobic coatings and surface modifications on biomaterials can make them more suitable for a range of biomedical applications. These can be achieved through diamond-like carbon (DLC) coatings and plasma-deposited fluoropolymer and siloxane modifications. The reliability and stability of these coatings and surface modifications depend on the selected monomer, the specifics of the processing route, the use of co-monomers, and the conditions during deposition. Studies of these modifications have highlighted the importance of surface physical–chemical–mechanical analysis and the requirement for surface-modified biomedical devices that are suitable for implant applications [19].

Newer technologies have made us think differently, such as microfluidics as well as the use of droplets and bubbles to evolve new generations of biomaterials. For example, about a decade ago, attention turned to the fact that the prevailing macroscale methodologies used to produce niche models failed to consider the spatial and temporal characteristics of native stem cell systems, which are complex and have to be mimicked by biomimetic structures. Microfluidic technologies can provide unprecedented control over the spatial and temporal structures of biological and biochemical signals, which allows for novel approaches to stem cell engineering and biomimetic cellular niches. The combination of biomaterials engineering with microfluids can result in numerous openings for stem cell biotechnology and biological applications. The micropatterning of biomaterials using microfluidics, for example, has opened up possibilities for the fabrication of physiological niche models in both two and three dimensions [20]. In native cellular niches, cells interact in a three-dimensional manner, and it is often seen that two-dimensional substitutions fail to elicit the same type of bioactive effect from these cells. Another study used microfluidics in a droplet-based fashion to generate highly monodisperse and responsive alginate-block–polyetheramine copolymer microgels. Through the use of droplet-based microfluidics, excellent control of both the physical dimensions and chemical properties of the grafted alginate microgels was achieved. The resulting microgels were comparable to isolated grafted alginate chains in the sense that they retained their amphiphilic and thermo-sensitive properties. Droplet-based microfluidics is also a promising tool for the generation of responsive biobased hydrogels for drug delivery applications, which have demonstrated potential as colloidal stabilisers for dispersed systems such as Pickering emulsions [21]. In addition, research has explored the utilisation of microbubbling to produce controlled protein-coated bubbles (bovine serum albumin, BSA) and manipulate them into the fabrication of a variety of structures that are suitable for many different biomedical applications. The application scope of these structures could extend to biosensor and tissue engineering scenarios. The single-step process of these technologies can benefit various fields, as the process is robust and exploits microbubbles as novel entities; other biomacromolecules, for example, can readily be substituted for the BSA protein, resulting in similar structures suitable for many biomedical uses [22].

An overriding theme within this field is environmental considerations, and many changes in the preparation and definition of biomaterials will have to be implemented to meet this demand. Many industrial organisations are already taking this matter very seriously and starting to accept it. For example, the biotechnology company Bolt Threads has developed two platforms for the sustainabe production of silk and leather. The materials produced are dubbed MICROSILK, which is characterised by a high-performance fibre produced though the both fermentation and traditional textile manufacturing techniques. This system utilises wet spinning to make micro silk fibres and has attracted much attention. The company is also able to manufacture a MYLO material, which 'looks, feels, and behaves' like handcrafted leather, but is produced from mycelia, the root structure of mushrooms, an attractive and sustainable alternative to animal leather [23]. With the advent of greener mass production preferences, the development of water-based silk deposition for biomedical engineering applications is being investigated with new vigour [24]. Very recently, a collection of special issues by MACRO journals provided a good literature database for renewed thinking on this topic [25].

Despite admiration for these more specific efforts to identify a narrow remit of new generations of composition-specific biomaterials, which have undoubtedly advanced the frontiers of biomaterials science and engineering, the content of this book will not add to this doctrine. Our focus is a distinctly different generation of biomaterials: bubbles, particles, capsules, and fibres at the nano- or microscale which are globally desired for many clinical applications that will improve healthcare and benefit patients. For example, microscale near-monodisperse stable bubbles that have diameters of 2–5 μm can improve ultrasound imaging of patients, but bubble production methods need to match the required microbubble characteristics very reliably, as coarser microbubbles can cause embolism in patients. Similarly, tailored microbubbles, including nanoparticles, microparticles, and capsules have enabled drug delivery to take place at a very advanced multifunctional level, thus allowing patients to be treated for multiple diseases with just one dose a day. This approach enables very targeted delivery of active pharmaceutical ingredients (APIs), which can therefore hugely minimise adverse effects to a patient's overall health and wellbeing. With respect to fibres at the nano- and microscale, their mass production in various morphologies such as scaffolds and meshes has enabled multiple healthcare innovations such as tissue engineering, wound healing (bandages), and microbial filtration at a level not hitherto possible.

This book gives a detailed description of the scalable production of microbubbles, particles, capsules, and fibres, which are a new generation of biomaterials hugely impacting modern healthcare.

Microfluidic devices are successfully used in the production of microbubbles, microparticles, nanoparticles, two-dimensional porous films, and three-dimensional tissue scaffolds. In addition to being a production technique, microfluidics also have diagnostic capability in point-of-care applications. Microfluidic devices play a role in wide-ranging applications from disposable biosensor applications, combined separation and analysis systems, and protein separation to omics technologies and genetic analysis. Microfluidic platforms, which are also used as miniaturised bioreactors, have carried cell culture studies to organs-on-chips and continue to progress in the field of human-on-a-chip applications. Studies in which electrohydrodynamic (EHD) systems are used as a production technique contribute to fibre and particle production in biomedical technologies. Fibre technologies play a major role in the biomedical industry in application-specific production; they have the effect of decreasing fibre diameters from the microscale to the nanoscale, thereby increasing the surface area. On the other hand, the EHD atomisation technique has allowed the development of controlled release systems with single- or multilayer applications of particles. Nanofibre production, in which EHD systems are used as the gold standard, is effectively used in many applications such as filtration materials, tissue scaffolds, wound dressings, and bandages in biomedical applications. In addition, they offer an adjustable and open-to-development potential to produce solutions to complex biomedical problems through drug loading, increased layers, and the design of composite/combined structures with different materials and structures.

One particular area of interest for the production of healthcare biomaterials is the scaling up of manufacturing technologies which are already available in the laboratory in order to meet the rising demands imposed by growing patient needs. Technologies such as electrospinning and microfluidic production routes are limited in their capacity for mass production; this is often a bottleneck in improving the availability of these materials for mass adoption, in addition to the high costs linked with batch processing. Centrifugal spinning has proven to be a technology that can produce large masses of fibre in a short timescale and has been used to produce fibres of various morphologies. In 2013, a novel method which married centrifugal spinning with solution blow spinning was devised [26]. Known as pressurised gyration, it is able to rapidly produce large amounts of nonwoven fibre and can easily incorporate a range of bioactive additions and pharmaceuticals to bring advanced biomaterials one step closer to mass adoption. Following the arrival of pressurised gyration, much work has gone into producing biomaterials for various healthcare applications such as drug-solubility-enhancing solid dispersions, tissue engineering scaffolds for cell seeding, and antimicrobial filters for hospital air and water filtration [24, 27, 28]. Since the inception of pressurised gyration, many iterations and sister technologies have been developed using the principle of combining a centrifugal force with an additional gas pressure to provide a greater range of control over the final fibre morphology. In this book, we look at gyration-based manufacturing techniques and list how we believe these technologies, in conjunction with all other biomaterial processing techniques, can be leveraged to realise the future of biomaterials for healthcare applications.

References

[1] Ene A and Mihai C 2006 New generations of resorbable biomaterials with textile structures *Medical Textiles and Biomaterials for Healthcare* (Amsterdam: Elsevier) 23–8

[2] Reddy S T, Swartz M A and Hubbell J A 2006 Targeting dendritic cells with biomaterials: developing the next generation of vaccines *Trends Immunol.* **27** 573–9

[3] Putlyaev V and Safronova T 2006 A new generation of calcium phosphate biomaterials: the role of phase and chemical compositions *Glass Ceram.* **63** 99–102

[4] Hasan J, Crawford R J and Ivanova E P 2013 Antibacterial surfaces: the quest for a new generation of biomaterials *Trends Biotechnol.* **31** 295–304

[5] Lv X, Feng C and Xu Y 2016 LB-S&T-30 the characterization of 3-D structure in the decelluarized urinary hollow organ: cues for new generation biomaterials of urinary hollow organ reconstruction *J. Urol.* **195** e348–9

[6] Farokhinejad F, Lane R E, Lobb R J, Edwardraja S, Wuethrich A, Howard C B and Trau M 2021 Generation of nanoyeast single-chain variable fragments as high-avidity biomaterials for dengue virus detection *ACS Biomater. Sci. Eng.* **7** 5850–60

[7] Kumar A 2008 New generation of polymeric biomaterials for biotechnological and bioengineering applications *J. Biotechnol.* **136** S118

[8] Cunningham A, Faircloth H, Jones M, Johnson C, Coleman T, Wicks G, Postma G and Weinberger P 2014 A reporter assay for the next generation of biomaterials: porous-wall hollow glass microspheres *Laryngoscope* **124** 1392–7

[9] Fernández J, Larrañaga A, Etxeberria A, Wang W and Sarasua J 2014 A new generation of poly (lactide/ε-caprolactone) polymeric biomaterials for application in the medical field *J. Biomed. Mater. Res.* A **102** 3573–84

[10] Ogueri K S, Ogueri K S, Allcock H R and Laurencin C T 2020 Polyphosphazene polymers: the next generation of biomaterials for regenerative engineering and therapeutic drug delivery *J. Vac. Sci. Technol.* B **38** 030801

[11] Ortiz-Arrabal O, Carmona R, García-García Ó-D, Chato-Astrain J, Sánchez-Porras D, Domezain A, Oruezabal R-I, Carriel V, Campos A and Alaminos M 2021 Generation and evaluation of novel biomaterials based on decellularized sturgeon cartilage for use in tissue engineering *Biomedicines* **9** 775

[12] Lopez-Lopez M T, Scionti G, Oliveira A C, Duran J D, Campos A, Alaminos M and Rodriguez I A 2015 Generation and characterization of novel magnetic field-responsive biomaterials *PLoS One* **10** e0133878

[13] Ni M and Zhuo S 2015 Second harmonic generation microscopy for label-free imaging of fibrillar-like mesostructured polysulfone biomaterials *Opt. Mater. Express* **5** 2692–7

[14] Molino P J and Wallace G G 2015 Next generation bioelectronics: advances in fabrication coupled with clever chemistries enable the effective integration of biomaterials and organic conductors *APL Mater.* **3** 014913

[15] Gungordu S, Edirisinghe E M and Tabish T A 2023 Graphene-based nanocomposites as antibacterial, antiviral and antifungal agents *Adv. Healthcare Mater.* **12** 2370026

[16] Revuelta J, Fraile I, Monterrey D T, Peña N, Benito-Arenas R, Bastida A, Fernández-Mayoralas A and García-Junceda E 2021 Heparanized chitosans: towards the third generation of chitinous biomaterials *Mater. Horizons* **8** 2596–614

[17] Lavik E and Rotello V 2022 *Bioconjugate Biomaterials: Leveraging Biology for the Next Generation of Active Materials* (Washington, DC: ACS Publications) 543–3

[18] Mousa H M, Tiwari A P, Kim J, Adhikari S P, Park C H and Kim C S 2016 A novel *in situ* deposition of hydroxyapatite nanoplates using anodization/hydrothermal process onto magnesium alloy surface towards third generation biomaterials *Mater. Lett.* **164** 144–7
[19] Siow K S 2018 Low pressure plasma modifications for the generation of hydrophobic coatings for biomaterials applications *Plasma Process. Polym.* **15** 1800059
[20] Kobel S and Lutolf M P 2011 Biomaterials meet microfluidics: building the next generation of artificial niches *Curr. Opin. Biotechnol.* **22** 690–7
[21] Karakasyan C, Mathos J, Lack S, Davy J, Marquis M and Renard D 2015 Microfluidics-assisted generation of stimuli-responsive hydrogels based on alginates incorporated with thermo-responsive and amphiphilic polymers as novel biomaterials *Colloids Surf.* B **135** 619–29
[22] Ekemen Z, Chang H, Ahmad Z, Bayram C, Rong Z, Denkbas E B, Stride E, Vadgama P and Edirisinghe M 2011 Fabrication of biomaterials via controlled protein bubble generation and manipulation *Biomacromolecules* **12** 4291–300
[23] Visjager J F, Bansal-Mutalik R and Patist A 2019 Developing the next generation of sustainable biomaterials *Chem. Eng. Prog.* **115** 30–5
[24] Heseltine P L, Bayram C, Gultekinoglu M, Homer-Vanniasinkam S, Ulubayram K and Edirisinghe M 2022 Facile one-pot method for all aqueous green formation of biocompatible silk fibroin-poly (ethylene oxide) fibers for use in tissue engineering *ACS Biomater. Sci. Eng.* **8** 1290–300
[25] Chen B, Ray S S and Edirisinghe M 2022 Sustainable macromolecular materials and engineering *Macromol. Mater. Eng.* **307** 2200242
[26] Mahalingam S and Edirisinghe M 2013 Forming of polymer nanofibers by a pressurised gyration process *Macromol. Rapid Commun.* **34** 1134–9
[27] Gultekinoglu M, Öztürk Ş, Chen B, Edirisinghe M and Ulubayram K 2019 Preparation of poly (glycerol sebacate) fibers for tissue engineering applications *Eur. Polym. J.* **121** 109297
[28] Raimi-Abraham B T, Mahalingam S, Davies P J, Edirisinghe M and Craig D Q 2015 Development and characterization of amorphous nanofiber drug dispersions prepared using pressurized gyration *Mol. Pharm.* **12** 3851–61

IOP Publishing

Biomaterials
Innovation for world healthcare
Mohan Edirisinghe, Merve Gultekinoglu and Jubair Ahmed

Chapter 2

Microfluidic manufacturing

Microfluidics has become a fundamental technology for the engineering and materials sciences. Microfluidic platforms are especially favourable due to their low minimum volume, high sensitivity, fast production, and analysis capabilities, especially in biomedical applications. Thanks to microfluidic reactors, microbubbles, nanoparticles, and microparticles can be prepared quickly and in custom sizes; this also provides the opportunity to prepare personalised products in addition to materials used in imaging, diagnosis, and treatment. The scientific background of microfluidics, its invention, development, and biomedical applications are discussed in detail in this chapter.

2.1 The principles of microfluidics

2.1.1 The history of microfluidics

Microfluidics is a multidisciplinary technology that emerged as the result of combining the disciplines of engineering, physics, chemistry, biochemistry, nanotechnology, and biotechnology. Microfluidics has a wide range of applications, from printers to electronic circuits and biomedical applications; it is based on the use of micro/nanoscale channels and flowing liquids. Microfluidic chip geometry, the material choice surface tension, viscosity, pressure, temperature, and flow rate are the basic parameters of microfluidic systems. Microfluidics also refers to miniaturised analytical technologies used in biomedical and chemical applications, as applications based on micro- and nanofluids are often used in biomedical and chemical analyses.

The history of the development of microfluidics started with the emergence of fluid mechanics marked by the development of the Hagen–Poiseuille equation in the 1800s. The Hagen–Poiseuille equation is a physical law that describes the pressure drop in an incompressible Newtonian fluid which exhibits a laminar flow profile through a cylindrical pipe with a constant cross-sectional area and whose length is greater than its diameter. On the other hand, the production of the first silicon in the 1940s, following the discovery of siloxanes in 1927, formed the cornerstone of the development of microfluidics. Following the discovery of photolithography in the 1950s, Siemens-Elena took the first steps towards commercialisation by obtaining the patent for the first inkjet printer in 1951. In this historical development process, the discovery of integrated circuits (ICs) took place in 1958, and in the 1960s, micro-electromechanical systems (MEMs) technology was introduced. Lab-on-a-chip (LOC) applications were developed for the first time by S Terry in 1979. Micro total analysis systems or micro TASs (μTASs) were developed by A Manz in 1990 following the discovery of soft lithography [1]. After μTAS technologies emerged, the American Defence Advanced Research Projects Agency (DARPA) started biological defence projects using LOC applications in the 1990s.

Microfluidics began to make significant advances in biomedical technologies in the early 2000s, when G M Whitesides produced the first polydimethylsiloxane (PDMS) microchips, R Fair introduced digital microfluidics, and S Quake developed pneumatic valves [2]. In light of these developments, microfluidic cell culture systems, organ-on-chip technology, and three-dimensional (3D) microfluidics-based bio-printers have been designed, paper-based microfluidic diagnostic systems have been developed, and studies of humans-on-chips were initiated in the 2010s (figure 2.1).

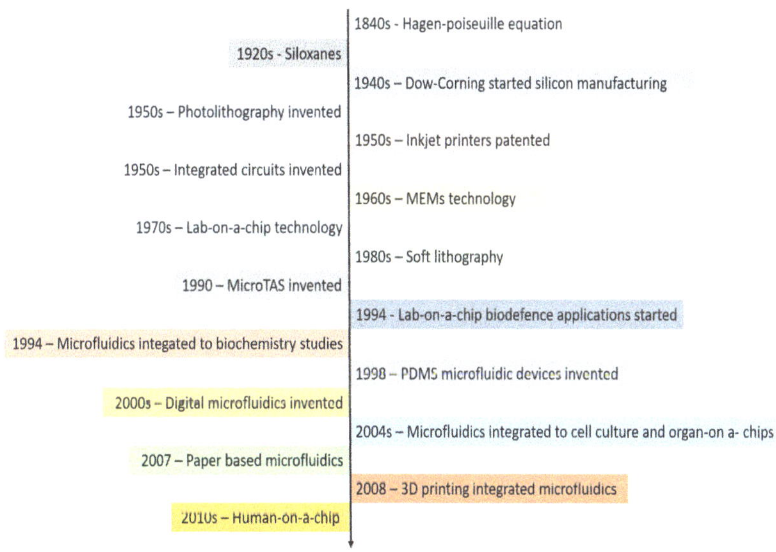

Figure 2.1. The historical development of microfluidics and scientific discoveries that contributed to its development between 1840 and 2010 [2].

G M Whitesides, one of the most important inventors of microfluidics technology, stated while defining microfluidics that 'molecular biology, molecular analysis, national security and microelectronics constitute the basic elements of microfluidics'. Affirming this definition, microfluidics has found a wide range of uses, from microelectronic analysis devices to crime scene investigations, single-cell analysis, bedside analysis kits, rapid diagnostic kits, and the development of systems to replace *in vivo* tests in microtissues.

Micro and nanofluids (μ-Nafls) are described by the laws of physics based on fluid mechanics, surface chemistry, heat transfer, mass transfer, and electrochemical and electrostatic properties. In light of this definition, microfluidic phenomena, techniques, and applications will be described in detail in the following sections.

2.1.2 Fluid dynamics in microfluidics

Fluids are liquid or gaseous substances that undergo deformation when exposed to shear stress and do not have a definite shape [3]. Fluid mechanics defines fluid behaviours in terms of the acting forces and the general physical principles. Fluid mechanics is closely related not only to physics but also to other basic sciences such as chemistry and biology, as well as engineering sciences such as mechanical engineering, electronics, construction, and geology. Different classifications are applied to fluids according to their different properties. When fluids are evaluated in terms of their physical properties, they are classified as liquids, gases, plasmas, or molten solids [4]. On the other hand, in terms of fluid mechanics, fluids are divided into Newtonian and non-Newtonian fluids. For Newtonian fluids, there is a linear relationship between the applied shear stress and the rate of deformation (shear rate). Therefore, the viscosity of Newtonian fluids at a constant temperature is also constant. For non-Newtonian fluids, the relationship between the applied shear stress and the shear rate is non-linear [5] (figure 2.2). Therefore, the

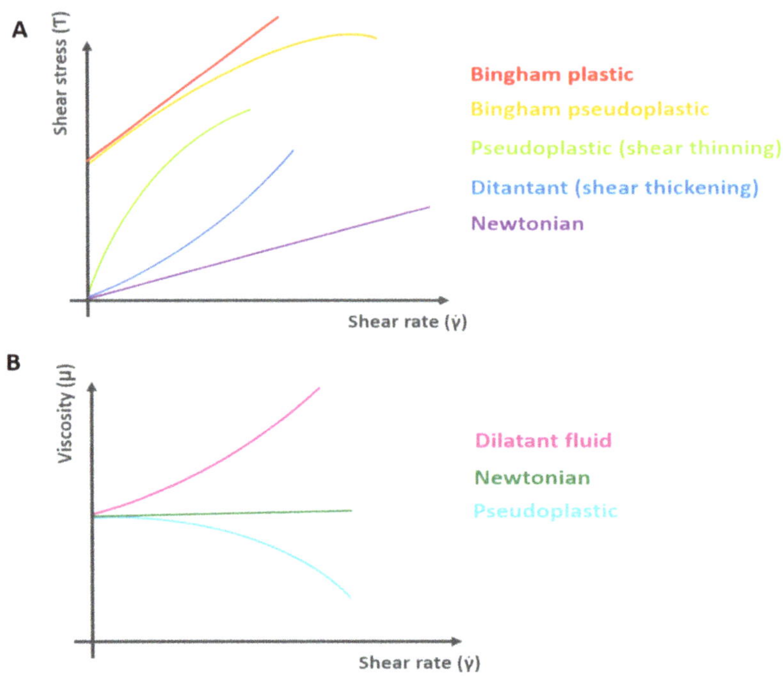

Figure 2.2. Time independent non-Newtonian fluids shear rate ($\dot{y}$) as a function of (A) shear stress (T, Pa) and (B) viscosity (μ, Pa s).

viscosity varies even at a constant temperature and is related to the speed gradient (equation (2.1)).

$$\mu(\text{viscosity, Pa s}) = \frac{\tau\ (\text{shear stress, Pa})}{\dot{\gamma}\ (\text{shear rate, } 1\ \text{s}^{-1})} \quad (2.1)$$

Non-Newtonian fluids are divided into two fundamental categories:

1. Time-independent non-Newtonian fluids
   (a) pseudo-plastic
   (b) shear thinning
   (c) Bingham fluids
2. Time-dependent non-Newtonian fluids
   (a) thixotropic,
   (b) rheopectic.

Microfluidics and microfluidic manufacturing technologies are closely related to fluid dynamics, which is a subdiscipline of fluid mechanics. Fluid dynamics is defined by various non-dimensional parameters that depend on parameters such as viscosity, surface tension, speed, flow distance, channel geometry, and frictional force. Examples of such non-dimensional parameters include the Reynolds number (Re) and the capillary number (Ca).

The Reynolds number is a dimensionless parameter used to characterise the flow regime. It is the ratio of the inertial force given by the velocity (or momentum) of the fluid to the viscous (or frictional) forces; it is calculated using equation (2.2). The Reynolds number is related to the density of the fluid (ρ), the velocity of the fluid (u), the diameter of the fluidic channel (D), and the viscosity of the fluid (μ). As the channel size decreases (i.e. as D decreases), the inertial forces decrease, resulting in a reduction in the Reynolds number.

The Reynolds number defines the flow characteristics in terms of laminar or turbulent flow. The critical Reynolds number defines the flow type of a fluid through a channel. At low Reynolds numbers, the viscous force is large enough to overcome inertia and keep the fluid in straight motion. A Reynolds number of less than 2300 ($Re<2300$) indicates laminar flow and a Reynolds number higher than 4000 ($Re<4000$) denotes turbulent flow (figure 2.3). If the Reynolds number is between 2300 and 4000, the flow is defined as an unstable (transition) flow type.

$$Re = \frac{\text{inertial forces}}{\text{viscous forces}} = \frac{\rho u D}{\mu} \quad (2.2)$$

The capillary number is a dimensionless quantity that defines the ratio of the viscous to interfacial forces. It can be calculated by taking the ratio of the product of the velocity (u) and viscosity (μ) to the interfacial tension (γ) (equation (2.3)). The capillary number is used to classify flow regimes such as squeezing, jetting, and dripping [6]. These regimes play an important role in the formation of fluid droplets inside microfluidic reactors.

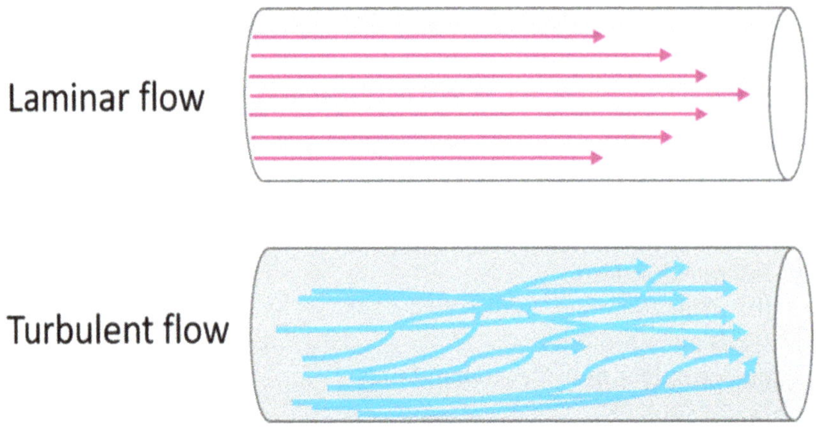

Figure 2.3. A schematic representation of Reynolds-number-related flow patterns of fluids: laminar flow and turbulent flow.

$$\mathrm{Ca} = \frac{\text{velosity} \times \text{viscosity}}{\text{interfacial tension}} = \frac{\mu u}{\gamma} \tag{2.3}$$

The Bond number (Bo) defines the ratio between gravity and the surface tension of the fluid. The Marangoni number (Ma) defines the ratio of the surface tension to the viscous forces in the presence of a temperature gradient. Although many dimensionless quantities describe flow conditions from different perspectives, the capillary and Reynolds numbers are the most important and prominent parameters in modelling, computation, and experimental studies of microfluidics.

Electro-osmotic flows (EOFs) and pressure-driven flows (PDFs) are implemented in microfluidic devices, and their flow patterns are described by Bernoulli's equation (equation (2.4)). Bernoulli's principle states that an increase in velocity along a non-viscous flow results in a concomitant decrease in either the pressure or the potential energy of the fluid. For Bernoulli's equation to be applicable, the flow must be stationary, the flow parameters (velocity, density, etc.) must not change over time, and the flow must also be incompressible. The density must remain constant along the streamline even as the pressure changes. The friction created by the viscous forces must be negligible.

Bernoulli's equation is given below:

$$P_1 + \rho \ \frac{v_1^2}{2} + \rho g z_1 = P_2 + \rho \ \frac{v_2^2}{2} + \rho g z_2. \tag{2.4}$$

The equation is defined by P, the pressure of the fluid at a cross-sectional point, ρ, the density of the fluid, v, the speed of the fluid, g, the acceleration due to gravity, and z, the elevation [7]. Bernoulli's equation states that the sum of the pressure and the potential and kinetic energies is constant. It is impractical to use pressure to direct flows in μ-Nafl systems. More commonly, a potential or applied voltage is used that produces an electric field. Electro-osmotic (EO) flows also obey Bernoulli's equation;

such flows are created by the application of an electric field. The connection between an electric and liquid field gives rise to an electrokinetic flow field. Electrokinetic pumping applications combine EO and pressure-driven flows [8].

Four basic types of electrokinetic conditions are important in μ-Nafl systems: electro-osmosis, electrophoresis, current potential, and sedimentation potential. Electro-osmosis is the movement of fluid relative to a constant charged surface. [9]. The directions of the electro-osmotic flow and the bulk flow may be different. Electrophoresis is defined as the movement of a charged surface, (typically charged particles) relative to a stationary fluid. If the charged particles have different charge-to-mass ($q\ m^{-1}$) ratios, this causes the particles to be separated into different groups according to their $q\ m^{-1}$ ratios [10]. Current potential is defined as the electric field induced when an ionic solution (e.g. an aqueous electrolyte) flows across the charged surface of a solid due to an external force such as pressure. This phenomenon is the opposite of electro-osmosis. The sedimentation potential is defined as the electric field induced when charged surfaces or particles move relative to a stationary fluid. This phenomenon is the opposite of electrophoresis.

The electric double layer (EDL) theory is important in adapting and applying fundamental descriptions of electrokinetic phenomena to μ-Nafl systems. The EDL first emerged in colloidal systems and electrode–solution interfaces [11]. An electric bilayer EDL consists of a sample substrate with a net negative charge that has positive counterions electrostatically attached to its surface [12]. This surface layer of counterions is considered to be an inert layer and is called the Stern layer [13]. The location of the first ionic layer, which is mobile, forms the slip or slip plane, and the potential zeta, ζ, in this plane is defined as the potential (figure 2.4). The zeta potential is defined by the potential difference between the dispersion medium and the stationary liquid layer adsorbed to the dispersed particles. In most μ-Nafl systems, aqueous electrolyte solutions are confined within channels or pores with critical micro- or nanoscale dimensions [14]. In such situations, it is necessary to evaluate the ionic concentrations and potentials that affect the convection phenomenon that is transferred to the solution starting from a wall.

2.2 Materials used in microfluidic chip development

Microfluidic chips create an opportunity to manipulate fluidics at the nano- to micro-volume levels with strict control over the precision. The type of fluid used in these systems should be compatible with the microfluidic chip in which it will be routed. It is of great importance for the accuracy and stability of the microfluidic system that the fluid system must not be in a solvent–solute relationship with the material of the microfluidic chip and that they are stable in each other's presence. The key points in the selection of the material used in the production of microfluidic devices are its interaction with the fluid, the effect of the device's material on the production method, and its compatibility with the techniques used in the application (characterisation, measurement, imaging). Advances in the microfluidics field, chemical synthesis, single-cell analysis, diagnostics, and electronics have triggered technological revolutions in

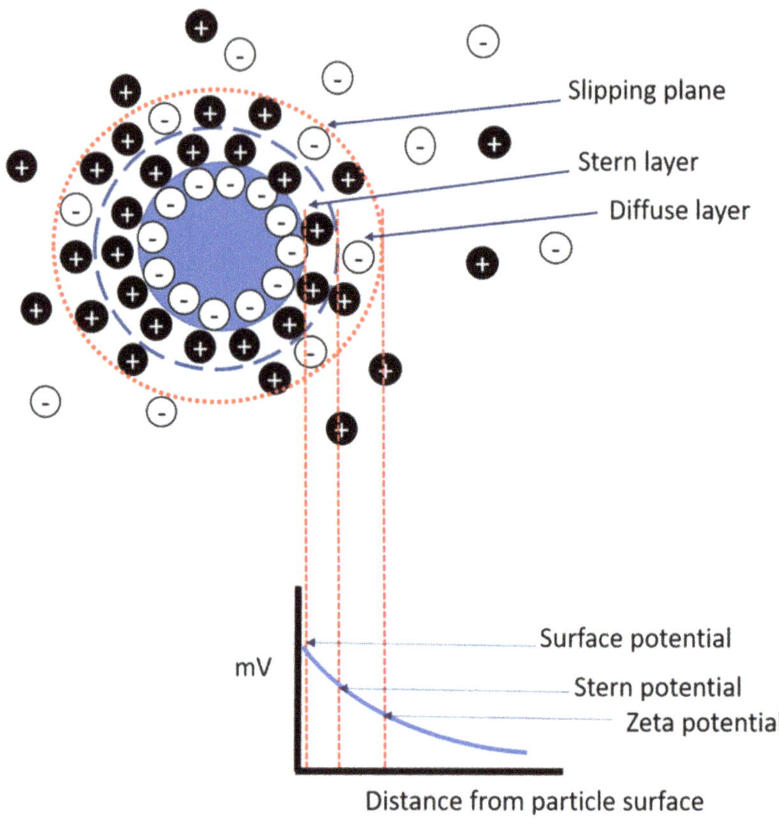

Figure 2.4. A schematic representation of EDL theory indicating the slipping plane, the Stern layer, and the diffuse layer.

many disciplines, including micro/nanofabrication, diagnosis, and pharmacology. Rapid growth in many of these areas is driven by increased synergies between materials development and newly developed microfluidics skills.

2.2.1 Inorganic materials

Inorganic materials are defined as materials that do not contain carbon–hydrogen bonds in their structure. Before the advent of the microfluidic concept, microchannels in the form of glass capillaries were used in gas chromatography. The earliest microfluidic systems originated in MEMs, which used inorganic materials such as silica and glass. In addition, inorganic materials were primarily used as substrates in the design of microfluidic systems due to their superior surface stability, adjustable thermal conductivity, and solvent compatibility.

2.2.1.1 Silicon

Silicon (Si) is a group 4 element which is widely found in nature. Si is a crystalline solid which can also behave as a semiconductor. As a result of these properties, Si has great importance in computing and MEMs technologies. Silicon-based microfluidic platforms have the advantages of being thermally and mechanically stable and resistant to organic solvents [15]. However, the high cost of these materials and the necessity of using expensive manufacturing techniques (photolithography, micromachining, laser ablation, chemical etching, etc.) to obtain the desired geometries stand out as significant disadvantages [16]. In addition, the requirements for specific production conditions and experienced personnel with long-term training increase the processing costs. Silicon is optically opaque, which limits its use in some biological applications that require optical measurements, imaging, and detection.

Considering its advantages and disadvantages, there are many applications that use silicon microfluidic platforms. Si microfluidic devices have been used for nucleic acid purification due to their robust nature, charged surface, and the intermolecular interactions of silicon [17]. Si-based digital microfluidic devices have been integrated into mass spectroscopy for ultra-sensitive analysis of analytes that requires only a single droplet [18]. In the last decade, due to the urgent need for more complex microfluidic systems, Si has been integrated into more complex microfluidic devices for analytical sensing and testing applications [19].

2.2.1.2 Glass

Glass is an amorphous solid composed of silicon dioxide (SiO_2), silicate, and carbonate compounds. Before the advent of the microfluidics concept, microchannels in the form of glass capillaries were used in gas chromatography [20]. Glass is optically transparent over a large wavelength range, chemically inert, stable, and well-defined in terms of surface chemistry. The optical properties of glass have led researchers to primarily use glass in the development of microfluidics, as it overcomes the limitations experienced with silicon (table 2.1). For example, glass is more compatible with electro-osmotic flows than silicon, as glass has lower

Table 2.1. A comparison of the advantages and disadvantages of the use of glass and polymers in microfluidic device materials. Reprinted by permission from Springer Nature [23], Copyright (2009).

	Polymers	Glass
Manufacturing costs	Low cost relative to glass, especially for mass production	Higher in cost, especially for relatively large-area substrates. Higher costs are also associated with clean-room facilities
Fabrication complexity	Fabrication steps are simpler than those of glass, and no wet chemistry is needed	Time-consuming and expensive, and wet chemistry is used
Clean-room facilities	Clean-room facilities are necessary for applications in which avoiding dust contamination is critical. Particles may	Clean-room facilities are needed to avoid contamination

	become pressed into the polymer during processing without affecting device functionality	
Properties	A wide selection of polymers, hence mechanical, optical, chemical, and biological properties can be tailored	Less variability in available properties relative to polymers
Operational temperature	Limited for polymers because of relatively low T_g compared to glass	A wider range of operating temperatures relative to polymers
Optical properties and fluorescence detection	Optical transparency is lower than that of glass. Except for special grades, polymers also have higher autofluorescence relative to glass	Excellent optical properties; autofluorescence levels do not affect detection capabilities
Bonding	Different bonding options are available; for example: adhesives, thermal fusion, ultrasonic welding, and mechanical clamping	Time-consuming relative to polymers. Bonding options include thermal, adhesive, and anodic bonding
Surface treatment	Surface treatment methods are available for polymers, but routine, well-established derivatization techniques are not available	Established chemical modification procedures for glass are available using organosilanes
Compatibility with organic solvents or strong acids	Except for some special grades, polymers are generally not compatible with most organic solvents and in some cases, strong bases or acids	Good resistance to organic solvents and acids
Joule heating	Subject to significant Joule heating because of low thermal conductivity	More resistant to Joule heating relative to polymers
EOF	Smaller EOF produced relative to glass because of a lack of ionisable functional groups	Higher EOF relative to polymers
Geometrical flexibility	Polymer processing techniques offer more flexibility for geometrical designs, including, for example, different cross-sections (curved, vertical, or V-groove), high-aspect-ratio square channels, channels with a defined but arbitrary wall angle, or channels with different heights	Limited to 2½-dimensional designs. Due to the isotropic nature of the etching process, only shallow, low-aspect-ratio, mainly semicircular channel cross-sections are possible in glass substrates
Permeability to gasses	Higher gas permeability relative to glass	Glass does not have the gas permeability required for some biological applications, such as living mammalian cells

electroconductivity than silicon [21]. In addition, glass has an inert surface chemistry for fluid interactions in microfluidic applications.

Glass microfluidic devices can be manufactured by laser, micro-milling, chemical etching (hydrofluoric acid, HF) etc [22]. The major disadvantage of glass in microfluidic device fabrication is the difficulty of preparing anisotropic structures with high aspect ratios through cost-effective techniques, as highly experienced personnel are needed. Recently, liquid glass has been produced in the form of light-curable amorphous silica nanocomposites. These developments have demonstrated advantages for prototyping and manufacturing glass-based microfluidics at lower cost, higher accuracy, and without the need for clean-room facilities or toxic chemicals.

2.2.2 Organic materials

The organic materials used in microfluidic device fabrication are generally robust and low cost. Organic materials have simple production processes for microfluidic devices. The most frequently used organic materials for microfluidic devices are poly (methyl methacrylate) (PMMA), polycarbonate (PC), polystyrene (PS), polyvinyl chloride (PVC), cyclic olefin co-polymers (COCs), and cellulose (paper). Compared with inorganic materials, organic materials—especially polymers—have many advantageous features such as easy surface modification, simple production techniques, cost-efficiency, low thermal conductivity, and high biocompatibility for biomedical applications. In addition to their advantages, organic materials also present challenges such as rapid aging, chemical resistance, and mechanical, thermal, and optical limitations.

2.2.2.1 Poly(methyl methacrylate) (PMMA)

PMMA (figure 2.5) is a cheap thermoplastic material with broad use in microfluidic devices. In addition to PMMA, PC, PS, PVC, and COCs are thermoplastics frequently used in microfluidic chip production. PMMA has superior properties over the other most frequently used polymer, PDMS, such as improved solvent compatibility, gas non-permeability, and greater hardness [24]. PMMA is particularly advantageous for disposable microfluidic chips due to its mechanical strength, optical transparency, compatibility with electrophoresis, and low cost. Reusable PMMA not only offers a lower cost but is also an environmentally

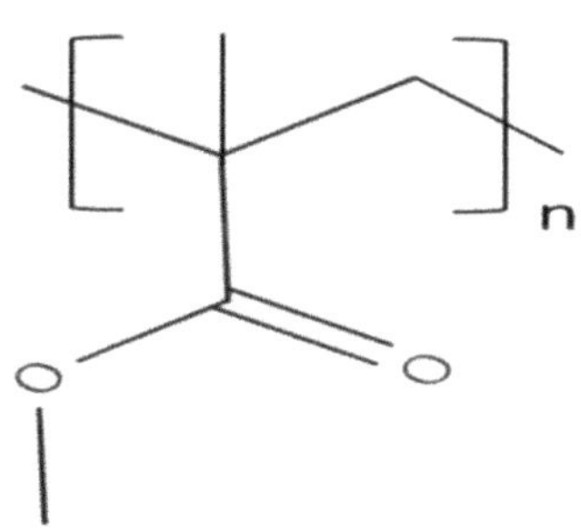

Figure 2.5. Molecular structure of PMMA.

friendly approach [25]. PMMA has additional advantages, such as its ease of fabrication and modification when used in microfluidic device production. Numerous methods can be used in the production of microfluidic PMMA devices, such as CO_2-laser micromachining, hot embossing, solvent printing, injection moulding, laser ablation, and micro-milling [24, 26, 27]. In addition, the surface chemistry of PMMA can easily be modified by solutions or plasma treatment to manipulate the surface energy and hydrophobicity/hydrophilicity parameters, which directly affect the fluid flow inside, depending on the intended use. For example, in a study of the use of PMMA microfluidic devices for blood cell filtration, channel surfaces were modified by an oxygen plasma treatment to increase surface energy and hydrophilicity [28].

After two-dimensional (2D) manufacture is applied for microfluidic channel production, there is a need to bond two layers of the chip to obtain a 3D microfluidic device without causing leakage. Several techniques can be used to bond the microchip layers, such as thermal bonding, solvent bonding, polymerisation bonding, microwave bonding, adhesive tape, etc [25]. PMMA has been used as a substrate for numerous microfluidic devices, such as fabrication chips, disposable biosensors, micromixers, DNA sequencers, and electrophoretic chips.

2.2.2.2 Polydimethylsiloxane (PDMS)

Polydimethylsiloxane (PDMS) (figure 2.6) is a hydrophobic and viscoelastic polymer. George M. Whitesides and his co-workers first described its use in microfluidic devices in 1995, and PDMS has since become the most widely used elastomer in microfluidic devices [29–31]. PDMS is optically transparent and has a UV cutoff value of 240 nm. PDMS is an insulating material in terms of electrical and thermal characteristics. PDMS is an inert, biocompatible (non-toxic) material which has a tunable Young's modulus (elastomeric) and is permeable only to gases and organic solvents (non-polar). In addition, PDMS has low surface energy and reactivity but can be oxidised by plasma for modification purposes [32]. The siloxane groups of PDMS make it versatile in terms of surface energy, hydrophilicity, and the bonding of new functional groups. Plasma treatment of the PDMS surface can impart a hydrophilic character to PDMS by reducing the contact angle of the water–PDMS interface. On the other hand, hydrophilic polymer grafting (using, for example, polyethylene glycol) can also induce a hydrophilic character and reduce nonspecific interactions with biological fluids and proteins [33].

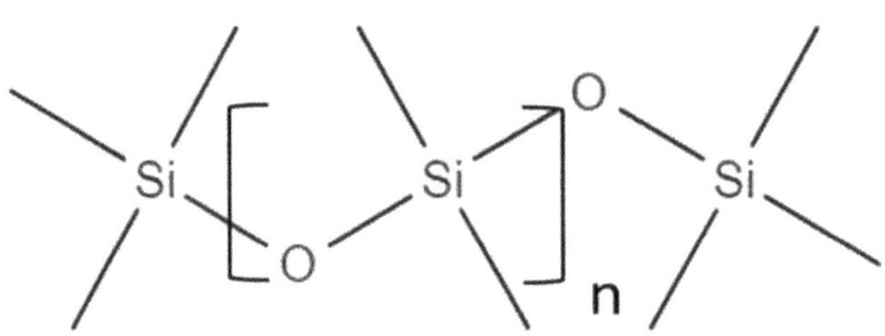

Figure 2.6. The molecular structure of PDMS.

PDMS is the most commonly used material in microfluidic devices. To fabricate microfluidic devices using PDMS, soft lithography (a non-photolithographic reproduction moulding strategy) is generally utilised. PDMS microfluidic devices can be produced via soft lithography using simple mixing, casting, and heating steps [34]. SU-8 is a very suitable and frequently used photoresist for microfluidic PDMS device fabrication [35].

PDMS has important advantages such as easy replication, low-cost fabrication, optical transparency, high gas permeability, elasticity, robustness, and biocompatibility, making it a particularly suitable material for microfluidic platforms designed for biomedical applications [36]. Microfluidics produced from PDMS have also contributed to the development of flexible electronics in the last decade. [37]. PDMS is permeable to gases due to its intermolecular spaces and can therefore support long-term cell culture applications that cannot be achieved using silicon or glass-based microfluidics. [38]. Although it is the most popular and widely used material for microfluidic devices, PDMS also has limitations and disadvantages. PDMS is incompatible with organic solvents. When it interacts with fluids that contain organic solvents, the channels of the microfluidic device deform and change their dimensional properties. Since PDMS is gas permeable, concentration changes can occur during liquid processing operations in microchannels due to evaporation [39]. PDMS can restrict short-wavelength fluorescence detection, resulting in the disadvantage of reduced measurement sensitivity compared to that of glass. Considering the advantages and disadvantages of PDMS, its potential for use in microchip production based on hybrid materials comes to the forefront.

2.2.2.3 Paper

Paper is a porous, economical, recyclable matrix produced by the compression of cellulose fibres from wood, cotton, and green plants. Litmus paper has been used as a scientific testing tool since the 1800s, according to the first well-known sample of literature [40]. Microfluidic paper-based analytical devices (μPADs) were first introduced by Martinez *et al* from the Whitesides Research Group in 2007 [41]. Paper has some unique properties, such as porosity and microstructure. These properties increase its passive transport of liquids due to its liquid capillary action, making it particularly suitable for microfluidic applications.

Paper can easily be functionalised by treating it with different liquids. Properties such as wettability, colour change, conductivity, and mechanical resistance can also be selected. μPADs have created an easy and inexpensive option for adapting laboratory-on-a-chip platforms, especially diagnostic applications. μPADs are cost-effective devices that can be produced with fast and inexpensive techniques using simple chromatography paper and are easily controlled by capillary forces without the need for additional pumping equipment. The main fabrication techniques used for μPADs are inkjet etching, plasma etching, wax printing, photolithography, cutting, and plotting [41].

The principal fluid flow phenomenon in paper-based microfluidics is based on capillary flow. The main parameters the affect capillary flow are the surface chemistry of the paper (wettability), the physicochemical properties of the grooves, and the pore size. The wicking-based flow that takes place on paper occurs at low Reynolds numbers due to micron-scale pores, and under these conditions, the flow is considered laminar [42]. For paper-based microfluidics (e.g. nitrocellulose) with constant cross-section and porosity, self-imbibition at narrow time intervals can be modelled by Darcy's law (equation (2.5)). The equation is defined using Q, the volumetric flow rate, κ, the paper permeability, A, the paper's cross-sectional area, μ, the dynamic viscosity, ΔP, the pressure drop over a channel length of L. Kinetic energy is ignored along the circular and straight microchannels [43].

$$Q = \frac{-\mathrm{K}A}{\mu L}\Delta P \tag{2.5}$$

μPADs are also defined by the Hagen–Poiseuille equation in terms of liquid flow characteristics and by the Laplace–Young equation, which defines the effect of the surface contact angle and the resulting surface wetting properties [42].

Due to their inexpensive paper-based starting materials and their potential for simple and large-scale production, μPADs are ideal platforms for point-of-care and rapid diagnostic kit applications. The most well-known and frequently used paper-based diagnostic kits are pregnancy tests, glucose sensor strips, and, in recent years, COVID-19 rapid diagnosis kits. The detection can be performed using colorimetric, electrochemical, luminescent, or electrochemiluminescent (ECL) techniques [42]. However, most paper microfluidic analytical instruments rely on colorimetric detection. The porous nature of the paper also allows for a combination of flow, filtration, and separation. Paper is biocompatible and its white background normally provides contrast for colour-based detection methods. Paper can also be easily disposed of or recycled, which is a huge advantage for disposable test kits. Paper-based microfluidics offers a promising platform for diagnostic bioassays to address global health issues due to their advantages of simplicity, rapidity, portability, and low cost, especially in the fields of health, environmental pollution, forensic science, and nutrition [44].

2.2.2.4 Hydrogels

Hydrogels are cross-linked polymer networks in which the majority of the total mass consists of water. Water-soluble polymers can be used as hydrogel matrices by controlling the degree of polymerisation of polymer chains. The highly porous structure of hydrogels, combined with their controllable pore size, allows for the diffusion of various molecules through the matrix. The macromolecular structure and the high water content of hydrogels allow them to mimic the extracellular matrix (ECM) and support molecular diffusion in biological systems [45, 46]. The main obstacle encountered in tissue engineering cell studies is the lack of vascularisation and the subsequent low diffusion in high-layer-thickness scaffolds (~500 μm) [47]. Microfluidics offers promising strategies with which to overcome the vascularisation and related problems encountered in tissue engineering studies. Through the use of hydrogel microfluidic devices, microchannels that function as vessels in the bulk structure can be created to provide nutrients and transfer oxygen to the cells. In addition, the inner surfaces of the channels of elastomer or thermoplastic microfluidic devices are coated with hydrogel, and vascular tissue engineering studies are carried out in the hydrogel layers [48, 49].

The inherent biocompatibility, tunable degradability, and high permeability of many hydrogels make them ideal for biomedical microfluidic applications. Due to their low density at the macromolecular scale, hydrogels can only support lower resolutions (on the micrometre scale) in microfabrication, while other polymers can support higher resolutions (on the nanometre scale). Two methods are adopted to create microchannels. The first is a method of direct writing that can generate random 3D structures at low speed; it involves gelling the gel solution from low-density water (LDW) and a moving head. The second is a two-step method that involves creating microchannels and seals. Hydrogels can be functionalised to respond to external stimuli (temperature, pH, or chemical concentration) [50, 51]. Swelling properties introduce mechanical changes (expansion or contraction) within the microchannels, where response times are determined by the diffusion rate. The stimulus-responsive behaviour of hydrogels also makes it possible to design them for modifiable surface wettability.

2.2.3 Hybrid materials

Hybrid materials are materials that result from the interaction of chemically dissimilar components (most often organic and inorganic in nature). They have specific structures that are different from those of the starting components but often retain some of their specific properties and functions. Following the initial use of silicon in microfluidic applications, microchannels were then fabricated from a variety of materials, such as glass, polymer, paper, and hydrogels. Each of these materials alone has limitations on its use in extended microfluidic applications [52]. The combination of different component materials and the use of composite materials are emerging strategies and offer approaches that can address these challenges.

Hybrid microfluidic systems are available that include combinations of Si, glass, PC, PMMA, hydrogels, paper, PDMS, and biodegradable materials. The combination of PDMS with other materials to fabricate hybrid microfluidic devices has been extensively studied in recent decades. [53]. PDMS and glass-layered hybrid microfluidic devices have also been regularly reported in the research literature. PDMS can be easily moulded with an SU-8 epoxy resin to produce microfluidic devices. The PDMS pattern obtained from the negative of the mould can be adhered to the glass by plasma or heat. The low-cost, easy fabrication procedures of PDMS–glass hybrid structures are examples of the advantageous features of hybrid structures [54].

Digital microfluidics is also a common example of a hybrid system. A glass bottom layer, a lithographically produced patterned electrode layer, and moulded PDMS layers are combined by plasma bonding [55]. Depending on the specific aim of the digital microfluidic device, the channel geometry, electrode material, and the combination of materials can be varied. Digital hybrid microfluidics yields miniaturised devices that offer easy-to-use and economical solutions that can combine chemical reaction, separation, and sensing steps in a single microfluidic device. In addition to solid-based hybrid and composite materials, liquid-based materials also offer new possibilities for microfluidics. For example, the idea of using a liquid liner to prevent fouling within a microchannel has revealed the antifouling microfluidics of liquid-infused porous membrane materials, which have exceptional stability when exposed to a variety of chemicals, particles, proteins, and blood [56].

Miniaturised paper/polymer hybrid microfluidic microplates (PMMA, PDMS, etc.) have been developed to reduce analysis time and cost [57]. They ensure rapid immobilisation of biomolecules and offer high performance over flow control. This is a feature that pure paper-based devices cannot offer. In some newly developed PDMS/paper hybrid microfluidic systems, paper can facilitate the on-chip integration of graphene-oxide-based nano-sensors without the need for complex surface treatment. These hybrid systems can facilitate highly efficient point-of-care diagnosis [58]. A summary of microfluidic device materials is given in table 2.2.

Table 2.2. A summary of microfluidic device material properties.

	Silicon	Glass	PMMA	PDMS	Hydrogel	Paper
Transparency	Opaque	Transparent	Transparent	Transparent	Transparent	Opaque
Surface hydrophilicity	Hydrophilic	Hydrophobic	Hydrophobic	Hydrophobic	Hydrophilic	Variable
Gas permeability	Poor	Poor	Variable	Good	Excellent	Good
Rigidity	Rigid	Rigid	Moderate to rigid	Soft	Soft	Variable
Chemical stability	High	High	Variable	Moderate	Low	Moderate
Thermal stability	High	High	Variable	Moderate to good	Low	Low
Thermal conductivity	High	Low	Low	Low	Low	Low
Biocompatibility	Good	Good	Good	Good	Good	Good
Running cost	High	High	Moderate	Moderate	Moderate	Low
Ease of manufacturing	Low	Low	Moderate to high	High	High	High

2.3 Microfluidic chip development technologies

Microfluidic devices provide advantages such as controlled heat and mass transfer in the realisation of chemical reactions, prevention of cross-contamination, and precision working that ensures high reproducibility. On the other hand, while providing these benefits, the key factors in microfluidic devices use are its size scale, low cost, and ease of manufacture. When microfluidic devices are being designed and manufactured, the material used and the procedure adopted should be the easiest and most economical combination for the target product (figure 2.7).

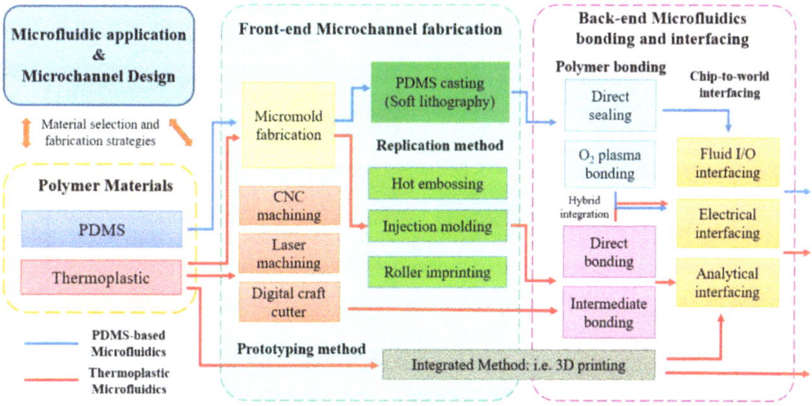

Figure 2.7. Microfluidic device fabrication chart for polymeric materials. Reproduced from [36]. CC BY 4.0.

When all these features are evaluated, machinability and processing techniques gain importance; consideration of the advantages and disadvantages of these factors allows the materials used in the microfluidic devices described in the previous section to move to the chip and application scales. In the following sections, photolithography, soft lithography, three-dimensional printing, and milling techniques, which are the main techniques used in the production of microfluidic devices, will be explained in terms of their methods, required equipment, operational costs, and ease of operation (figure 2.8).

2.3.1 Photolithography

The words 'photo', 'litho', and 'graphy' are all of Greek origin, meaning 'light', 'stone', and 'writing', respectively. Photolithography is a process used in microfabrication to model parts on a thin film or a large portion of a substrate (wafer). Photolithography is the most frequently used lithographic technique commonly found in literature. It is the process of shaping photoresist that covers a silicon wafer using a photomask. Since its invention, photolithography has greatly promoted the development of ICs and MEMs technologies. Photolithography, which also contributes to the production of the masks used in soft lithography, has maintained its importance as a technique that forms the cornerstone for its various uses in microfluidic devices today.

The first step in microfluidic device fabrication via photolithography involves transferring the designed channel geometry to the photomask. There are numerous drawing programs that can be used in the design of channel geometries, such as AutoCAD, CADopia, Adobe Illustrator, Cadence, CorelDRAW, Layout Editor, etc [59]. The photomask thus produced is used to transfer the channel patterns to the photoresist substrate. The photoresist can be produced by two different strategies, namely positive photoresist and negative photoresist. The negative photoresist becomes insoluble in the solvent processing step as a result of cross-linking when the polymer resist is exposed to ultraviolet (UV) radiation. This allows a negative

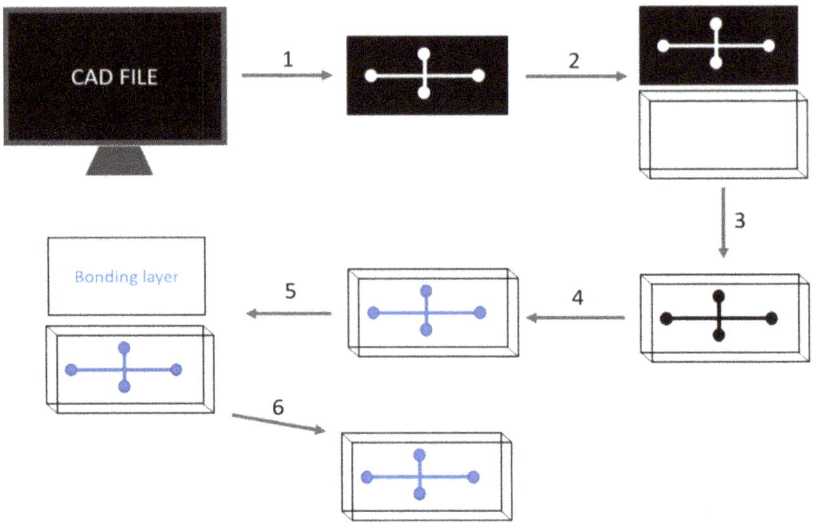

Figure 2.9. A schematic representation of the steps of PDMS microfluidic device fabrication using the soft lithography technique. (1) CAD-based photomask production (e.g. SU-8), (2) the production of photoresist on a silicon wafer using photolithography, (3) PDMS moulding on a silicon wafer replica, (4) PDMS replica removal, (5) bonding the second layer (glass, PDMS, etc.) to the top of negative PDMS replica, and (6) the final product, i.e. the microfluidic device.

rapidly so that the reaction medium is free of contamination, smooth, and free of gaps. Plasma sealing can also be supplemented with heat (70 °C) to increase durability [32]. Another irreversible sealing method, fusing, is applied by curing the excess monomers and curing agents of polymers in the sealing area [68]. Polymeric double-sided tape is also used as an inexpensive and easy method to reversibly seal surfaces together [32]. The smoothness of the surfaces that are reversibly interconnected by secondary van der Waals interactions is important for the strength of the bonding. [68]. When choosing the method to be used for bonding the surfaces together, the type of surface materials to be bonded, the type of working fluid in the channels, and the pressure should be considered. The success of bonding the surfaces to each other is important in terms of ensuring the tightness of the bond and the effective operation of the microfluidic device.

2.3.3 Three-dimensional printing

The number of fields using 3D printing technologies and its technological developments has increased, especially in the last decade. Three-dimensional printing, also called additive manufacturing (AM) or rapid prototyping (RP), has been incorporated into new technologies used for the fabrication of microfluidic devices [69]. The printing of 3D microfluidic devices has become a cost-effective and easy alternative to traditional fabrication methods. Three-dimensional printers have been developed since the 1980s and have since been used in the production of microfluidic devices, especially those produced to meet the needs of biomedical technologies, cell culture systems, and tissue engineering applications [70, 71].

Three-dimensional printing was first used to produce microfluidic devices via the stereolithographic (SL) technique. The SL technique consists of the 3D printing of a prepolymer (photosensitive resin) with the aid of pneumatic valves and the process of forming a pattern by curing the prepolymer with a UV laser at the time of printing. Cured polymer resins are collected layer by layer. Uncured prepolymers are washed away from the structure to create a pattern in the targeted geometry [72]. Two-photon polymerisation (2PP) is another class of lithography-based 3D printing that uses femtosecond laser pulses to cure a photosensitive resin [73]. Stereolithography enables production at the micrometre scale. The micro-stereolithography technique (digital light processing, DLP), which is customised using micro-mirror arrays as a dynamic mask, allows the resolution to be reduced to less than 100 μm [74, 75].

Extrusion 3D printing (fused deposition) technology is based on creating 3D structures by heating thermoplastic polymer coils or filaments and positioning them layer by layer in 2D for microfluidic device manufacturing [76]. The polymer is melted by heat in the printer's nozzle/chamber and written directly onto the collecting layer (figure 2.10) [75]. The extrusion-printed polymer hardens as it cools. The surface on which the underlay is placed moves along the x and y axes and the 3D structure is built up layer by layer, thus achieving 3D positioning. Extrusion 3D printing is used not only for the manufacture of microfluidic devices but also for the manufacture of valves, connectors, and fittings used in microfluidic devices [73]. The extrusion 3D technique is a cheap, fast, and direct production method that can be adapted to microfluidic device fabrication [77].

Photopolymer jetting, also called multi-jet modelling (MJM), is another 3D printing technique used to fabricate microfluidic devices [73]. The main difference between the photopolymer jetting 3D printing technique and stereolithography is

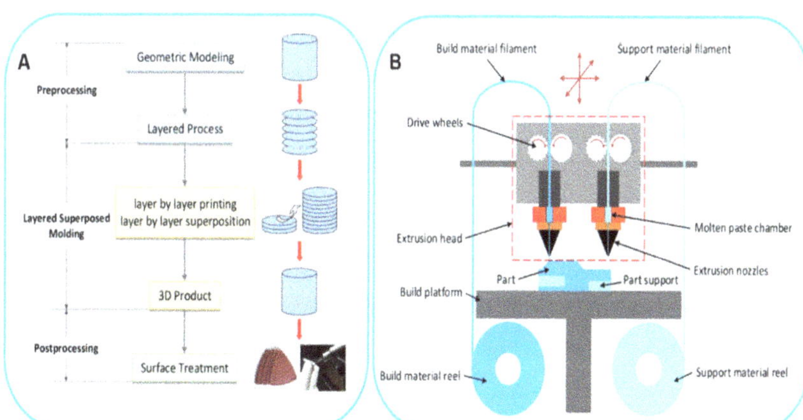

Figure 2.10. (A) A step-by-step view of the 3D printing procedure. (B) A schematic representation of 3D printing by fused deposition modelling [75] John Wiley & Sons. [2016].

that curing is done during the printing process in stereolithography, while the curing process is carried out after the printing layer is complete in the photopolymer jetting technique. In this technique, different materials can be used in different layers. When the printing process is complete, the sacrificial wax layer must be removed from the printed 3D structure [78].

Inkjet 3D bioprinting is dedicated to the biological applications of microfluidics, especially for cells, microtissues, organs, and drug screening. This technique relies on direct writing of the microfluidic device or replica moulding. Hydrogels are the most commonly used inks for bioprinting, as they can satisfy the requirements of oxygen and nutrient transport [79, 80]. Hydrogel ink can also be cross-linked by light [81].

2.3.4 Milling

Micro-milling is a top-down, subtractive manufacturing technique applied with the aid of a rotational cutting unit. Micro-milling allows microfluidic devices to be produced with channels of differing geometries at the micron scale using the abrasion/cutting method and can be applied to materials ranging from polymers to metals. The basic equipment required to apply the micro-milling technique consists of a workbench, a spindle for positioning the material to be milled, a cutting device with a rotary head, and a computer to manage the operation and design (figure 2.11) [82]. Micro-milling systems operated by computer commands are also known as computer numerical control (CNC) micro-milling devices. The operational capability and precision of CNC micro-milling devices are affected by the resolution of the CAD, the motion accuracy of the milling device in the *x*–*y*–*z* axes, and the geometry and dimensions of the milling rotary insert.

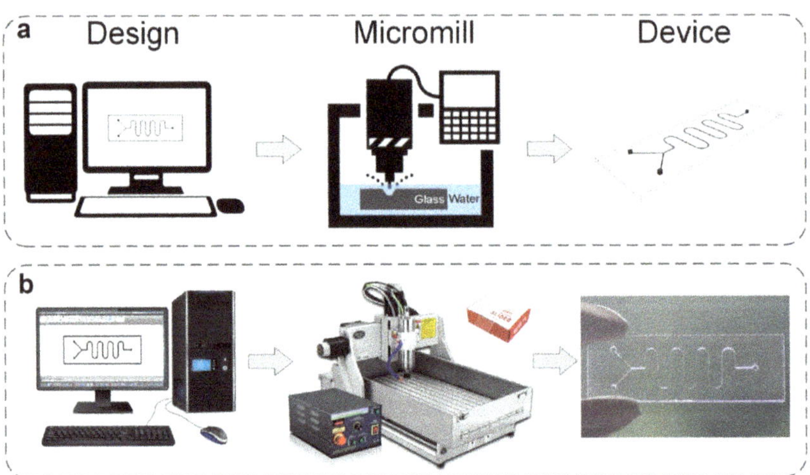

Figure 2.11. The process used to fabricate of glass microfluidic devices by micro-milling. (a) Schematic diagram, (b) photo of the corresponding setup. Reprinted by permission from Springer Nature [82] Copyright (2018).

Micro-milling has certain advantages in terms of producing microfluidic devices. The most important advantage is that the final product can be produced in a single step. In addition, the technique offers ease of manufacture and fast application that does not require preprocessing as a preparatory step [83]. The micro-milling technique is a simple and advantageous technique with a wide range of uses that include not only direct production but also mould fabrication. When evaluated in terms of production cost, the cost of each product is identical regardless of the number of produced items.

CNC milling devices have come to the forefront as capable systems in terms of precision, speed, and automation features for the production of microfluidic platforms. CNC mills enable production to scale from the micron to the metre scale. Therefore, they can manufacture microfluidic platforms with high scalability. Important factors in producing microfluidic patterns with targeted geometry and resolution are the material, geometry, and dimensions of the end mill [84].

To summarise, the CNC micro-milling technique is dependent on CAD design, spindle resolution, the materials used (thermoplastic, thermoset, elastomer, wax, metal, glass, etc.) and the end mill that directly shapes the resulting microfluidic product. The end mills used in micro-milling setups can consist of high-speed steel, cobalt, or carbide with coatings of titanium nitride (TiN), titanium carbo-nitride (TiCN), titanium aluminium nitride (TiAlN), or diamond [83]. Among the above materials, high-speed steel and carbide are the most preferable end mill materials due to their ability to resist heat and wear stress [85]. In addition, the end mill characteristics (fluting, helical angle, length, diameter, etc.) directly contribute to the resulting microfluidic channel geometry. The resulting channel shape can be manipulated to be square, ball-nosed, bull-nosed, tapered, drill bit shaped, etc. depending on the end mill shape fitted (figure 2.12) [83].

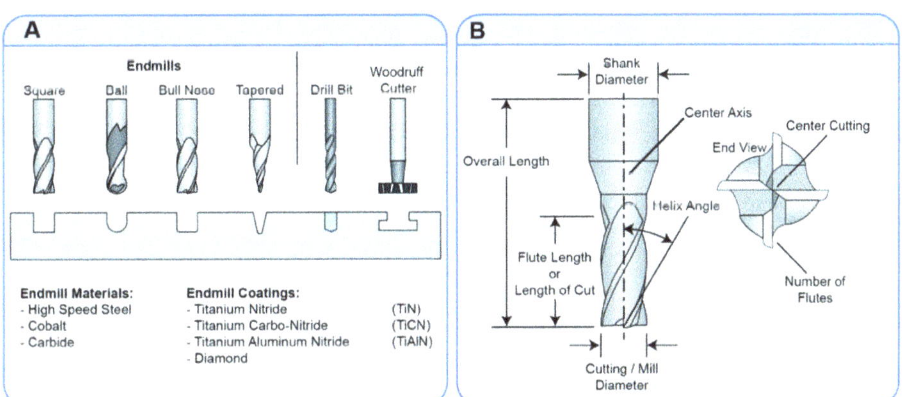

Figure 2.12. Representative images of micro-milling end mills. (A) End mill geometries, the resulting abraded (milled) surfaces, the materials used, and details of the coating materials. (B) End mill design details including diameter, fluting, helix angle, and length characteristics. Reproduced from [83] with permission from the Royal Society of Chemistry.

Microfluidic devices produced using the micro-milling technique allow for the inexpensive, easy, and fast production of prototype polymer-based microfluidic devices, especially for biological applications. Cell separation [86], macrophage culture [87], polymeric microparticle production [88], blood flow simulation [89], cancer modelling [90], etc. can easily be performed using microfluidic devices that have been specifically designed and produced with a target application in mind.

2.3.5 Hot embossing

Hot embossing is a simple, easy, and fast technique for microfluidic device fabrication. Thermoplastics are preferred materials for hot embossing technique applications, as they are suitable for shaping through temperature manipulation. However, hot embossing is applied not only to thermoplastics in the manufacture of microfluidic devices but also to wax, thermosets (uncured), elastomers (thermoplastic only), glasses/ceramics with polymeric top layers, and metals. Metal surfaces can be heat embossed, but the ability to manipulate them is limited to high temperatures and thin layers [91]. The hot embossing technique is based on the moulding of a negative copy of the microfluidic channel geometry by heat and pressure onto the desired surface. Hot embossing moulds can be composed of glass, metal (Ni), silicon wafers, etc [92].

Another advantage of hot embossing, apart from its ease of production at high accuracy, is the reduction in production costs as the number of products produced increases (economies of scale). Due to the use of a main mould that is produced once, manufacturing costs decrease inversely as the number of devices manufactured increases. PC and PMMA are the materials most frequently used for the manufacture of microfluidic devices by the hot embossing technique. The glass transition temperatures (T_g) of PC and PMMA polymers are 150 °C and 105 °C, respectively [93]. For this reason, these materials are commonly preferred, given the economic benefits, ease of production and energy savings.

The hot embossing technique is used to produce both negative and positive patterns. As an example, microfluidic cell culture platforms were fabricated by the hot embossing technique using a patterned SU-8 silicone master mould to obtain a negative PDMS replica. The resulting negative PDMS copy was first used to produce the epoxy master mould, and then COC microfluidic cell culture devices were fabricated from the negative of the epoxy copy (figure 2.13) [94].

In a study conducted with the aim of producing a PMMA microfluidic device by hot embossing (a Ni–Co stamp), the effects of embossing temperature and pressure on pattern accuracy were investigated. The microfluidic device pattern, which emerged as the temperature–pressure parameters were increased from 180 °C—20 kN to 200 °C—25 kN, was investigated comparatively. As a result, it was determined that increasing the pressure and temperature parameters provide higher accuracy and resolution in production [91].

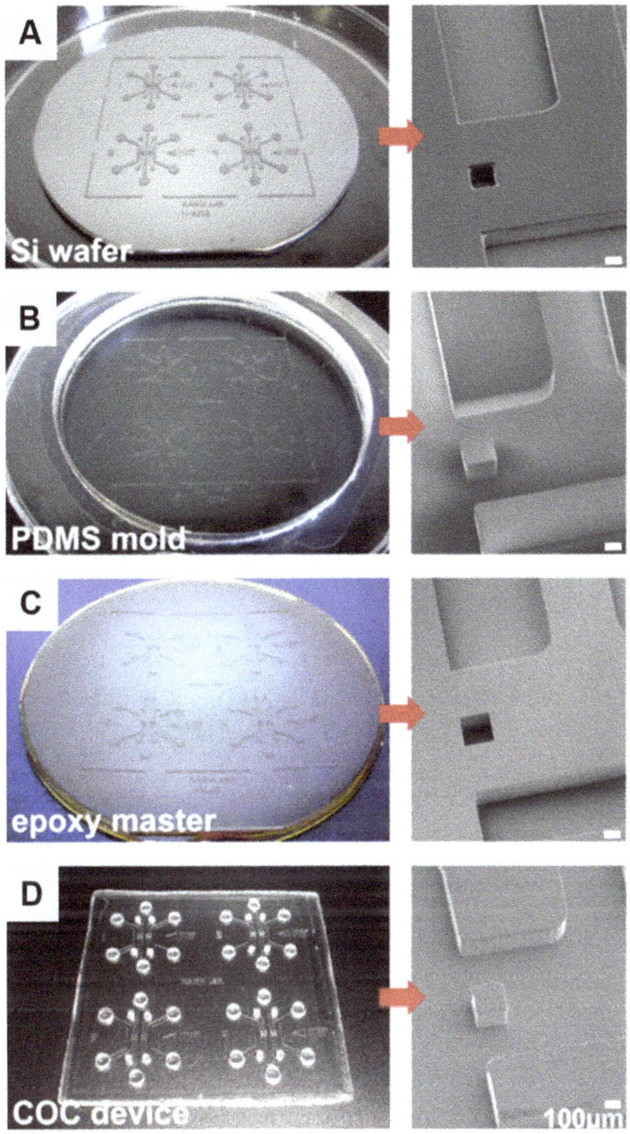

Figure 2.13. The steps of microfluidic device manufacture by the hot embossing technique. (A) Si wafer, (B) PDMS, (C) epoxy resin master, (D) COC microfluidic device. Reprinted by permission from Springer Nature [94], Copyright (2011).

2.3.6 Injection moulding

Although injection moulding is a well-known and frequently used method, the required production infrastructure creates high initial costs [95]. On the other hand, once the mould is produced, economy of scale reduces the running costs further down the line. The accuracy and the resolution parameters are dependent on the mould used. Reproducibility, accuracy, reduced cost, and an easy automation procedure are the key advantages of the injection moulding technique. In addition, the possibility of production using various polymers such as thermoplastics, thermosets, and elastomers creates an increasing variety of possibilities for the manufacture of microfluidic devices (figure 2.14).

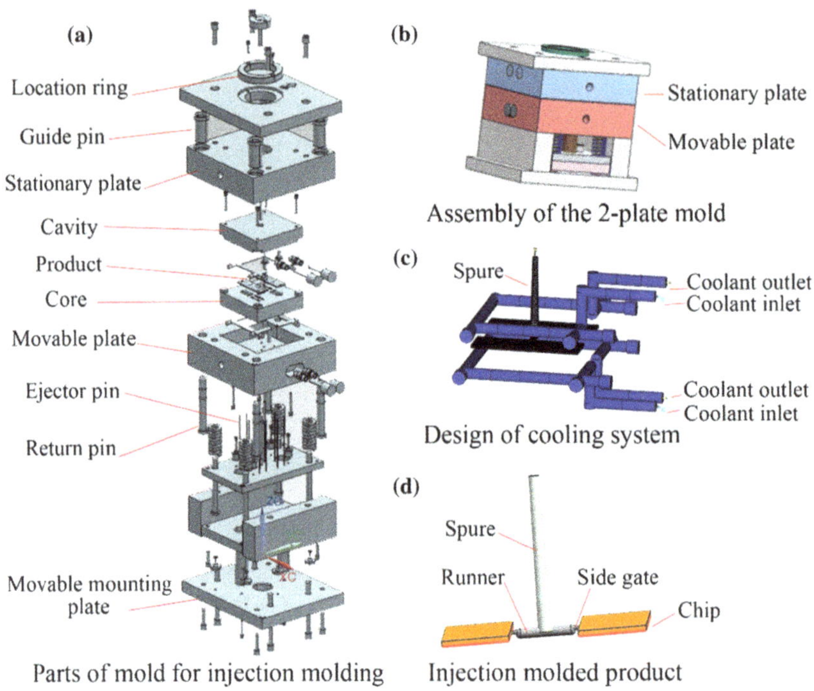

Figure 2.14. The steps in the production of microfluidic devices by micro injection moulding. (A) The parts of the mould used for injection moulding, (B) the assembly of the two-plate mould, (C) the design of the cooling system, and (D) the injection-moulded final product. Reprinted by permission from Springer Nature Customer [26], Copyright (2020).

The injection moulding technique can be divided into three main sub-groups as follows:

(I) Microinjection,
(II) Reactant injection, and
(III) Compression injection [96].

Microinjection moulding is the process of melting and moulding thermoplastics, non-cross-linked elastomers, or thermoset polymers from their granule or powder forms by heat treatment. Microinjection can include microstructure-manufactured microfluidics, depending on the pre-designed moulds used. The T_g of the polymer is an important parameter to consider when solidifying the molten polymer. When the temperature of the mould falls below the T_g value of the polymer, the polymer solidifies and the product can easily be removed from the mould [23].

Reactant injection requires at least two different molten polymers to be injected simultaneously into the mould, where they react. Compression injection consists of the injection of the molten polymer into the mould in the presence of applied pressure. Therefore, the mould pressure and temperature, injection speed and pressure, holding pressure and time, and cooling/reacting time are the working parameters that define the standard operational procedure (SOP) [97]. Figure 2.15 summarises a comparative evaluation of microfluidic device fabrication methods in terms of their technical capabilities and cost [83].

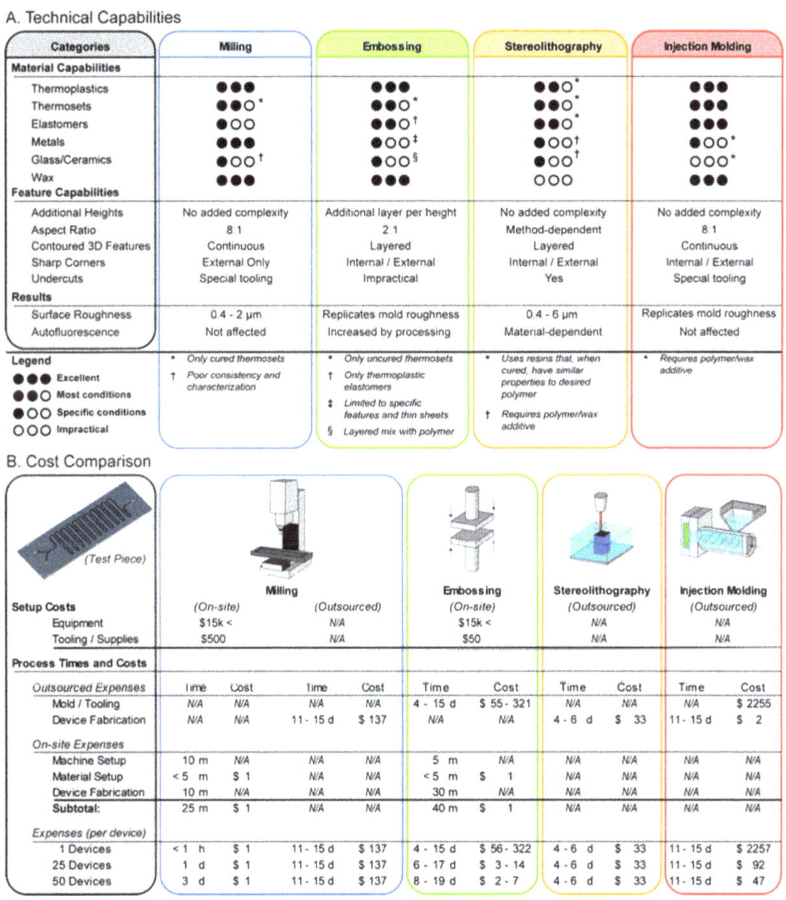

A. Technical Capabilities

Categories	Milling	Embossing	Stereolithography	Injection Molding
Material Capabilities				
Thermoplastics	●●●	●●●	●●○*	●●●
Thermosets	●●○*	●●○*	●●○*	●●●
Elastomers	●○○	●●○†	●●○*	●●●
Metals	●●●	●○○‡	●○○†	●○○*
Glass/Ceramics	●○○†	●○○§	●○○†	○○○*
Wax	●●●	●●●	○○○	●●●
Feature Capabilities				
Additional Heights	No added complexity	Additional layer per height	No added complexity	No added complexity
Aspect Ratio	8:1	2:1	Method-dependent	8:1
Contoured 3D Features	Continuous	Layered	Layered	Continuous
Sharp Corners	External Only	Internal / External	Internal / External	Internal / External
Undercuts	Special tooling	Impractical	Yes	Special tooling
Results				
Surface Roughness	0.4 - 2 μm	Replicates mold roughness	0.4 - 6 μm	Replicates mold roughness
Autofluorescence	Not affected	Increased by processing	Material-dependent	Not affected
Legend ●●● Excellent ●●○ Most conditions ●○○ Specific conditions ○○○ Impractical	* *Only cured thermosets* † *Poor consistency and characterization*	* *Only uncured thermosets* † *Only thermoplastic elastomers* ‡ *Limited to specific features and thin sheets* § *Layered mix with polymer*	* *Uses resins that, when cured, have similar properties to desired polymer* † *Requires polymer/wax additive*	* *Requires polymer/wax additive*

B. Cost Comparison

(Test Piece)	Milling				Embossing		Stereolithography		Injection Molding	
Setup Costs	*(On-site)*		*(Outsourced)*		*(On-site)*		*(Outsourced)*		*(Outsourced)*	
Equipment	$15k <		N/A		$15k <		N/A		N/A	
Tooling / Supplies	$500		N/A		$50		N/A		N/A	
Process Times and Costs										
Outsourced Expenses	Time	Cost	Time	Cost	Time	Cost	Time	Cost	Time	Cost
Mold / Tooling	N/A	N/A	N/A	N/A	4 - 15 d	$ 55 - 321	N/A	N/A	N/A	$ 2255
Device Fabrication	N/A	N/A	11 - 15 d	$ 137	N/A	N/A	4 - 6 d	$ 33	11 - 15 d	$ 2
On-site Expenses										
Machine Setup	10 m	N/A	N/A	N/A	5 m	N/A	N/A	N/A	N/A	N/A
Material Setup	< 5 m	$ 1	N/A	N/A	< 5 m	$ 1	N/A	N/A	N/A	N/A
Device Fabrication	10 m	N/A	N/A	N/A	30 m	N/A	N/A	N/A	N/A	N/A
Subtotal:	25 m	$ 1	N/A	N/A	40 m	$ 1	N/A	N/A	N/A	N/A
Expenses (per device)										
1 Devices	< 1 h	$ 1	11 - 15 d	$ 137	4 - 15 d	$ 56 - 322	4 - 6 d	$ 33	11 - 15 d	$ 2257
25 Devices	1 d	$ 1	11 - 15 d	$ 137	6 - 17 d	$ 3 - 14	4 - 6 d	$ 33	11 - 15 d	$ 92
50 Devices	3 d	$ 1	11 - 15 d	$ 137	8 - 19 d	$ 2 - 7	4 - 6 d	$ 33	11 - 15 d	$ 47

Figure 2.15. A comparative evaluation of microfluidic device fabrication methods in terms of (A) technical capabilities and (B) cost comparison (N/A = not applicable). Reproduced from [83] with permission from the Royal Society of Chemistry.

2.4 Microfluidic reactors

2.4.1 Mixing microfluidic reactors

Mixing microfluidic reactors are used for the rapid and homogeneous mixing of two or more samples in reactors with micron-scale channel sizes. For microfluidic reactors that provide mixing by the diffusion effect, two basic strategies are applied to ensure that mixing takes place. The first of these is 'active' mixing, in which an external force (pressure, electricity, ultrasound, etc.) is applied to ensure that proper mixing occurs. On the other hand, applications in which mixing is achieved using only the channel design/geometry of the microfluidic reactor (without the application of an external force) are defined as 'passive' mixing [98].

Reducing the volume and increasing the volume-to-surface ratio with the aid of micron-sized channels in microfluidic mixing reactors offer the possibility of using such reactors in applications that call for precise manipulation. In addition, a reduction in the channel's cross-sectional area in microfluidic mixer reactors also reduces the Reynolds number. Reducing the channel diameter while increasing the surface area is an important way to ensure homogeneous and highly efficient mixing of the medium. On the other hand, the channel length can be increased by preparing the channel geometry in the chip with S- or U-shaped curves (as opposed to a linear geometry) to increase the mixing time. Microfluids with low Reynolds numbers provide a controlled, linear mixing environment that does not exhibit turbulence [98]. Microfluidic mixer reactors are of great importance in providing solutions with high precision and efficiency for complex LOC applications. The use of these reactors in the food, chemical, biomedical (table 2.3), and pharmaceutical industries, especially in the fields of diagnosis, determination, and micro-/nano-production, is increasing day by day.

Table 2.3. The mechanisms of mixing microfluidic reactors and their biomedical applications. Reprinted by permission from Elsevier [99], Copyright (2019).

No.	Mechanism	Applications	Ref.
1	Acoustically driven mixer	Improving immunosensor performance	[100]
2	Multi-laminar flow	Following enzymatic bioreactions	[101]
3	Cilia reactor	Enhanced bioreaction efficiency (biotin–avidin assay, immunoassay, DNA hybridisation assay)	[102]
4	Chaotic micromixers	Luminol–Horseradish peroxidase (HRP) chemiluminescence reaction, tracking the early folding kinetics of human telomere G-quadruplex	[103–105]
5	Three-dimensional focusing	Studies of fast protein dynamics	[106]
6	Ultra-rapid hydrodynamic focusing microfluidic mixer	Microsecond protein folding events	[107]

(*Continued*)

Table 2.3. (*Continued*)

No.	Mechanism	Applications	Ref.
7	Hydrodynamic focusing microfluidic mixer	Self-assembly of liposomes	[108]
8	Coaxial turbulent jet mixer	Nanoparticle (NP) synthesis	[109]
9	Staggered herringbone micromixer (SHM)	Lipid nanoparticle (LNP) formation	[110]
10	Bubble-driven mixer	Cancer biomarker detection (enzyme-linked immunosorbent assay, ELISA)	[111]
11	Micro balloon mixers on centrifugal microfluidic platforms	Enhanced biosensing of dengue virus	[112]

2.4.1.1 One-dimensional streamline

The most common example of one-dimensional (1D) streamline microfluidic mixing is hydrodynamic flow focusing (HFF) (figure 2.16). HFF consists of an internal flow and an external flow that surrounds it like a sheath [114]. This core–shell-like enveloping flow pattern is usually described by the Péclet number (Pe, Jean Claude Eugène Péclet), which characterises the diffusion of flows that have two layers. The Péclet number is a dimensionless number defined as the ratio of the advective transport rate to the diffusion transport rate in the continuum. At the time of mass transfer, the Péclet number can be calculated by taking the product of the Reynolds number and the Schmidt number ($Pe = Re \times Sc$). T_{diff} is the diffusion time, T_{conv} is the convection time, U is the fluid velocity, D_h is the size of the microchannel's cross-section, and D is the precursor's diffusivity [115] (equation (2.7)).

$$Pe = \frac{T_{\text{diff}}}{T_{\text{conv}}} = \frac{U \quad D_h}{D} \tag{2.7}$$

A 1D streamline microfluid mixer was developed that contained a coaxial capillary fluid (figure 2.17A) [116]. The increased flow rate ratio, accompanied by high concentration and a high surface-to-volume ratio at the core–sheath fluid interface, decreased T_{diff}, thereby improving the mixing. The reduction of the overall flow rate also allowed T_{conv} to act longer in the microchannel, providing an improved mixing medium. In light of this information, 1D streamline microfluidic reactors based on HFF have great design and application potential. In particular, the use of 1D streamline reactors can produce nanoparticles with a narrow size distribution in a highly efficient manner [117].

2.4.1.2 Two-dimensional vortex

Two-dimensional vortex microfluidic mixing reactors allow 2D chaotic flow mixing to take place at low Reynolds numbers through the use of specifically pre-designed channel geometries. Mixing based on a 2D vortex flow provides a rapid mixing

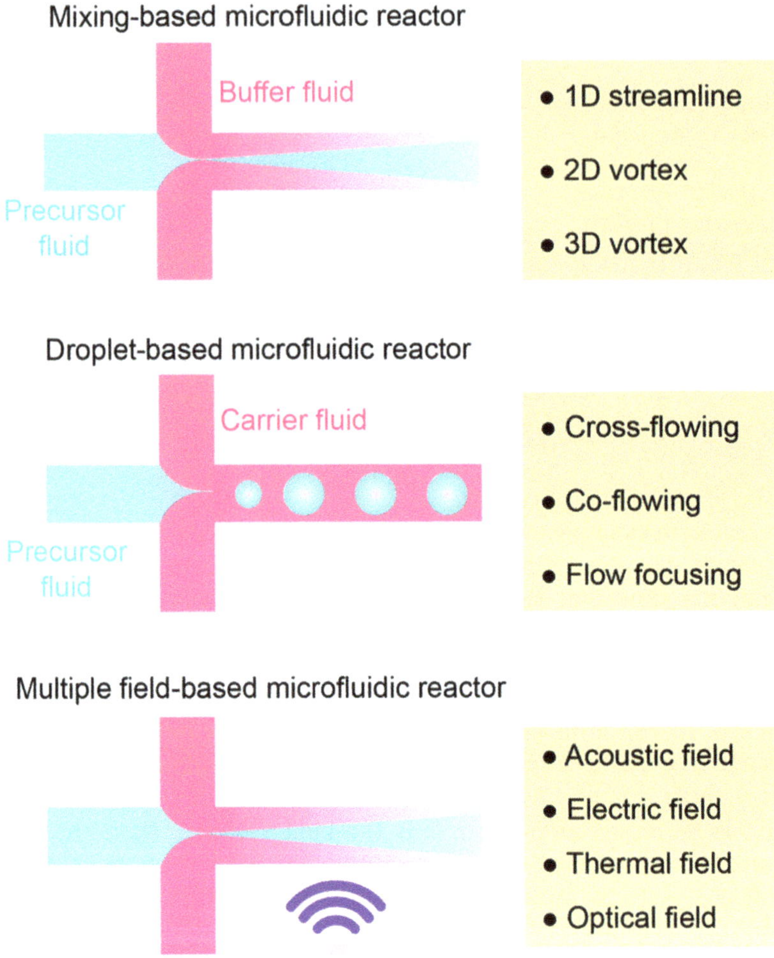

Figure 2.16. Microfluidic reactors and their action mechanisms. Reproduced from [113] with permission from the Royal Society of Chemistry.

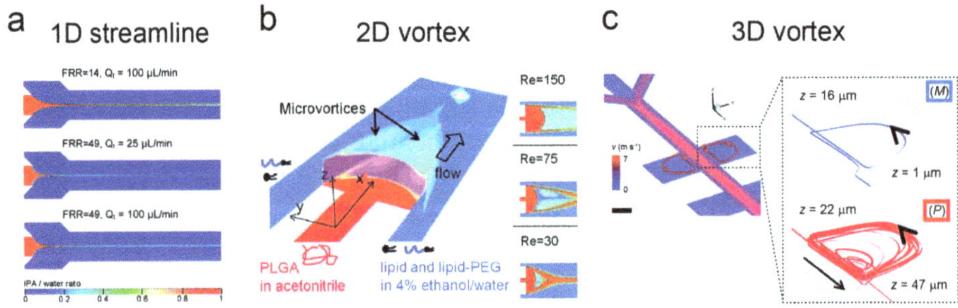

Figure 2.17. Mixing microfluidic reactors. (A) 1D streamline [116], (B) 2D vortex [119] (C) 3D vortex [122]. Reproduced from [113] with permission from the Royal Society of Chemistry.

environment with chaotic advection. Chaotic advection is related to the sequential repetition of stretching and folding of the fluid volume [118]. The flow circulating in the cross-section is provided by the induction of anisotropic flow resistance and by placing designed protrusions in the channel at an oblique angle to the main flow direction (figure 2.17B) [119]. Protrusions of the appropriate geometry are designed to repeatedly stretch and fold the liquid volume by increasing the surface-to-volume ratio and the concentration gradient [120]. The Dean vortex is another inertia-based mixing strategy, which is seen in microfluidics channels with curved geometries. In equation (2.8), De is the Dean vortex, Re is the Reynolds number, D_h is the radius of the channel, and the R is the curvature radius of the channel [113].

$$De = \mathrm{Re}\sqrt{D_h/2R} \tag{2.8}$$

The Dean vortex is caused by a mismatch between the central flow and the secondary surrounding flow interacting with the wall. Inertial forces are the main factor in this mismatch. The outward movement in the central flow mixes with the inward movement in the circumferential flow, resulting in the formation of a Dean vortex due to opposing movements [121].

2.4.1.3 3D vortex

Three-dimensional (3D) vortices have the potential and efficiency to mix the reaction medium more effectively than 1D streamlines and 2D vortices. Three-dimensional vortexes have a particular sign, which is determined by the rotation sense. This causes them to have helical chirality, which has a special effect on the way molecules self-assemble. Chiral 3D vortices can be produced by a micro-chamber with inclined geometry, which can be designed by placing notches along the sidewall of the microchannel (figure 2.17C) [122]. A difference between the flow rates of the main channel and the microchambers is obtained through the formation of counter-clockwise (CCW) and clockwise (CW) laminar flows that allow mixing to take place on opposite sides of the microfluidic chamber [123].

2.4.2 Droplet-based microfluidic reactors

Over the last few decades, droplet-based microfluidic reactors have gained great significance in many different fields. Biomedical applications stand out from other applications due to the huge research and application potential of droplet-based microfluidic reactors in, for example, drug delivery systems, gene therapy, tissue engineering products, and sensor applications. In particular, droplet-based micro-fluidic reactors have the potential to become the gold standard for the production of microbubbles and micro–nanoparticles. Droplet-based microfluidic reactors are based on co-flow, crossflow, and flow-focusing techniques. In the following sections, these systems will be explained in detail with conceptual and application examples.

2.4.2.1 Co-flows

The reaction mechanism of the co-flows that take place in droplet-based microfluidic reactors is provided by the co-flows of immiscible liquid phases. In a co-flow reactor, two separate fluids move in the same direction through a microfluidic device that has coaxially positioned capillary systems. In a co-flow capillary system, the liquids injected in separate phases cause droplets to form, accompanied by a downstream jetting or dripping regime at the end of the formed jet (figure 2.18). The droplet formation induced when a jet reaches a critical length is described by the Rayleigh-Plateau instability [124]. In conditions under which the jet length is sufficient, the axisymmetric changes occurring in the jet line induce contraction and expansion in certain regions of the jet. In both the jetting and dripping regimes, the axisymmetric geometry can be varied to obtain a co-flow, co-flow focusing, or non-embedded co-flow focusing [125].

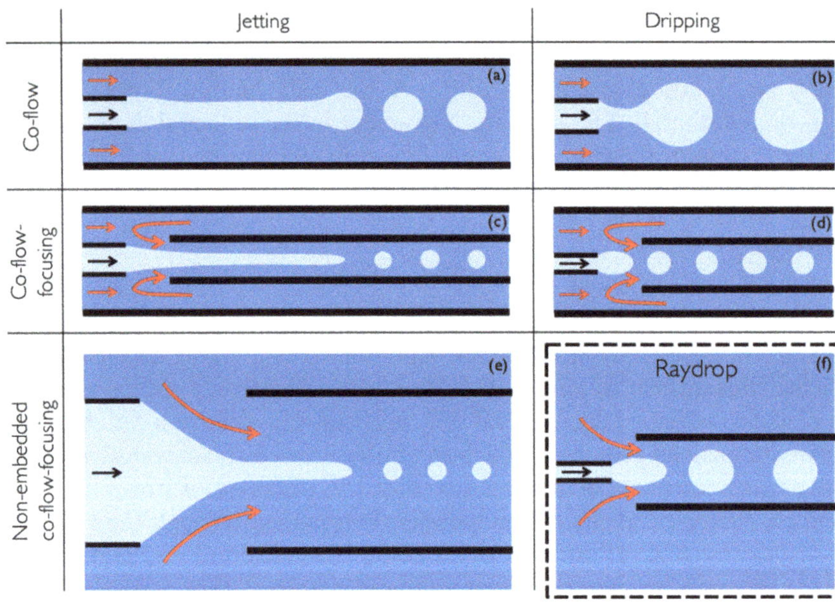

Figure 2.18. Droplet-based microfluidic reactors with axisymmetric designs. In the reactor schematics, the capillary channel walls are shown in black. (A) Jetting co-flow, (B) dripping co-flow, (C) jetting co-flow focusing, (D) dripping co-flow focusing, (E) jetting non-embedded co-flow focusing and (F) dripping non-embedded co-flow focusing. Reprinted by permission from Springer Nature [125], Copyright (2020).

The local pressure difference and the surface tension between the two liquid interfaces in the tapering regions of the jet are explained by Laplace's theorem. The resulting pressure difference causes droplets to form following the thinning of the jet along its axis. Droplet formation is achieved under conditions in which the surface tension between the fluids in the flow system and the viscous drag caused by instability are balanced and the Reynolds number is less than one [126]. The drip regime is a type of co-flow obtained by injecting liquids into the inner and outer fluids at low flow rates. Under low flow rates, the surface tension between the liquids is overcome by the drag force created by the outer phase and at the end of the jet. As a result, the liquid in the inner layer is separated and droplet formation is achieved.

Therefore, the formation of the dripping regime is related to the capilliary number due to the effect of the surface tension between two immiscible liquids on the viscous drag forces. In addition, the size of the droplets in the dripping regime is also related to the capilliary number. If the flow rate of the outer liquid layers increases, the capilliary number decreases and the droplet size increases. Under conditions in which Ca≈1, droplets are separated at the end of the jet and droplet formation is induced in the jetting regime [127].

2.4.2.2 Crossflows

Crossflows are another fluid-fluid interaction-based droplet manufacturing technique. A crossflow (or T-shaped flow) is similar to a co-flow in that it causes droplet formation due to the effect of Rayleigh-Plateau instability caused by a pressure difference at the liquid–liquid interface and an imbalance of inertial and viscous forces. Crossflow microfluidics have two main components: the main continuous phase in the straight channel and the side channel of the microfluidic device (figure 2.19). Crossflow microfluidic devices are most frequently designed with a T-junction geometry [128]. T-junction geometries have of a minimum of two side channels that are perpendicular to each other.

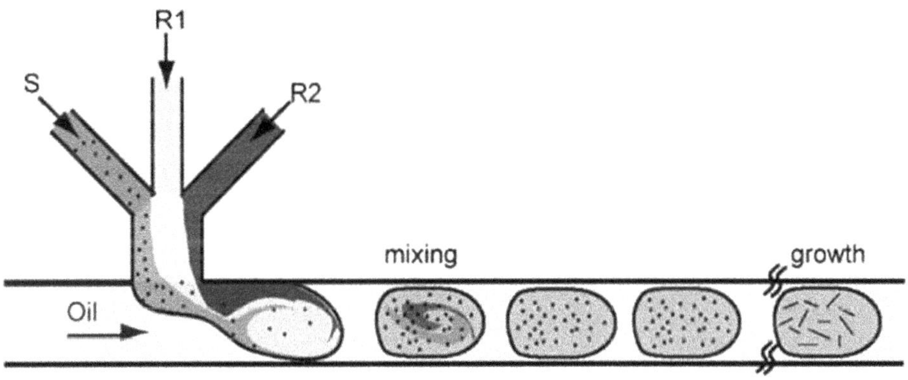

Figure 2.19. A representative image of a crossflow induced by a T-junction microfluidic device. The representation shows the initiation of gold nanoparticle growth in a seed solution (S), aqueous solutions (R1 and R2), and an oil phase [129] John Wiley & Sons. [2009].

Side-chain T-shaped microfluidics provides a practical and easy tool for droplet generation that uses crossflows for oil-in-water and water-in-oil emulsion systems [130]. Due to the partial blocking of the continuous phase by the dispersed phase, a shear gradient is produced, which causes the dispersed phase to extend and finally fragment into droplets. The shear stress has a significant impact on the droplet size [131]. It can provide very precise control in production, which allows the formation of structures from emulsion droplets to micro- and nanoparticles and liposomes in monodisperse and targeted sizes [129, 132, 133].

2.4.2.3 *Flow focusing*

The simplest description of hydrodynamic focusing is that it consists of squeezing the target sample fluid with another fluid, commonly referred to as the sheath fluid. In microfluidic systems which use the flow-focusing (FF) technique, the dispersed and continuous phases coaxially flow through a shrinkage region in the system to form an elongation filament. This filament then splits into droplets in a narrow region. The hydrodynamic focusing technique is categorised as two-dimensional (2D) or three-dimensional (3D) flow focusing, depending on the scale at which the sample fluid is compressed [134].

The 2D flow-focusing technique is a less complex technique compared to the 3D alternative. In the 2D flow-focusing approach, one dimension of the sample fluid remains constant while the other decreases due to the compression effect produced using a sheath fluid [135]. On the other hand, 3D flow-focusing systems include systems that are more complex and difficult to design and implement, since they have multiple sheath insertion and alignment steps. The tight focus zone makes it possible to manage the creation of particles/droplets with a narrow size distribution. The main parameters affecting particle size are as follows: the geometry of the microfluidic capillary channels, the flow rate, and the fluidic chemistry (viscosity, surface tension, charge, additives, etc) [133]. Flow-focusing devices are specified with different geometric designs to suit the target application/production purposes. Examples of the device geometries are illustrated in figure 2.20. The geometries

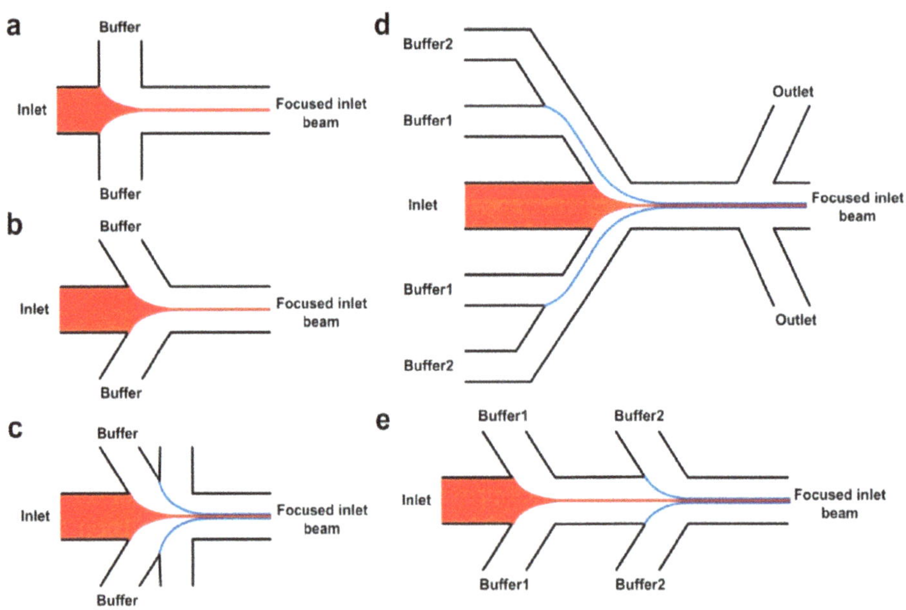

Figure 2.20. Flow-focusing microfluidic device designs. (A) Central flow with perpendicular sheath flows, (B) central flow with tilted angle sheath flows, (C) central flow with perpendicular and tilted angle sequent sheath flows, (D) an outlet bifurcation design used to concentrate products, and (E) serial sheath flows used to implement multistep processes. Reprinted from [136], Copyright (2016), with permission from Elsevier.

can be varied and include perpendicular, tilted, and complex serial combinations. In particular, applications that require more stable flows or more complex multistep production can be realised using serial sheath flow solutions [136].

Flow-focusing microfluidic systems offer manufacturing potential in a wide variety of particle and drug delivery applications based on materials such as metals, polymers, and lipids. In addition, FF is a technique frequently used in LOC and point-of-care (POC) applications such as cell separation and rapid diagnosis kits [135, 137, 138]. These applications are explained in detail with examples in the following sections.

2.4.3 Multiple-field microfluidic reactors

Multiple-field reactors combine the abovementioned reactor types with integrated externally applied fields (table 2.4). Compared to mixing and droplet-based microfluidic reactors, multiple-field microfluidic reactors have superior application potential to produce complex structures with better functionality when integrated with externally applied acoustic, electrical, thermal, and optical fields.

Table 2.4. A comparison of microfluidic reactors based on their advantages and challenges. Reproduced from [113] with permission from the Royal Society of Chemistry.

Microfluidic reactors	Advantages	Challenges
Mixing-based	Easy device fabrication	Inhomogeneous synthetic conditions in parabolic flow
	Scalable NP production	Prone to channel fouling
Droplet-based	Homogeneous synthetic conditions	Difficulty in generating droplets in micro-reactors
	Compatible with extreme synthetic conditions	Sophisticated flow control
Multiple-field-based	Complex NP structures with improved functionalities	Use of external force fields
	Complicated device fabrication	On-demand and active mixing

2.4.3.1 Optical fields

Microfluidic reactors integrated with optical fields can be used in fabrication and detection technologies in the fields of photoresponsive synthesis or point-of-care (POC) devices. Photopolymerization can be applied in a precisely controlled manner to produce microbubbles and micro/nanoparticles in a microfluidic reactor. The ultraviolet-light-induced photopolymerization of polymeric materials can easily be applied by microfluidic reactors [139]. In addition, photoresponsive nanoparticles such as plasmonic, photoluminescent, and shape-changeable nanoparticles can be easily synthesised by optical field microfluidic reactors [140]. The material used for the microfluidic device must be permeable to the wavelength used. The increased surface area and short light penetration depth of optical field-sourced microfluidic reactors make them highly desirable for use in fabrication.

Microfluidic biosensors use various optical field-based sensing techniques, such as fluorescence, chemiluminescence, surface plasmon resonance, and absorbance [141]. Though it becomes more difficult at smaller length scales, optical detection typically requires expensive hardware that is challenging to miniaturise [142]. On the other hand, expensive and complex biomolecular detection assays can be adapted to simple microfluidic systems that have reduced costs and fewer analytes. Optofluidics, which pioneered the combination of photonics and microfluidics, is a technology that is now coming to the fore, especially in the field of biosensors, and is expected to have wider application in the coming years [143].

2.4.3.2 Acoustic fields

A type of mechanical wave called an acoustic wave is propelled along as a longitudinal wave by an acoustic source. Such waves are created by the mechanical stress produced by a piezoelectric transducer. Surface acoustic waves and bulk acoustic waves are two distinct forms of sound waves [144]. In the field of microfluidics, both have been extensively utilised to manage microlitre volume solutions. Particle, bubble, and cell manipulation and separation using label-free techniques have been widely applied using microfluidic platforms in conjunction with acoustic fields [145, 146].

Utilising acoustic-wave-induced pressure in an acoustic resonator, acoustic standing wave technology can move and spatially localise cells and particles [147]. Since acoustophoresis is frequently carried out in a continuous flow, a separation mechanism is required that can split up particles with various acoustic physical properties. In addition, acoustophoresis can be used to aggregate particles or retain them against the flow in specific places, which is frequently accomplished using acoustic traps/tweezers. Microfluidics systems must be built with clearly defined acoustic resonators as a fundamental prerequisite to operating in an acoustic field mode [148].

2.4.3.3 Thermal fields

Thermal field-controlled microfluidic reactors allow for the fabrication and sensing of materials with precise manipulation and control capabilities that are provided by the temperature parameters [149]. The heat-controlled reactions of nanoparticles synthesised by the thermal effect in microfluidic reactors provide ultra-sensitive and uniform production at low volumes. Thermal-field-induced applications also include optothermal and thermoelectric microfluidic devices, especially biosensors [150–152]. Particle generation that uses an optothermal effect is accomplished by capturing and combining colloidal particles one at a time using heat generated by a light source. On the other hand, thermoelectric biosensors allow for the detection of biomolecules at lower analyte volumes and provide higher sensitivity compared to monofunctional electrochemical or calorimetric biosensors [153].

2.4.3.4 Electric fields

Electric-field-driven systems are useful for numerous biological applications and can be easily adapted to microfluidic devices using dielectrophoresis (DEP), electro-osmosis, and electrothermal induced-charge electro-osmotic (ICEO) flow mechanisms. Fluid flow and reaction processes are carried out in microfluidic devices with the help of the electrokinetic phenomena. Electric field-controlled microfluidic systems can use direct current (DC) or alternating currents (AC) [154].

The fluids that are used can act as conductors, insulators, or capacitors depending on their chemical structure and ionic strength. When an exemplary flow-focusing microfluidic setup is examined, it can be seen that when a DC-voltage-driven electrical field is applied to the electrodes placed in the microfluidic device, the water phase of the water and oil phases used acts as a conductor, the oil phase acts as an insulator, and the interface between the two phases acts as a capacitor. Particle and droplet generation and their sizes can easily be manipulated using the voltage and electric field parameters [155]. In addition to DC voltages, AC voltages are also effective for droplet generation. The effect of AC voltages on droplet generation is founded on electrowetting based on the dielectric (EWOD) principle. EWOD is mainly related to the contact angle gradient between the conductive fluid and the channel.

2.4.3.5 Magnetic fields

Magnetic-field-driven microfluidic reactors are produced by combining microfluidic devices, reactants, magneto fluids, and magnets. Magnetic particles take a leading role in these reactors, as they help to transport and localise materials [156]. The advantageous features of these systems include versatility, targetability, controllability, and non-contact mobility. In addition, magnetic manipulation in microfluidic reactors can perform both internal and external positioning, or a mixture of them [157]. This results in increased sensitivity and scope for a wider range of applications. Biomolecular separation, cell sorting, gene delivery, drug delivery, and magneto-mixing reaction environments are the main application areas of magnetic field-induced microfluidic devices.

2.5 Applications of microfluidic bio-fabrication

2.5.1 Microbubbles

Microbubbles are essentially scientific balloons made of an outer layer of polymer, protein, or lipid that is filled with gas. Microfluidics are the most practical and important tool for the facile and precise production of microbubbles. Microbubbles produced using precise production parameters and under well-defined conditions have seen wide use in the biomedical field within the last few decades. Microbubbles were initially used in the biomedical field as ultrasound imaging contrast agents. This use depends on the density difference between the gas layer inside the microbubbles and the host tissue (figure 2.21). Albunex® (Molecular Biosystems, now part of Mallinckrodt Inc. Hazelwood, MO, USA) pioneered a commercial contrast agent microbubble with an albumin outer layer which is used for myocardial echocardiography imaging [158, 159]. In addition to their ultrasound imaging applications, microbubbles have great potential for use in applications such as drug delivery, gene therapy, micro-mixing, microrobotics, micropumping, rotators, transporters, bio-assemblers, and chemical switchers (figure 2.22) [160].

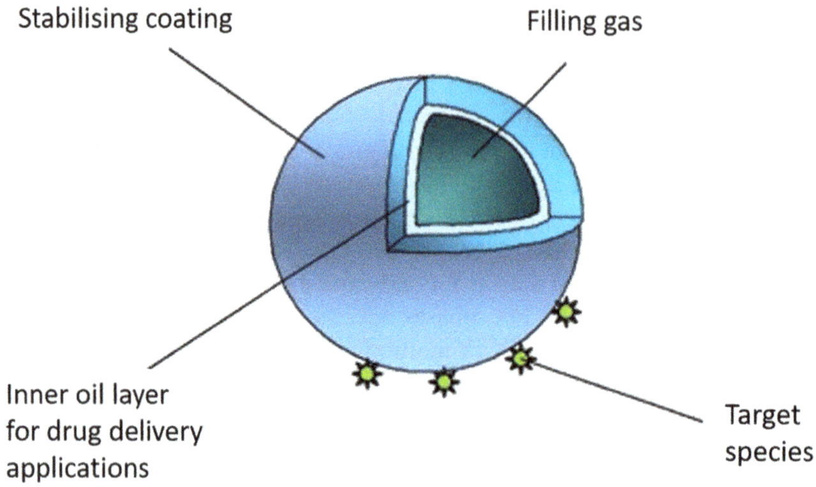

Figure 2.21. A schematic representation of a multilayered microbubble with a gas-filled core, an inner oil layer, a stabilising coating, and the target species. Reproduced from [159] with permission from the Royal Society of Chemistry.

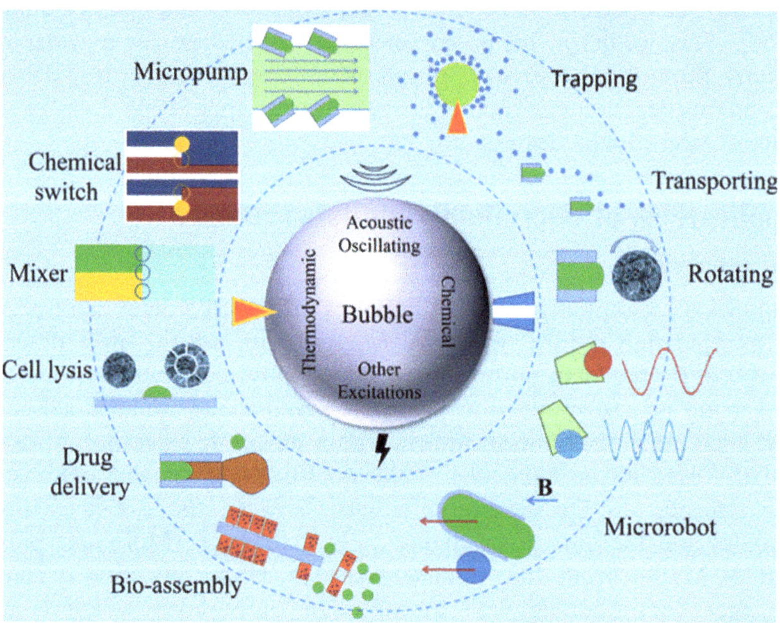

Figure 2.22. A schematic representation of the microfluidics-assisted generation of microbubbles and their respective application areas. Reproduced from [160] with permission from the Royal Society of Chemistry.

Microbubbles exhibit a wide range of use in biological applications because they can disappear from biological systems after fulfilling their intended purpose without causing any adverse side-effects. In addition, microfluidics aids in producing stable microbubbles with reduced size and high throughput. A microbubble's lifetime in a liquid is inversely proportional to the size of the microbubble. If the microbubble size decreases, the stability of the bubbles in a liquid system increases due to the reduction in the buoyant force [161].

Microbubbles have an outer shell layer which can be composed of polymers, proteins, or lipids. The outer shell can also consist of more than one layer. Multilayered microbubble structures create the opportunity for greater stability or versatile biological applications in just a single step. Multiple drugs can be delivered by different layers due to their physicochemical characteristics. Moreover, theragnostic applications, which include both therapeutics and diagnostics, can be implemented using microbubbles, which can perform both imaging and the transport of drug payloads. In the last few decades, microfluidic devices have been used to produce small and monodisperse microbubbles with precise control [162]. The main limitations of microfluidic devices are the pressure and flow rate conditions (figure 2.23) [159]. The microfluidic device's inner channel geometry, its length and diameter, the applied gas pressure, liquid flow rate, viscosity, and surface tension are the key parameters for microbubble production. The microfluidic device geometry is directly related to the microbubble production technique.

Microfluidic devices are categorised as T-junction, flow-focusing, and co-flow microfluidic devices, depending on their channel geometries. Table 2.5 gives brief

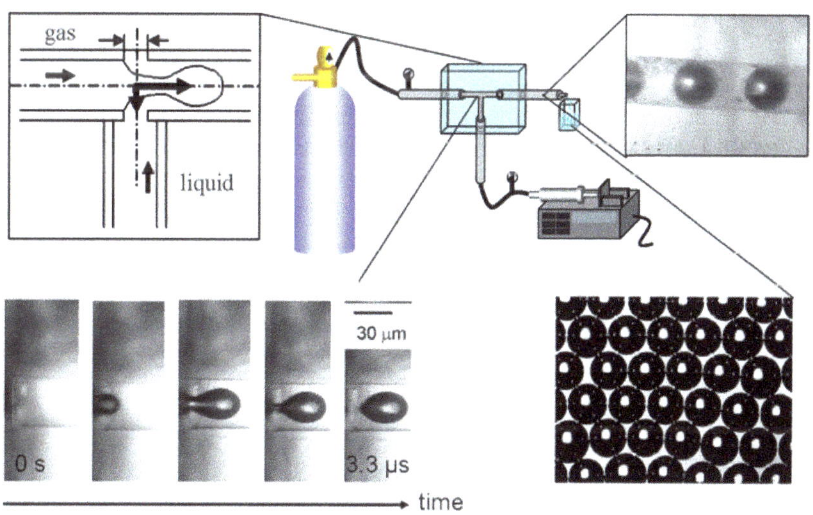

Figure 2.23. Representative images of the T-junction microfluidic device setup and microbubble fabrication. High-speed camera images of microbubble production inside the T-junction microfluidic device and its corresponding resulting structures. Reproduced from [159] with permission from the Royal Society of Chemistry.

Table 2.5. Classification of commercial microbubbles according to the gas they contain, their outer-layer structure, and manufacturer. Reproduced from [159] with permission from the Royal Society of Chemistry.

Name(s)	Manufacturer	Stabilising coating	Filling gas
SonoVue®	Bracco Diagnostics, Inc.	Phospholipid	Sulphur hexafluoride
Definity® *Aerosomes*™ *MRX115* *DMP115*	Bristol-Myers Squibb Medical Imaging Inc.	Phospholipid	Octafluoropropane
Optison™	Amersham Health plc. (GE Healthcare Inc.)	Cross-linked human serum albumin	Octafluoropropane
Filmix™	Cav-Con Inc.	Phospholipid	Air
Imavist™ *Imagent®*	Alliance Pharmaceutical Corp. Schering AG	Surfactant	Perfluorohexane and air
Albunex®	Molecular Biosystems (Mallinckrodt Inc.)	Sonicated human serum albumin	Air
Sonazoid™	Amersham Health plc. (GE Healthcare Inc.)	Phospholipid	Perfluorocarbon
Bisphere™	Point Biomedical Corp.	Polymer–protein bilayer	Air
Quantison™	Quadrant Healthcare plc.	Spray-dried serum albumin	Air
Echovist®	Schering AG	None	Air
Levovist®	Schering AG	Palmitic acid	Air
Sonavist™ *SHU 563 A*	Schering AG	Cyanoacrylate	Air
Echogen®	Sonus Pharmaceuticals Inc.	Surfactant	Dodecafluoropentane

information about commercial microbubbles, including the gas they contain, their outer-layer structure, and manufacturer [159]. In the following sections, the microfluidics-induced production of polymeric, lipid, and multilayered microbubbles is discussed in detail, including its manufacturing parameters and the target biological applications (ultrasound imaging, drug delivery, tissue engineering, etc).

2.5.1.1 Polymeric microbubbles

Polymeric microbubbles consist of at least two different layers, namely a polymeric material that forms the outer layer and a gas-filled inner layer. The outer layer can be composed of a wide range of different polymers, from natural to synthetic polymers. Polymeric microbubbles can have direct or indirect application potential. In direct applications, microbubbles with an intact gas-charged polymeric outer layer have the potential for direct application as contrast ultrasound imaging agents. However, when the gas charge is removed by detonating the microbubbles following production, the remaining polymeric patterns are deposited in films or bulk structures, which have potential uses ranging from wound dressings to surface coating materials and tissue engineering products (tissue scaffolds).

Many polymers can be used as the shell material in the production of microbubbles. Microbubbles with a polymer outer layer are harder, thicker, and more durable than protein or lipid outer layers. Microbubbles with a polymer outer layer are preferred in therapeutic applications because they have high stability. Sonavist® (Schering AG, Berlin, Germany) and BiSphere™ (POINT Biomedical Corp. San Carlos, CA, USA) products are commercial examples of microbubbles in which a cyanoacrylate polymer is used as the outer layer [159]. Examples of commercialised microbubbles are detailed in table 2.5.

Microfluidic setups offer uniform production and a high degree of control over the size distribution of microbubbles compared to techniques such as traditional sonication and foaming. The geometry of the microfluidic device (a Y, T, S, or W shape), its channel aspect ratio, the flow rate, the gas pressure, the molecular weight of the gas, and the physicochemical properties of the polymer solution (molecular weight, concentration, viscosity, surface tension, etc.) have direct effects on the size and stability of the produced microbubbles. The microfluidic device design (specifically, its inner geometry and the angle between the channels) directly affects the flow type and the microbubble production parameters. In figure 2.24, the T-junction, axisymmetric, and asymmetric flow-focusing geometries are illustrated in detail.

In a study that developed porous tissue scaffolds, microbubbles with a natural polymer 'gelatine' shell layer and a nitrogen inner layer were produced. In an application in which PDMS microfluidic chips are used, the channel size was 200 μm

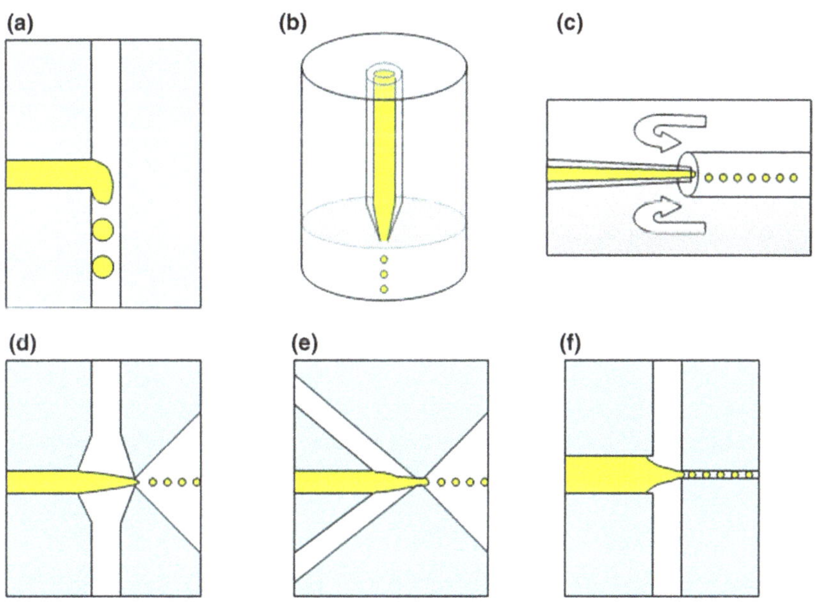

Figure 2.24. A schematic representation of the microfluidic device geometries used for microbubble fabrication: (a) T-joint (junction), (b) and (c) axisymmetric flow focusing, (d), (e) and (f) asymmetric flow focusing. Reprinted by permission from Springer Nature [163], Copyright (2016).

and the chosen geometry was a T-junction where the gas-polymer solution flows intersected each other at a 90° angle. While the gas pressure and polymer solution concentration were kept constant, the effect of the flow rate of the polymer solution on the microbubble size was investigated (figure 2.25).

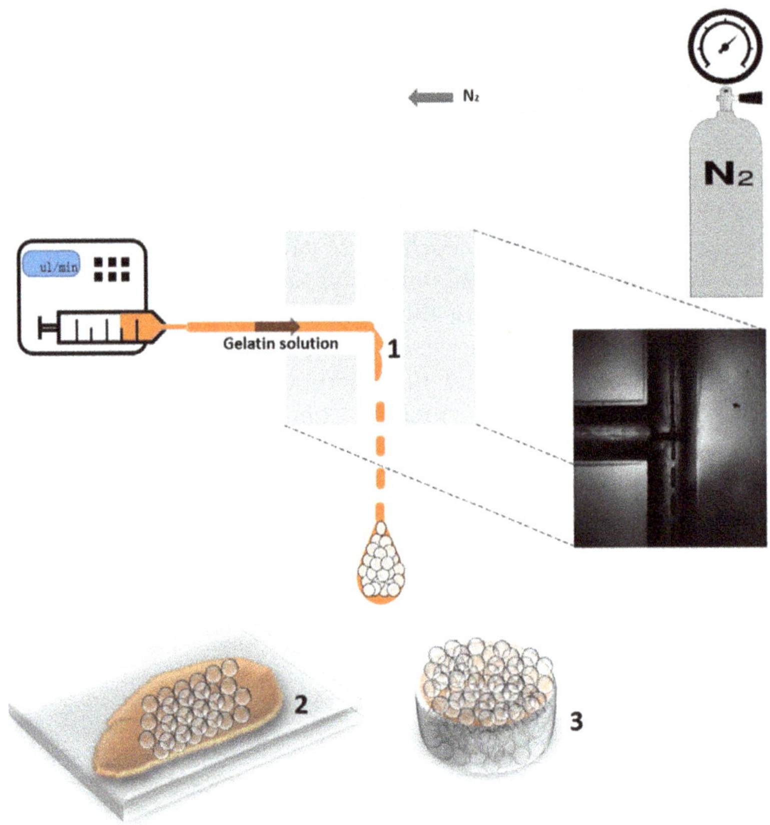

Figure 2.25. Steps in the formation of microbubbles and the manufacture of a gelatine tissue scaffold by a T-junction microfluidic device [164] John Wiley & Sons. [2019].

It was determined that the microbubble diameter decreased with increasing flow rate. In addition, the microbubbles produced were collected in layers at the outlet of the microfluidic chip. The porous structure obtained from the residues of the burst microbubbles was cross-linked with glutaraldehyde, and its stability was increased as a result. The cell viability and spreading properties of the porous gelatine scaffolds deposited in layers were examined. The results showed increased cell viability, proliferation, and spreading. Microbubble-based gelatine scaffolds with controllable pore sizes and outer-layer thickness have been identified as promising materials (figure 2.26).

Microbubbles produced by microfluidic devices have been widely used for ultrasound imaging. However, in recent decades, ultrasound-sensitive microbubbles have

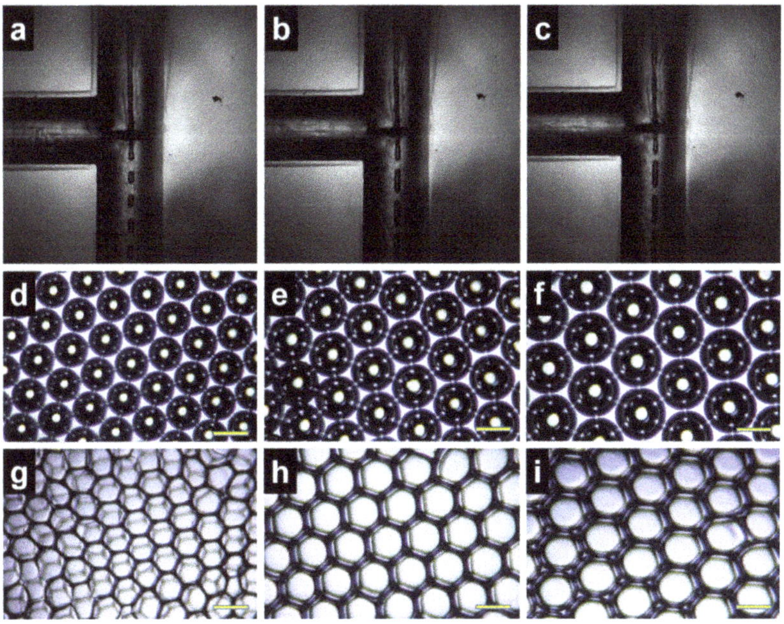

Figure 2.26. (a–c) High-speed-camera images of microbubble production. (d–f) Microbubble collection on glass slides. (g–j) Porous residue following the complete bursting of the microbubbles (scale bar=100 μm) [164] John Wiley & Sons. [2019].

not only been used in imaging but also in therapeutic applications. The use of polymer outer layers for microbubbles has also gained importance because of their mechanical strength; they are stronger than outer layers produced using other materials such as lipids and proteins. For example, in a study of the treatment of pancreatic tumours, Huang *et al* prepared microbubbles from a shell of poly(N-isopropyl acrylamide) (PNIPAM)/alginate hybrid polymers as the core content of gemcitabine/hydrogen sulphide [165]. The hydrogen sulphide (H_2S) gas used was chosen not only for microbubble production but also for its anticancer activity. The aim of this drug/gas combination was to prevent cancer cells from developing drug resistance.

In this microfluidic system, the alginate/PNIPAM was the continuous phase, while the H_2S, which formed the gas layer in the core, was the dispersion phase (figure 2.27). Polyvinyl alcohol (PVA) was used to stabilise the interfacial tension between the two phases. In the production of microbubbles, the flow rate of the gas was kept constant at 10 μl min^{-1}, while the flow rate of the liquid phase was optimised by working with different flow rates in the range of 5–40 μl min^{-1}. As an electrical voltage was applied to the liquid phase to induce Taylor cone formation, the droplet sizes decreased. It was reported that multi-drug carrier microbubbles with dimensions of approximately 400 μm were produced by this microfluidic system using a liquid flow rate of of 40 μl min^{-1}, a gas flow rate of 10 μl min^{-1}, and a voltage of 5 kV.

While *in vitro* release studies reported that improved/increased drug release capacity was achieved using ultrasound, *in vivo* studies also proved that the increased drug release capacity contributed to the shrinkage of tumour sites. The fact that ultrasound-assisted treatments do not exhibit the side effect of surrounding tissue

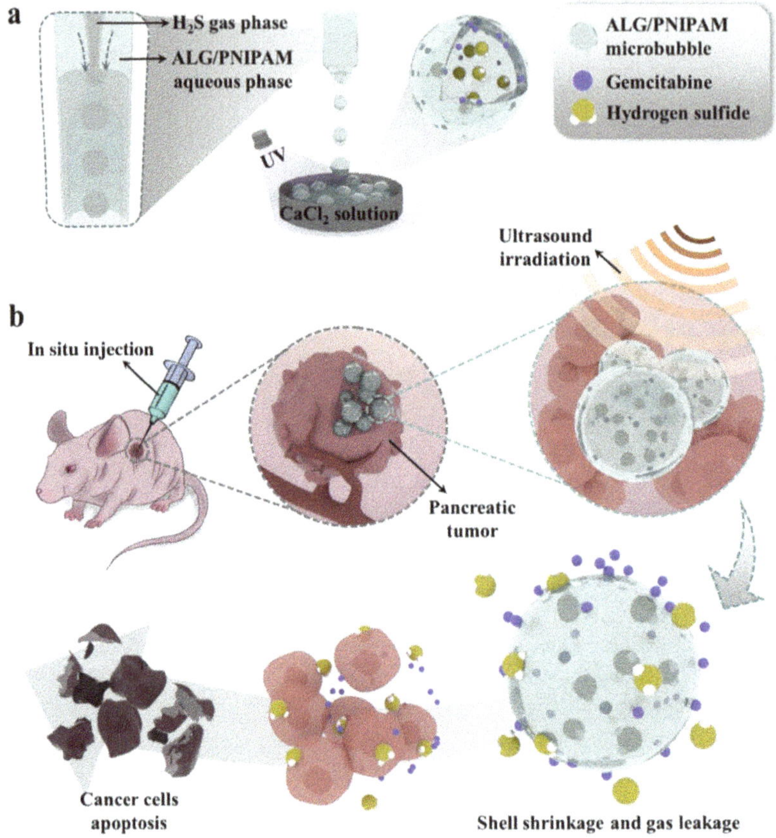

Figure 2.27. A schematic representation of ultrasound-sensitive microbubbles: (a) production and (b) application and action mechanisms [165] John Wiley & Sons. [2021].

destruction encountered in techniques such as radio-frequency ablation, stand out as a strong advantage of microbubble drug delivery systems [165–167].

Microbubbles with polymer-based shell structures are used in ultrasound imaging, ultrasound-sensitive treatment, the production of multilayer scaffolds, as well as in the preparation of porous polymeric film surfaces (figure 2.28). In a study, gas-charged homogeneous microbubbles were produced using alginate in a microfluidic device with a T-junction internal geometry [168]. To optimise the microbubbles produced, polyethylene glycol-40-stearate (PEG-40S) (as a surfactant) and phospholipids (L-α-phosphatidylcholine) were added to the polymer solution at differing concentrations to vary the viscosity and surface tension parameters. After the bubbles had burst, porous films with equidimensional pores were obtained.

Viscosity is an important parameter in microbubble production. Viscosity, which directly increases with an increase in the polymer concentration, also increases the bursting resistance of the microbubbles [169]. Increasing the amount of surfactant by keeping the polymer concentration constant reduces the surface tension formed in the shell of the microbubbles. This promotes the explosion of the microbubbles and the formation of film surfaces.

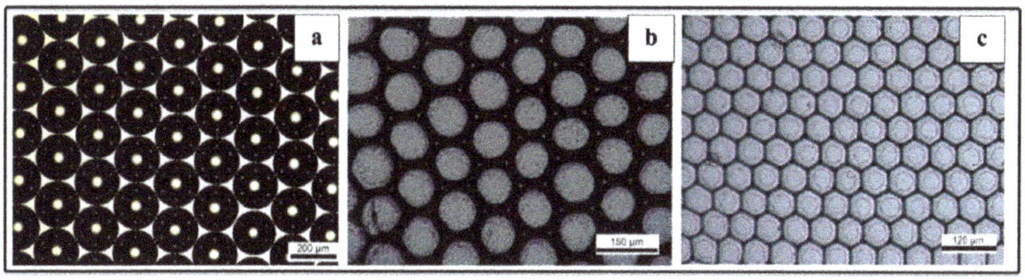

Figure 2.28. Optical microscopy images of microbubbles at different stages: (a) production, (b) before bursting, and (c) after bursting to form a porous film. Reprinted with permission from [168]. Copyright (2016) American Chemical Society.

In addition to the importance of the polymer solution and the surfactant concentration, other parameters affect the bursting that follows microbubble formation and shell thinning. The length and diameter of the capillary channels of the microfluidic device, the flow rate of the solution, and the gas pressure parameters are also important parameters for the porous film surfaces obtained by microbubble formation and explosion (figure 2.29).

Following the bursting phase, microbubbles produced by microfluidics can not only produce uniform porous membranes but can also produce nanoparticles. In several studies, nanoparticles with diameters of less than 100 nm were produced by the bursting of microbubbles; this was made possible by the precision control of microfluidic techniques.

In an example study, microbubbles were produced by T-connected microfluidic devices; nanoparticles were then produced by bursting the bubbles by loading nitrogen gas into the alginate shell. The study aimed to imitate the marine ecosystem, which is the source of alginate, by using the water interface as a collection unit [170]. A schematic illustration of the bursting of microbubbles by the jetting and microfluidic device, as performed in the marine environment, is shown in figure 2.30. In a microbubble study by Elsayed *et al*, the gas pressure was first optimised at a constant flow rate [170]. While keeping the amount of surfactant constant, the alginate solution concentration was then optimised by considering the viscosity and surface tension. The effect of gas pressure while keeping the flow rate constant, and the effect of flow rate on the microbubble size while keeping the gas pressure constant were investigated separately. As a result of the optimisation trials, it was determined that an increase in pressure caused an increase in the diameter of the microbubble, while an increase in the flow rate caused a decrease in the diameter of the microbubble. When the nanoparticles formed by the explosion of microbubbles with the same diametric distribution on the water surface were examined, it was determined that the nanoparticle size increased due to the increase in the viscosity of the alginate solution. As a result, it was reported that nanoparticles in the range of 80–200 nm can be produced by bursting alginate microbubbles.

The production of nanoparticles by bursting microbubbles has also been carried out for biomedical applications in combination with drug loading. Nanoparticles were prepared for the treatment of type 2 diabetes mellitus (T2DM) by loading metformin

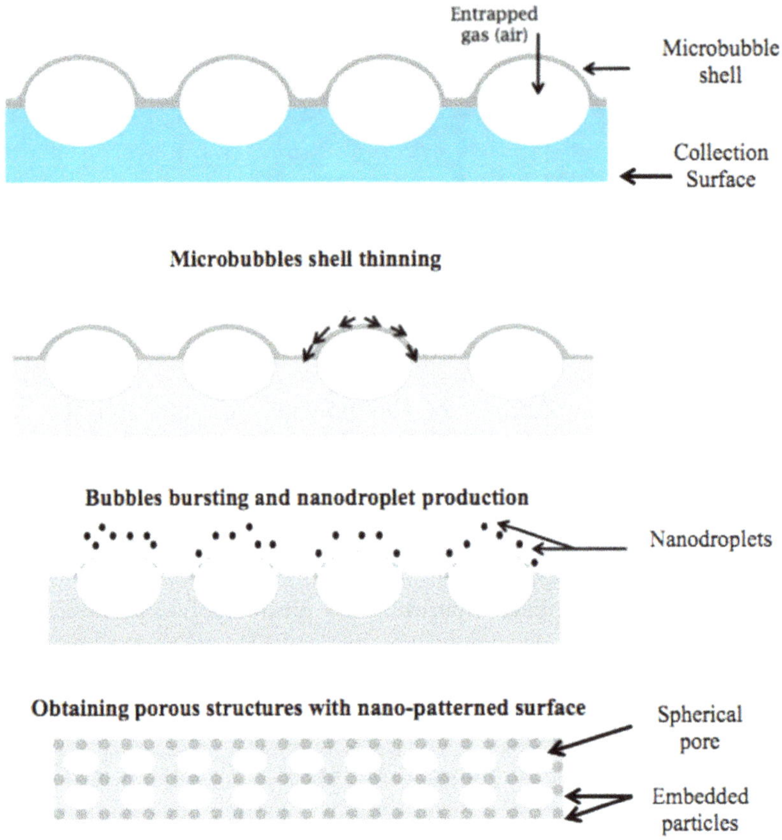

Figure 2.29. A step-by-step schematic illustration of the fabrication of porous structures with nano-patterned surfaces obtained by bursting microbubbles. Reprinted with permission from [168]. Copyright (2016) American Chemical Society.

into microbubbles prepared using polyvinyl alcohol–sodium alginate (PVA-SA) as a dual polymer system [172]. While PVA/SA microbubbles were produced with diameters of ~100 nm, ~70 nm nanoparticles were obtained as a result of bubble detonation. The produced nanoparticles thus exhibited a controlled release profile for up to 60 min at an acidic pH and up to 240 min at a neutral pH and thus have the potential to function as a next-generation drug carrier for the treatment of T2DM.

2.5.1.2 Lipid microbubbles

Microbubbles are used in a wide range of fields from ultrasound imaging to drug delivery systems and tissue engineering products. In accordance with the increasing usage domains and applications, the materials that make up the shell can also vary. For this reason, studies using lipid molecules in the shells of microbubbles are becoming more and more common. Lipids are preferred in targeting studies and imaging because they can easily pass through biological structures and do not have a toxic effect on the biological environment when they lose their integrity. Lipid microbubbles, which can

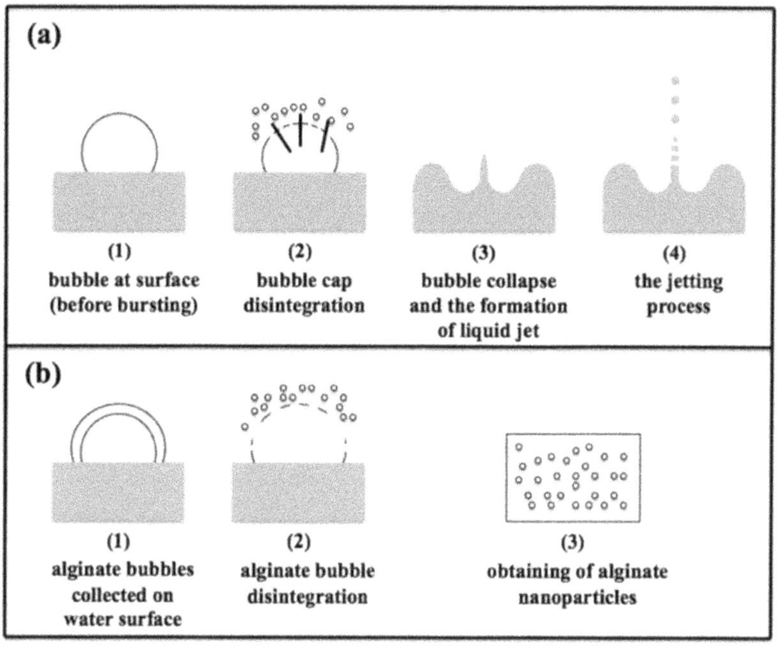

Figure 2.30. A schematic illustration of the bursting of microbubbles by a jetting and microfluidic device; this parallels the bursting of microbubbles in the marine environment. Reprinted from [170], Copyright (2015), with permission from Elsevier.

be produced in a precise and controlled manner by microfluidics, are also affected by liquid flow rate, gas pressure, microfluidic device geometry and dimensions; in this respect, they are similar to polymeric microbubbles. In recent years, the effects of the concentration of the lipid solution and post-production shrinkage as well as stabilisation on microbubble sizes have been investigated [173, 174].

Microbubbles with lipid shell structures can be prepared with very low polydispersity indices using microfluidic devices. In a study by Hettiarachchi *et al*, perfluorocarbon (PFC)-loaded lipid shell microbubbles were successfully prepared as ultrasound imaging agents using the flow-focusing technique in PDMS microfluidic devices (figure 2.31) [175]. 1,2-dipalmitoyl-sn-glycero-3-phosphocholine (DPPC), 1,2-dipalmitoyl-sn-glycero-3-phosphate (DPPA), 1,2-dipalmitoyl-sn-glycero-3-phosphoethanolamine-N-[methoxypoly(ethylene glycol)-5000] (lipid conjugate DPPE-PEG_{5000}) and 1,2-distearoyl-sn-glycero-3-phosphocholine (DSPC) were used as lipid shell layers. The designed microfluidic device and the adjustable lipid microbubble size range offered a wide range of opportunities for targeted biomedical imaging (via the production of ultrasound agents) and therapeutic designs.

In another study using lipid (1,2-dibehenoyl-sn-glycero-3-phosphocholine (DBPC), DPPA, 1,2-dipalmitoyl-sn-glycero-3-phosphoethanolamine (DPPE), and 1,2-distearoyl-sn-glycero3-phosphoethanolamine-N-[carboxy(polyethylene glycol)-2000] (DSPE-mPEG-2000)) shell layered microbubbles, it was reported that the distribution of the microbubble diameters produced by microfluidic devices

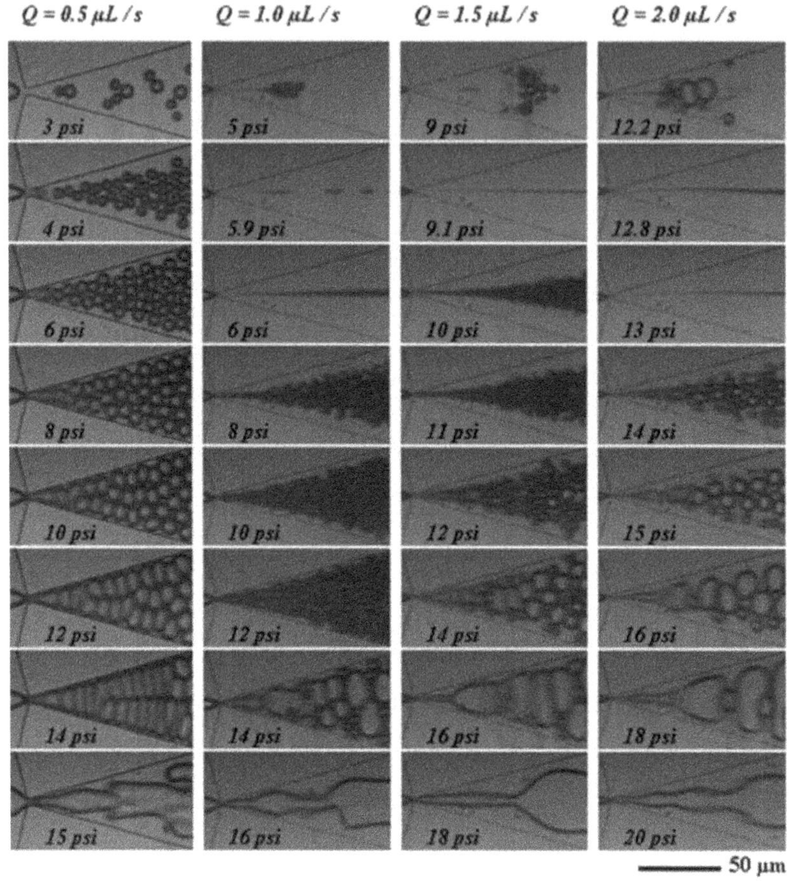

Figure 2.31. High-speed camera images of a comparative study of the effects of different flow rates (0.5–2.0 ml s^{-1}) and pressures (3–20 psi) on size in lipid microbubble production. Scale bar=50 μm. Reproduced from [175] with permission from the Royal Society of Chemistry.

decreased compared to their initial size as the bubbles contracted (figure 2.32) [174]. It was determined that the shrinkage of the microbubbles was independent of the gas mixing ratio but dependent on the lipid concentration.

After the microbubbles were produced, a more stable morphology was obtained by shrinking the microbubbles via a decrease in their internal pressure, and their diameters were reduced by a factor of two to seven times. In addition, the diameters that decreased as a result of shrinkage decreased proportionally to their original sizes. It has been determined that microbubbles, which are produced in a controlled manner inside microfluidic devices and whose stability is increased by the shrinking and stacking of lipid structures, have great potential for use in biomedical applications.

2.5.1.3 Multilayered microbubbles

Multilayered microbubbles have come to the forefront in biomedical applications as a result of the enhanced effects that can be realised when they are produced with

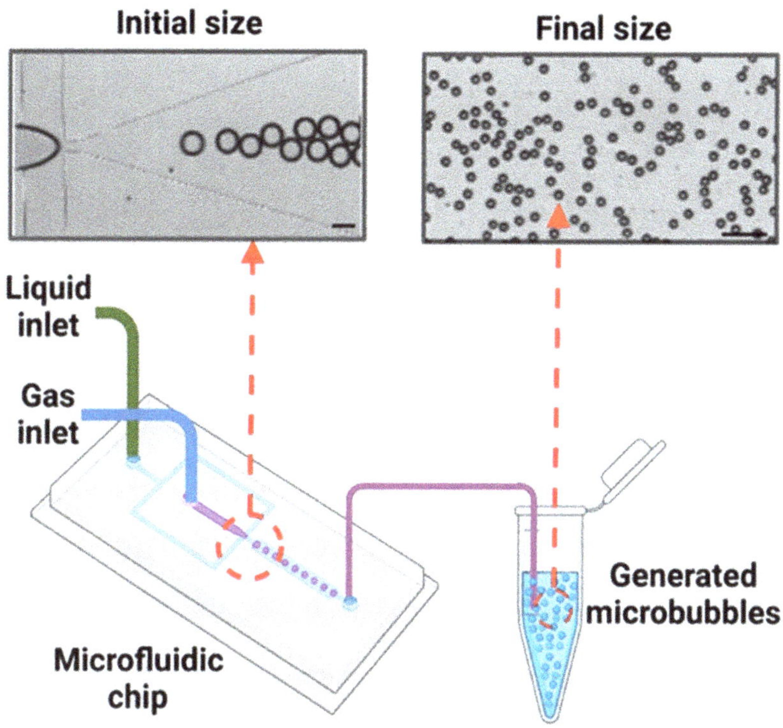

Figure 2.32. Illustration of lipid microbubble production by the microfluidic device and high-speed camera images at the times of manufacture and post-shrinkage. Reprinted with permission from [174]. Copyright (2022) American Chemical Society.

different layers. With an increase in the number of layers in microbubbles, it becomes possible to combine features such as acoustic imaging, drug targeting, and combined diagnostics and treatments in a single application. By designing the channel geometries of microfluidic devices or connecting microfluidic chips in parallel to prepare different layers, operations that require complex and difficult procedures to prepare with conventional methods can be performed quickly and reliably in a single step. In addition, the use of optically transparent microfluidic chips such as PDMS and PMMA provides great advantage in terms of monitoring and control during the production process.

A study in which two T-junction microfluidic chips were connected in parallel produced microbubbles with a gas-charged core composed of layers of bovine serum albumin (BSA) and silicone oil [176]. While the treatment of triple-negative breast cancer (TNBC) with curcumin and doxorubicin using two-layer microbubbles was the objective, acoustic imaging could also be performed thanks to the gas-charged core. Drug release was induced by the application of ultrasound (figure 2.33). Although doxorubicin exhibits anticancer activity at high doses, in order to prevent damage to healthy tissues, the dosage of doxorubicin was reduced and supported with curcumin and acoustic ultrasound waves. The results obtained proved that the dual active substance system showed higher anticancer activity even though the

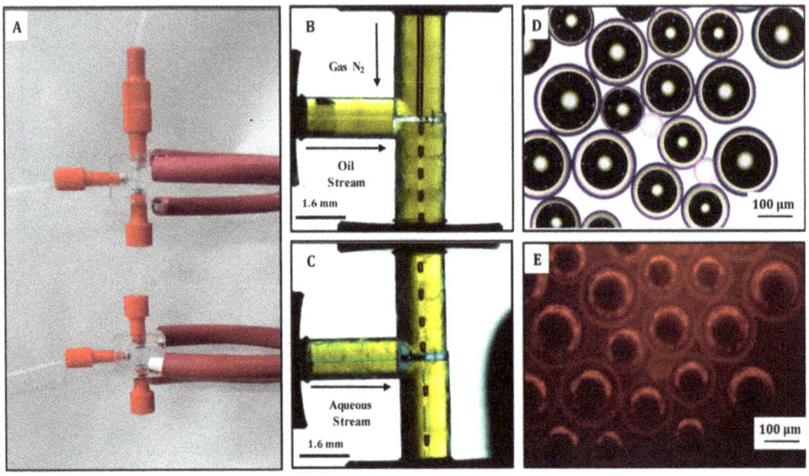

Figure 2.33. (A) An image of serially connected T-junctions. (B) Gas and oil streams. (C) A high-speed camera image of microbubbles produced inside the T-junctions by an aqueous stream. (D) An optical microscope image of core–shell microbubbles. (E) A fluorescent microscope image of core–shell microbubbles. Reprinted with permission from [176]. Copyright (2020) American Chemical Society.

amount of doxorubicin used was five times lower. The synergistic effect created by the application of ultrasound also increased the anticancer activity in both 2D and 3D cell culture studies.

The dimensions of microbubbles are directly related to parameters such as the liquid flow rate, gas pressure, solution concentration, and diameters of the capillary channels in the microfluidic system. The stability and lifetime, which are the other important features in microbubble applications, are affected by the shell thickness, elasticity, and gas permeability parameters of the microbubbles. The shell thickness and elasticity can be modified by different solution concentrations and the type of material used in the shell. In addition, increasing the shell layers and using different materials and thicknesses have come to the forefront as alternative solutions in recent years.

In a study that compared data produced using theoretical modelling and experimental studies of multilayer microbubbles, microfluidic-supported T-junction assemblies were used. A photoluminescent agent was added to the shell structure of microbubbles to form a BSA shell and N_2 core structure [177]. Microbubbles have gained the ability to support photofluorescent imaging in addition to ultrasound imaging through the use of Si quantum dots (SiQDs). The size and stability of microbubbles produced by single, double, and triple-series microfluidic setups were evaluated. In addition, the effects of flow rate, BSA concentration, and SiQD concentration on microbubble size and lifetime were separately examined and compared for the different microfluidic device combinations.

For a constant BSA concentration, it was determined that as the microfluidic capillary diameter decreased, the microbubble diameter also decreased. It was found that increasing the flow rate decreased the microbubble size inversely. The microbubble size decreased as the number of serially connected T-junctions increased.

When the flow rate was kept constant and the BSA concentration was varied, the microbubble diameter decreased when the BSA concentration and the number of serial T-junctions increased. The microbubble diameter also increased as the capillary diameter increased (figure 2.34).

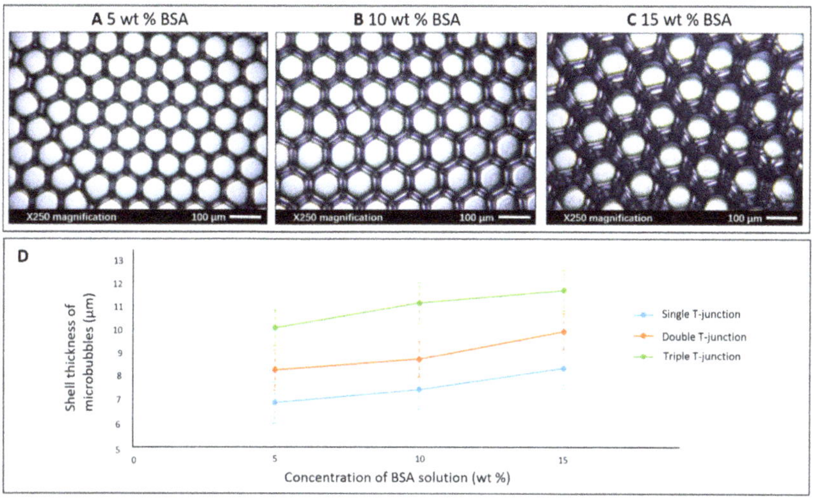

Figure 2.34. (A–C) Optical images of dried microbubbles produced by a triple T-junction setup (scale bar 100 µm). (D) A graphical representation of the shell thickness of microbubbles at different BSA solution concentrations for single, double, and triple T-junctions (100 µm capillary size, 800 µl ml^{-1} liquid flow rate and 80 kPa gas pressure). Reprinted with permission from [177]. Copyright (2022) American Chemical Society.

On the other hand, the effects of the BSA concentration and the number of serial T-junctions on the microbubble lifetime were investigated by keeping the flow rate and gas pressure constant. Increasing the BSA concentration and the number of serial T-junctions decreased the diameter of the microbubbles and increased their lifetime. In the triple-series T-junction system, the lifetime of the microbubbles produced in a 5 wt. % BSA solution with a 100 µm capillary channel, an 800 µl min^{-1} flow rate, and a pressure of 80 kPa was 15 min, while it was 30 min with 10 wt.% BSA and 40 min with 15 wt.% BSA. When 15 wt.% BSA was used in double and single T-junction systems under the same conditions, the lifetimes decreased to 35 and 25 min, respectively. When the shell thicknesses were examined, it was determined that increased numbers of serial T-junctions decreased the microbubble diameter and increased shell thickness and lifetime. In addition, increasing the SiQD concentration also had the effect of increasing the lifetime. As a result, it was determined that increasing the number of layers and the shell thickness is an important approach in the production of equidimensional, stable microbubbles with extended lifetimes.

As an example of a theranostic application, microbubbles containing growth factor (basic fibroblast growth factor (bFGF)) were prepared. The microbubbles were intended to be noninvasively triggered by ultrasound and used in the treatment of myocardial infarction (MI) (figure 2.35) [178]. In this study, the microparticles

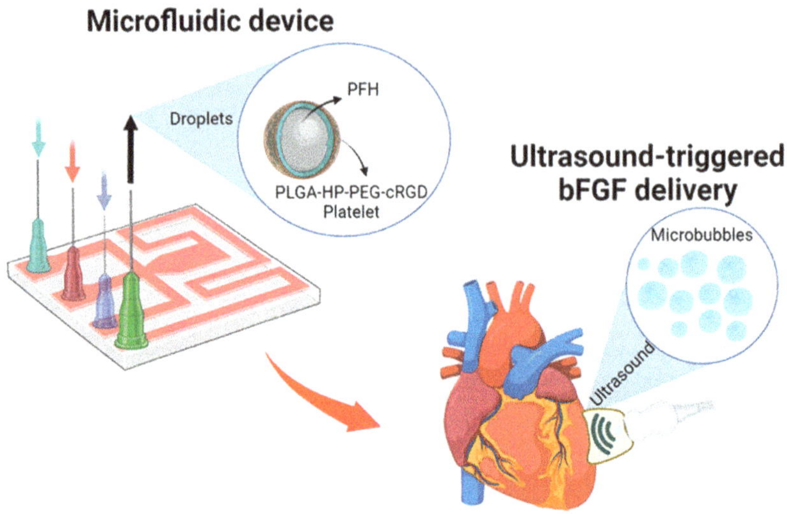

Figure 2.35. Illustration of the production of bFGF-loaded multilayer microbubbles in the microfluidic device, followed by the ultrasound triggering step in the MI region. Reprinted with permission from [178]. Copyright (2023) American Chemical Society.

had a core consisting of perfluorohexane (PFH) and a shell consisting of poly(lactic-co-glycolic acid)-heparin-polyethylene glycol-cyclic arginine-glycine-aspartate-platelet (PLGA-HP-PEG-cRGD-platelet), bFGF, and gold nanoparticles. These microparticles were prepared using a microfluidic setup. The microbubbles were then obtained by the transition of the PFH in the core from the liquid phase to the gas phase, which was triggered by ultrasound. This induced the release of bFGF into the MI region and also made it possible to perform ultrasound imaging in the region without the need for an invasive procedure.

2.5.2 Nanoparticles

The definition of 'nanoparticle' refers to particles that have diametric distributions in the range of 1–100 nm, but it is also used to describe larger particles (of more than 100 nm) up to the micron level. Nanoparticles, one of the cornerstones of nanotechnology, can be produced from different types of materials, such as polymers, lipids, ceramics, and metals. These particles, which have low size and high surface area, have a wide range of uses, especially in the biomedical field. They have a usage potential that ranges from drug delivery systems to imaging agents and even targeting applications. Nanoparticles are intended to have small sizes and narrow size distributions; however, there are various disadvantages of their synthesis by conventional methods. The advantages and challenges of nanoparticle synthesis, their characterisation, their *in vitro* and *in vivo* applications, and large-scale production with a focus on the translation to clinical applications are discussed in detail in table 2.6. In addition, the positive effect of microfluidic systems on potential difficulties is also presented comparatively. Nanoparticles are

Table 2.6. A comparative assessment of the advantages and challenges of nanoparticles that are candidates for clinical use in terms of their synthesis, characterisation, *in vitro* and *in vivo* applications, and large-scale synthesis. Reprinted by permission from Springer Nature [179], Copyright (2012).

	Advantages	Disadvantages/challenges	Stage of development	Potential impact
Synthesis	• Tunable nanoparticle size • Narrower size distribution • Reproducible synthesis • Potential for high-throughput synthesis and optimisation of nanoparticles	• Solvent and high-temperature incompatibility for low-cost polydimethylsiloxane microchannels • Higher costs and complexities in the fabrication of glass and silicon microdevices	*****	Rapid combinatorial, controlled, and reproducible synthesis of libraries of distinct nanoparticles for a specific application, and/or reference nanoparticles for toxicology studies
Characterisation	• Label-free characterisation • Potential for feedback control and real-time nanoparticle optimisation	• Current methods do not apply to all classes of nanoparticles • Not all properties can be characterised, such as drug encapsulation and release and signal-to-noise ratio	*	In-line rapid characterisation and optimisation of nanoparticles
In vitro	• Biological conditions closer to *in vivo* microenvironments • Potential for high throughput screening of a large number of nanoparticles at different concentrations	• Higher costs and complexities of fabrication and operation compared with well plates • Might not be reusable; if reusable, they would be difficult to keep sterile	****	High-throughput studies of nanoparticle toxicity, efficacy, tumour penetration, and organ distribution using 'organ-on-a-chip' systems

In vivo	• Large numbers of organisms could be used for a single measurement • High-throughput evaluation of toxicity for a large number of nanoparticles	• Lack of methods to translate data from small-scale organisms to other species • Pharmacokinetics or biodistribution cannot be determined	**	Real-time tracking of the distribution or toxicity of nanoparticles on small-scale organisms
Large-scale synthesis	• Continuous synthesis • Bench scale to clinical scale reproducibility • Parallelisation allows the scale of production to be tuned	• Difficult to build systems at a low cost that are comparable to a batch reactor able to prepare grams or kilograms of nanoparticles	***	Synthesis of nanoparticles for human administration using stackable parallel microfluidic units

Rank: Most advanced in development (*****) to least advanced in development (*), based on the amount of research carried out on each category as well as the potential ease of adoption by industry.

undoubtedly of great importance in the biomedical field due to their low size, high surface area, suitability for surface modification and targeting applications, and desirable properties in dose control and controlled release systems. Microfluidics have played an important role in nanoparticle production as a result of their adjustable properties (chip channel diameter, geometry, flow rate, solution, etc.), which allow the production parameters, conditions, and products to be precisely controlled. In the following sections, microfluidics-assisted nanoparticles will be classified according to material type and examined in detail with examples of biomedical applications.

2.5.2.1 Polymeric nanoparticles

Whitesides and co-workers, who made the greatest contribution to the development of microfluidics in the biomedical field by developing PDMS microchips in the early 2000s, subsequently started to produce microparticles using microfluidics for the first time [180]. Researchers later continued the developments in microfluidic technologies with the production of polymeric nanoparticles. Unlike microbubbles produced by feeding liquid and gaseous phases to the flow system, nanoparticle production is achieved by incorporating two or more liquid phases into the flow within a microfluidic device. Microfluidics has also become an important technique for the production of polymeric nanoparticles. In addition to microfluidic technologies, there are many other nanoparticle production methods available, such as the mini-emulsion, double-emulsion, nanoprecipitation, and micro-milling methods. However, it is quite challenging to obtain a narrow size distribution, perform shape-controlled production, and use a wide range of materials (gels, polymers, metal hybrids, etc.) using traditional methods. The properties (hydrophilicity, hydrophobicity, amphiphilicity, molecular weight, solubility, etc.) of polymers, drugs, and active substances used in the production of drug-loaded particles in conventional methods are effective in obtaining the desired particle size. In microfluidic setups, polymeric nanoparticle production based on flow-focusing, co-flow, or crossflow-based models is very convenient for producing nanoparticles with narrow size distributions quickly, economically, and under sterile conditions (figure 2.36). The solubility and surface tension differences between the polymer and the solvent are effective in nanoparticle production in the microfluidic channel. In addition, depending on the type of polymer, cross-linking techniques such as heat, light, and radiation can be used in the production of nanoparticles. The permeability and durability of the microfluidic chip material when exposed to solvents, heat, or light are also important at this stage. In addition, multilayered and multi-drug-carrier polymeric nanoparticles can easily be produced through the use of parallelisation in the microfluidic setup, which will be examined in detail in the following sections.

In 2008, Karnik *et al* first reported a polymeric nanoparticle production model for a microfluidics-induced nanoparticle formation process (figure 2.37) [182]. Poly (lactic-co-glycolic acid)-*b*-poly(ethylene glycol) (PLGA-*b*-PEG) was dissolved in acetonitrile and added to the water stream. Nanoparticles were then synthesised by using two adjacent water flow streams to focus the organic polymer phase in the

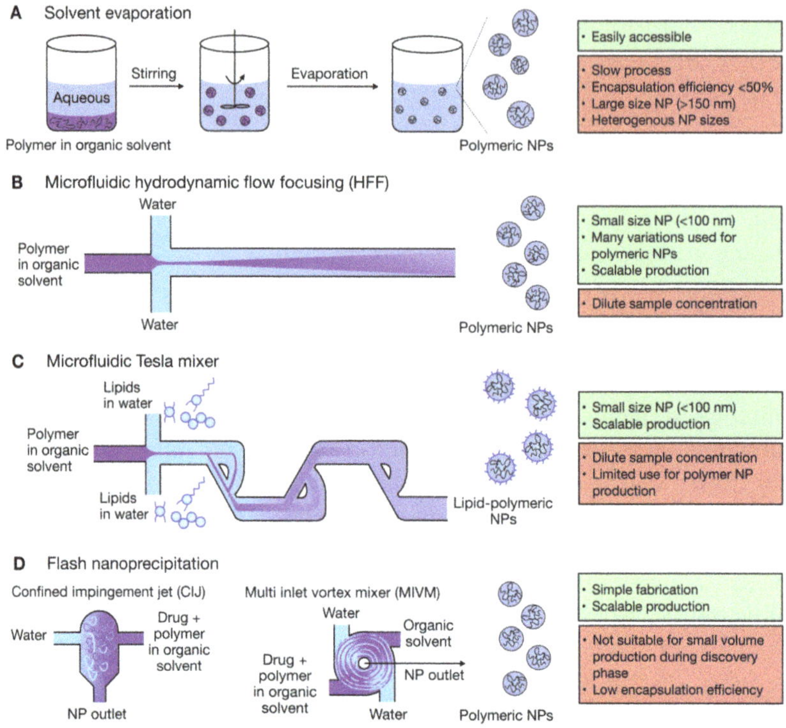

Figure 2.36. Polymeric nanoparticle production techniques with their advantages (green) and disadvantages (red). (A) Solvent evaporation, (B) microfluidic hydrodynamic flow focusing, (C) microfluidic Tesla mixer and (D) flash nanoprecipitation setups. Reprinted from [181], Copyright (2021), with permission from Elsevier.

microfluidic chip (figure 2.38). In the microfluidic system, PLGA-*b*-PEG nanoparticles were produced and optimised using the flow rate, concentration, and polymer combination parameters. PLGA-*b*-PEG has been selected as a biocompatible and biodegradable U.S. Food and Drug Administration (FDA)-approved model polymer that has the potential to be used in multiple-drug delivery applications. In addition, docetaxel was used as a model drug to test drug loading and release tests. Simultaneously, nanoparticles produced from the same polymer using the nanoprecipitation method were comparatively examined in terms of their properties such as size, polydispersity, zeta potential, and drug loading-release.

Conventional bulk nanoprecipitation is based on the relationship between a polymer, a solvent, and a non-solvent. The polymer is dissolved in a suitable organic solvent and then dropwise added to a non-soluble solvent and rapidly mixed. Surfactants can be added to manage the surface tension between the polymer and the solvent. Although it is possible to produce particles less than 100 nm in size via this method, the polydispersity index (PDI) cannot approach the sort of uniform size distribution obtained using microfluidic systems. In addition, while the drug loading capacity of the nanoparticles produced by the bulk nanoprecipitation method is poor, the release profile usually results in a rapid release. Using the microfluidic

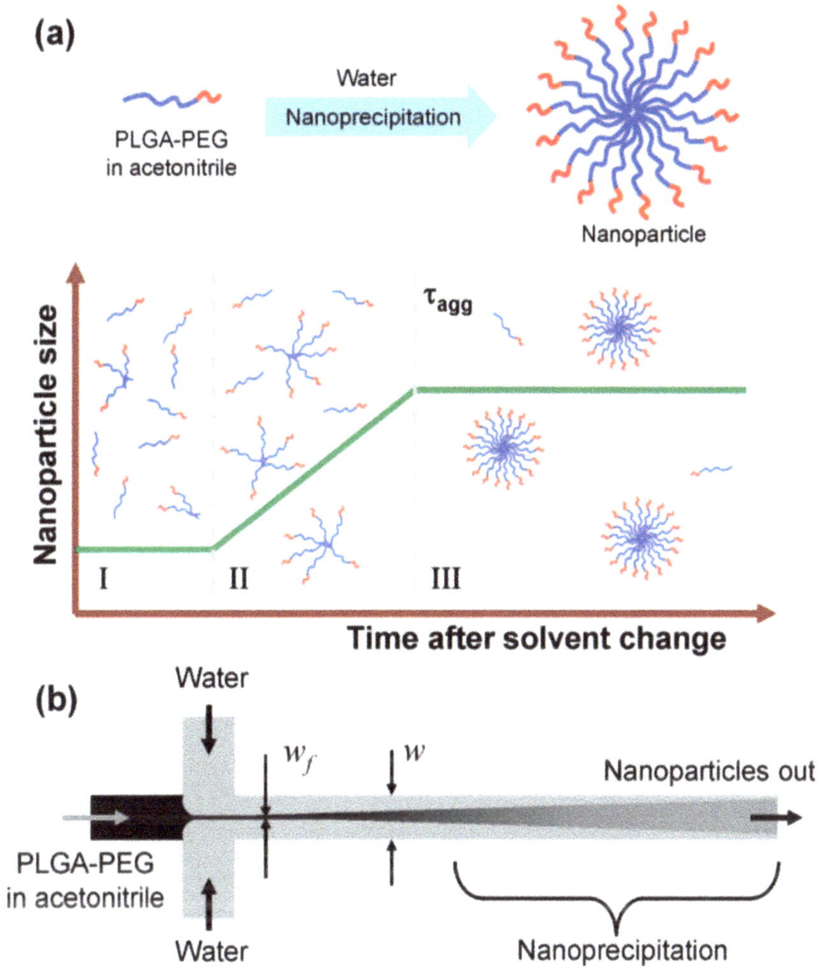

Figure 2.37. The PLGA-*b*-PEG nanoparticle production mechanism: (A) nanoprecipitation assembly of the di-block amphiphilic copolymer, (B) microfluidic flow-focusing setup. Reprinted with permission from [182]. Copyright (2008) American Chemical Society.

system and precise control of the flow rate and mixing speed, a balance of a high drug loading capacity and a controlled release profile can be established in a controlled manner in nanoparticles with a narrow size distribution, increased surface area, and low volume.

In another study, PLGA-*b*-PEG nanoparticles were produced by a T-junction microfluidic device. The polymer was dissolved in acetonitrile. The polymer concentrations used were 2.5%, 5%, and 10%. The PEG content of the PLGA-*b*-PEG polymer was also varied (10% and 15% PEG) in the block polymer chain [183]. A 10% PEG content gave rise to smaller nanoparticles with a lower polydispersity index. Solutions of 5% PLGA-*b*-PEG polymer at a water:oil flow ratio of 3:1 produced nanoparticles with a size of 108 ± 1 nm and a PDI of 0.04 ± 0.02.

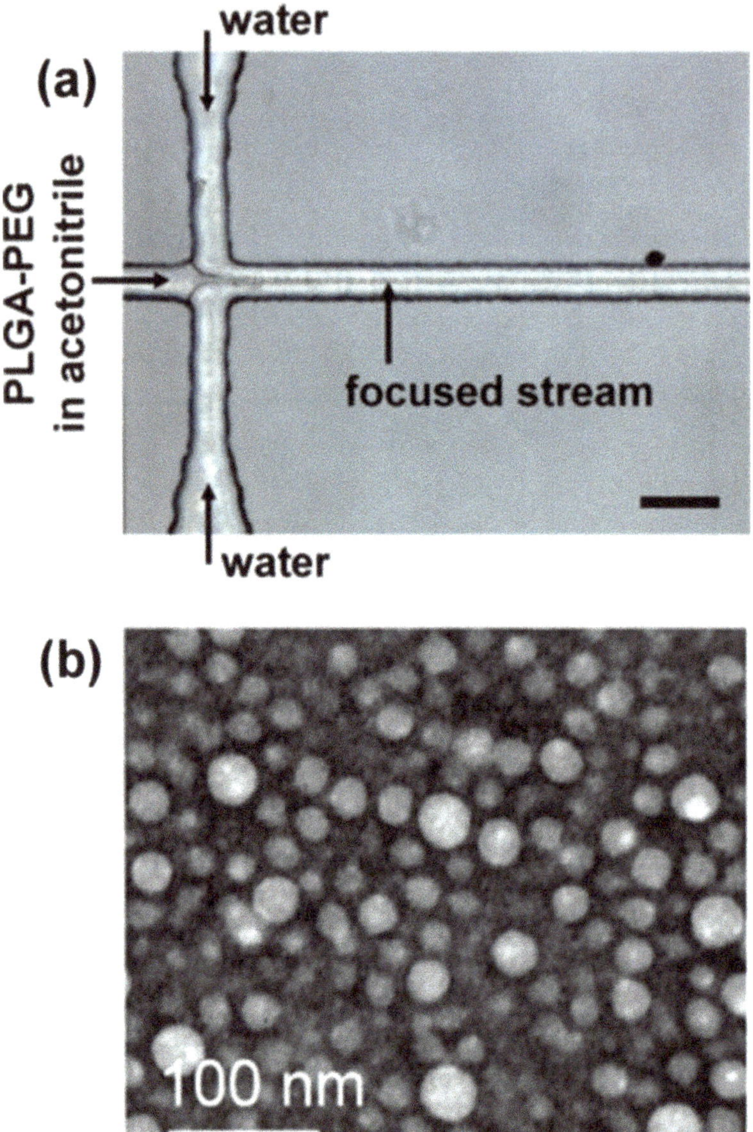

Figure 2.38. (A) Microfluidic device inner channel micrograph taken during nanoparticle synthesis (scale bar: 50 μm). (B) Scanning electron microscopy (SEM) image of PLGA-*b*-PEG nanoparticles produced by the microfluidic chip (scale bar: 100 nm). Reprinted with permission from [182]. Copyright (2008) American Chemical Society.

The results show that uniform nanoparticle fabrication can be performed quickly and easily using microfluidic chips.

Another example of drug loading studies of nanoparticles produced with microfluidics is the production of sorafenib drug-loaded poly(ethylene glycol)-block-(ε-caprolactone) (PEG-*b*-PCL) nanoparticles [184]. PEG-*b*-PCL nanoparticles were developed for anticancer drug loadings in cancer therapy applications. Sorafenib, a hydrophobic drug, was used with an amphiphilic PEG-*b*-PCL polymer and drug-loaded nanoparticles were synthesised by nanoprecipitation using the co-flow technique in a microfluidic device. The nanoparticle size was determined to be ~80 nm and the PDI was found to be less than 0.2. In addition, the drug loading capacity was measured and found to be 16% ± 1%, and the encapsulation efficiency was approximately 54% ± 1%. The drug delivery system was developed to address the solubility problem of hydrophobic drugs; it showed a drug-carrying capacity ~20 000 times higher than the solubility of the free drug. The advantages of microfluidics in nanoparticle design and production for biomedical applications were displayed yet again in this study, which showed that the nanoparticles had small sizes, a narrow size distribution, and a high drug loading efficiency.

2.5.2.2 Liposomes

In the research literature, liposomes have been shown to have a range of uses as drug carriers and targeting agents as a result of their cell-membrane-like structures and biocompatible nature. Liposomes can be obtained in sizes between 20 and 1000 nm, depending on the lipid used, the drug that is loaded, and the production method. As in the production of polymeric nanoparticles, liposomes can be produced with the help of microfluidic chips. Liposomes have a wide range of potential uses in the biomedical field, from drug delivery systems to immunotherapy and from gene transfection to vaccines. For this reason, liposomes constitute more than half of the nanoparticles approved by the FDA for clinical applications [181]. The production of liposomes using bulk extrusion, microfluidic hydrodynamic flow focusing (MHFF), microfluidic staggered herringbone micromixers (MSHMs), bifurcating mixers, baffle mixers, and T-junction mixing is shown schematically in figure 2.39 and the advantages/disadvantages of these methods are indicated in detail.

As a result of the sudden needs that have arisen in recent years, studies in which microfluidic chips are used to produce nanoliposomes that can be conjugated with SARS-CoV-2 spike mutations or genomic sequences have gained importance. The objectives of this approach are to facilitate the screening of SARS-CoV-2 variants and determine the side-effects of COVID-19 [185].

On the other hand, most of the vaccine studies used during the 2019 pandemic are liposome-based. For example, the Pfizer/BioNTech and Moderna vaccines are based on the production of liposome vesicles in microfluidic reactors [186, 187].

Liposomes have a similar structure to that of the cell membrane and can easily transfer their cargo to the interior of the cell. In addition to their vaccine applications, liposomes are also very efficacious drug carriers for cancer therapy. The adverse effects of conventional anticancer drugs, which have high toxicity for both cancerous and healthy cells, can easily be eliminated by liposome shells that cover these drugs. Khorshid and co-workers fabricated liposomes with and without a sucrose cover using a 3D-printed microfluidic device with two different inner microchannel geometries (zigzag and circle)(figure 2.40). Berberine hydrochloride was loaded with liposomes to obtain an anti-proliferative effect on triple-negative breast cancer cells (MDA-MB-231) [188]. A cytotoxicity evaluation was conducted

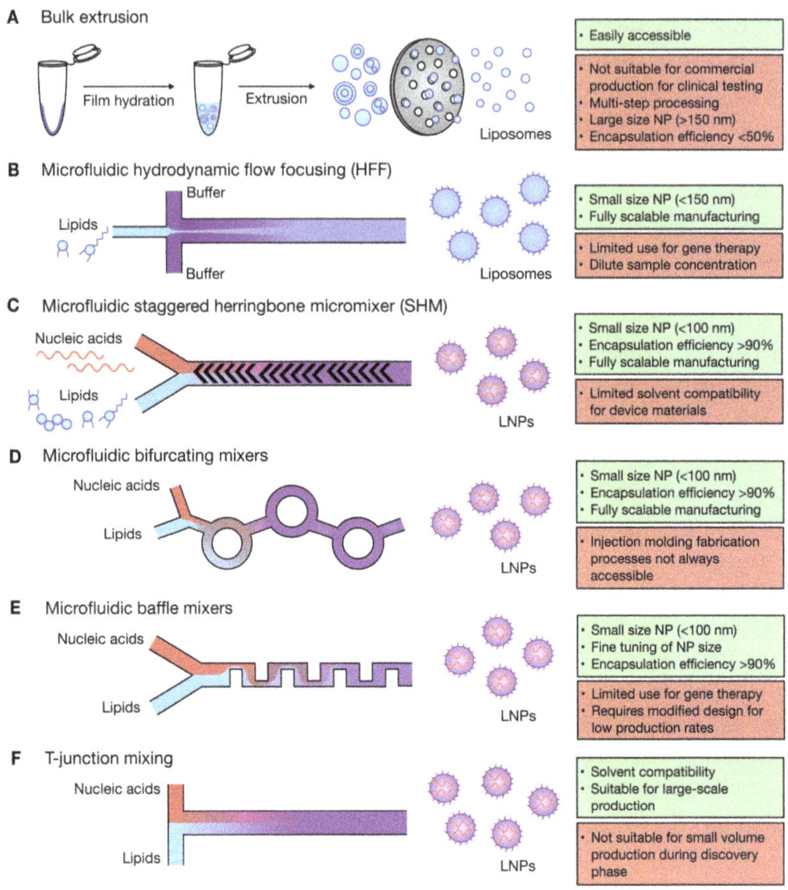

Figure 2.39. Liposome production techniques with their advantages (green) and disadvantages (red). (A) The production of liposomes by bulk extrusion, (B) the production of liposomes by microfluidic hydrodynamic flow focusing (MHFF), (C) the production of lipid nanoparticles (LNPs) by microfluidic staggered herringbone micromixers (MSHMs), (D) the production of LNPs by microfluidic bifurcating mixers, (E) the production of LNPs by microfluidic baffle mixers, and (F) the production of LNPs by T-junction mixing. Reprinted from [181], Copyright (2021), with permission from Elsevier.

to compare healthy cells with AC16 cardiomyocyte cells. The nanoliposome size was approximately 140 nm, and the nanoliposome PDI was extremely low (~0.06). A sucrose decoration added to the liposomes increased their anti-proliferative effect on the MDA-MB-231 cell line by actively targeting the cancer's sugar efficiency without having a cytotoxic effect on healthy cells.

Paclitaxel-loaded liposome formulations were also fabricated by a microfluidic device [189] (figure 2.41). Liposomes were prepared with four different types of phospholipids; 1,2-dimyristoyl-sn-glycero-3-phosphocholine (DMPC), DPPC, DSPC, 1,2-dioleoyl-sn-glycero-3-phosphocholine (DOPC), and cholesterol. The phospholipid:cholesterol ratios were varied in empty liposome manufacture to control the targeted size and PDI limits (<200 nm, low PDI $\leqslant$ 0.25). DMPC and

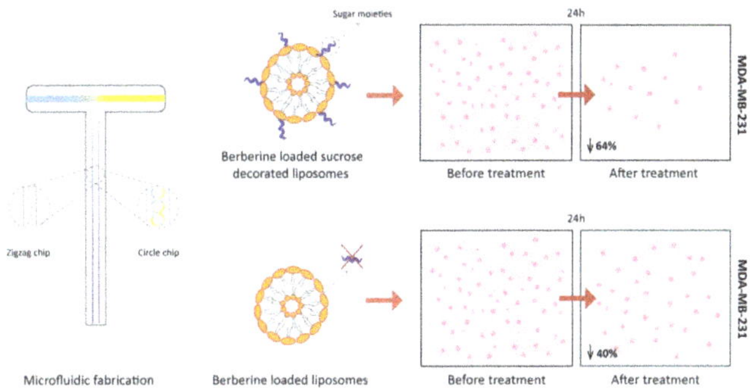

Figure 2.40. An illustration of the fabrication of berberine-loaded liposomes and their anti-proliferative effect on the MDA-MB-231 triple-negative breast cancer cell line. Reprinted from [188], Copyright (2022), with permission from Elsevier.

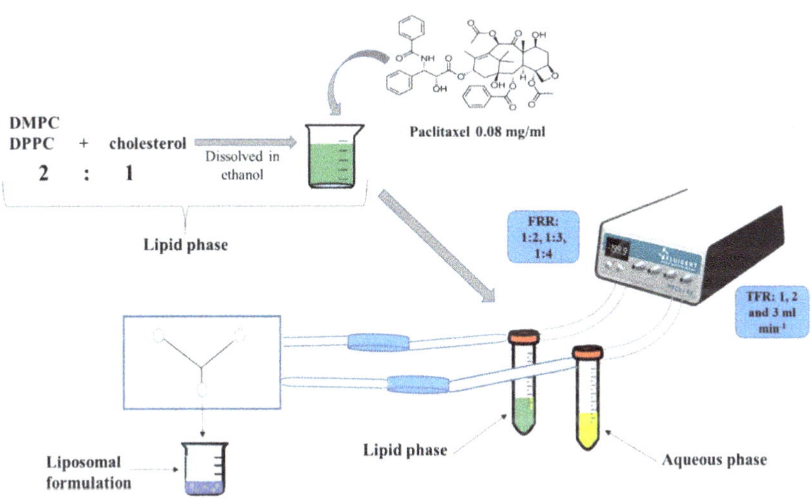

Figure 2.41. The production scheme used to obtain paclitaxel-loaded nanoliposomes. Reprinted from [189], Copyright (2022), with permission from Elsevier.

DPPC exhibited lower particle sizes corresponding to their shorter chain lengths. Optimised cholesterol rates increased the stability of the paclitaxel-loaded liposomes fabricated by a microfluidic device, and the liposomes showed increased encapsulation efficiencies of up to 88% for DMPC and 91% for DPPC. As in the case of the encapsulation efficiency results, the highest drug release profile was obtained using the DPPC liposomes.

2.5.2.3 Metallic (inorganic) nanoparticles

Metallic nanoparticles can be produced by bulk mixing techniques. It is also possible to produce more precise and controlled metallic particles with narrow size distributions using microfluidic chips. Bulk mixing and microfluidic droplet mixing techniques are schematically represented and discussed in terms of their advantages and disadvantages in figure 2.42. Silver, gold, and iron nanoparticles are the most frequently fabricated inorganic nanoparticles. The material of the microfluidic chip inner wall should be inert to the inorganic material to inhibit coagulation inside the microfluidic device. Microfluidic reaction channels decrease the reaction volume and increase the stability and polydispersity of the produced nanoparticles [181]. In addition, channel geometries can be varied from linear to zigzag to increase mixing efficiency.

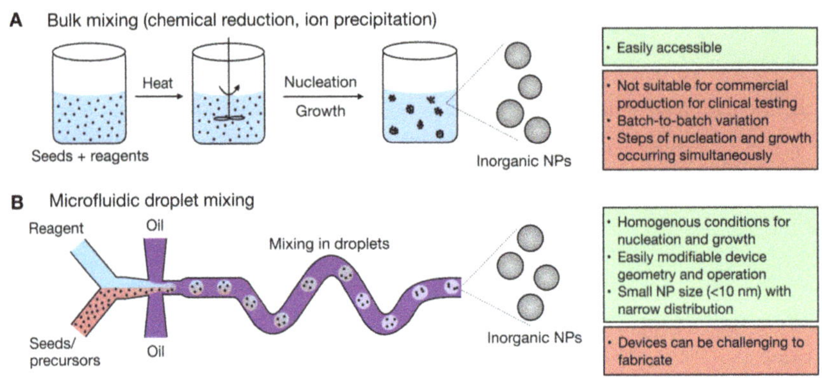

Figure 2.42. Metallic nanoparticle production techniques with their advantages (green) and disadvantages (red). (A) Bulk mixing (conventional) and (B) microfluidic droplet mixing. Reprinted from [181], Copyright (2021), with permission from Elsevier.

Microfluidic devices have many advantages for the synthesis of metallic nanoparticles. These advantages include the small size and narrow size distribution of the particles, the use of standard operating conditions, and a reaction-specific device design capability. On the other hand, it has been reported that there are still some difficulties in the device design and fabrication steps [181]. Over the last decade, 3D printers have offered fast and versatile solutions to eliminate the disadvantages arising from the design and production of microfluidic chips.

In a recent study, a 3D-printed poly(lactic acid) (PLA) microchannel layer was fabricated and then connected to a PMMA slide to obtain an optically transparent microfluidic device for silver and gold nanoparticle synthesis [190]. Mineral oil has been used for both gold nanoparticle (AuNp) and silver nanoparticle (AgNp) synthesis to reduce fouling inside the microfluidic channels and to develop the synthesis reaction into a continuous flow. The AuNp synthesis reaction was applied at 90 °C and at flow rates of 40–100 μl min^{-1}. AuNp particle size measurements showed sizes of 20 ± 9 and 34 ± 12 nm for flow rates of 40 and 100 μl min^{-1}, respectively (figure 2.43). AgNps were synthesised at a temperature of 20 °C with flow rates in the range of 30–120 μl min^{-1}. The AgNps had a size distribution of 5 ± 2 nm to 8 ± 3 nm, respectively. The reaction temperature and flow rate parameters were precisely controlled at low volumes in the microfluidic channel, thus obtaining metallic nanoparticles with a narrow size distribution. AuNps and AgNps have been reported to maintain their stability for up to three

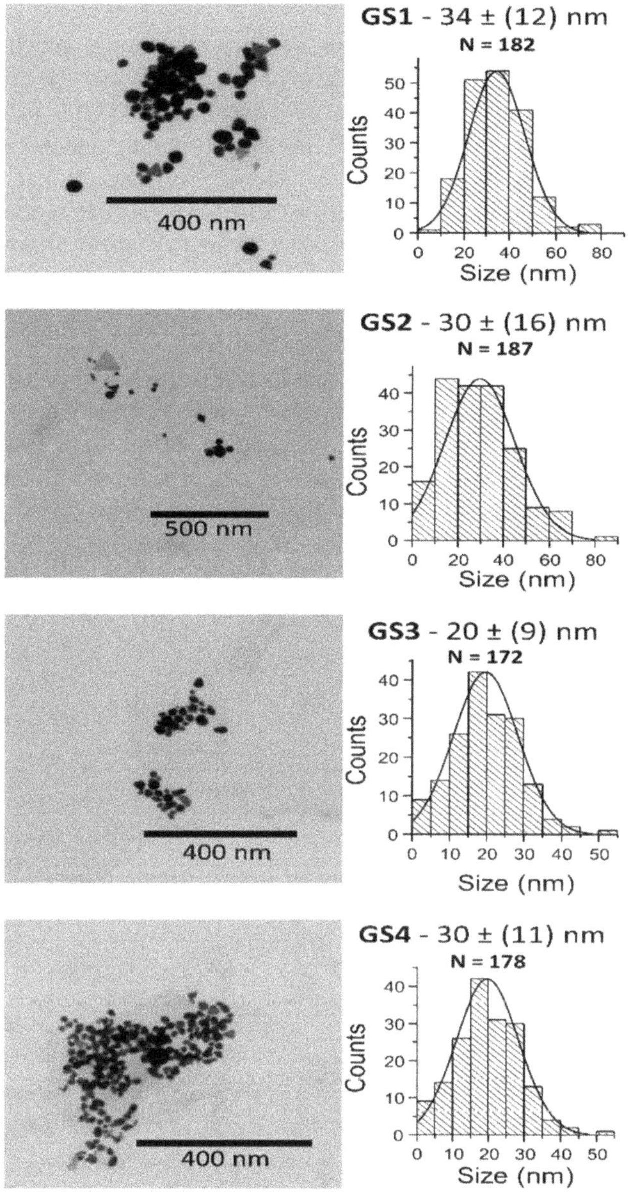

Figure 2.43. Field-emission SEM micrographs and size distribution graphs of AuNps produced by a 3D-printed microfluidic device. Reprinted from [190], Copyright (2019), with permission from Elsevier.

weeks. Given that 3D printers offer easy, fast, economical, and versatile solutions for microfluidic chip production, it is predicted that in the coming years, studies of the production of AuNps and AgNps in cubic, bar, and triangular morphologies and even in core–shell structures over spherical morphologies will become increasingly widespread.

2.5.2.4 Core–shell nanoparticles

The requirement for improved diagnosis, imaging, targeting, and treatment in the biomedical field is increasing every day. As a result of the development of application areas and the vast potential of microfluidic devices in the biomedical field, nanoparticles used as drug carriers, imaging, targeting agents can be produced quickly, economically, and reliably. It is also very important that multiple treatment/diagnostic applications are made in a single particle system. Core–shell nanoparticles have gained great importance in health applications because they offer multiple or sequential release steps that can be applied to drugs loaded into different layers of multilayer nanoparticles. This enables the treated area to be imaged and allows targeted treatment to be localised.

Core–shell nanoparticles can be produced from polymer, lipid, silica, metal, and metal oxide materials (figure 2.44). Biomedical applications in which these materials are produced as a single layer via microfluidic processes have been examined in detail in the previous sections. This section will examine how multilayered particles, which have an importance in combined diagnosis, treatment, and imaging applications, are produced and used through microfluidic means.

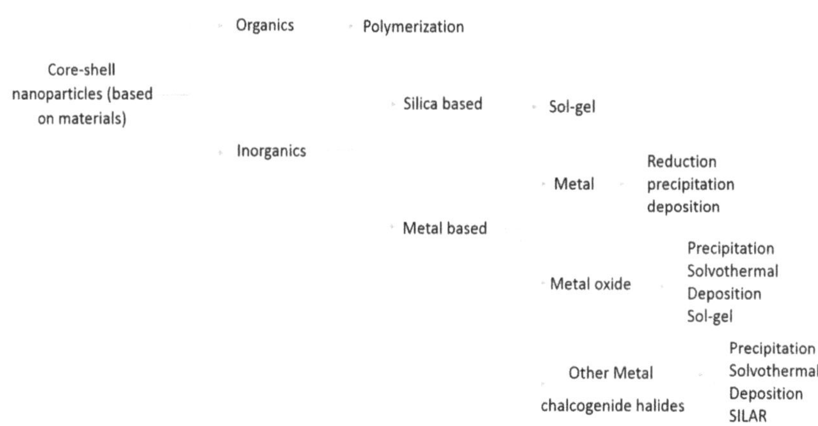

Figure 2.44. The classification of core–shell nanoparticles by material type and method of synthesis. Reproduced from [191] with permission from the Royal Society of Chemistry.

Core–shell nanoparticles have been widely used in several forms as drug carriers in the biomedical industry. Core–shell nanoparticle types were illustrated in figure 2.45. Microfluidic technologies are very useful in the production of core–shell structures; these depend on the flow types of liquids and parallelisation. Double- or multi-emulsion particles can easily be prepared using flow focusing, co-flows, and micro-mixing. In addition, serially connected microfluidic chips make it possible to increase the number of shell layers and to add specific design geometries. The drug release mechanisms of core–shell structures consist of temperature-triggered, pH-triggered, and/or sustained sequential release. Temperature-triggered core–shell nanoparticles aim to deliver their cargo to the targeted area via

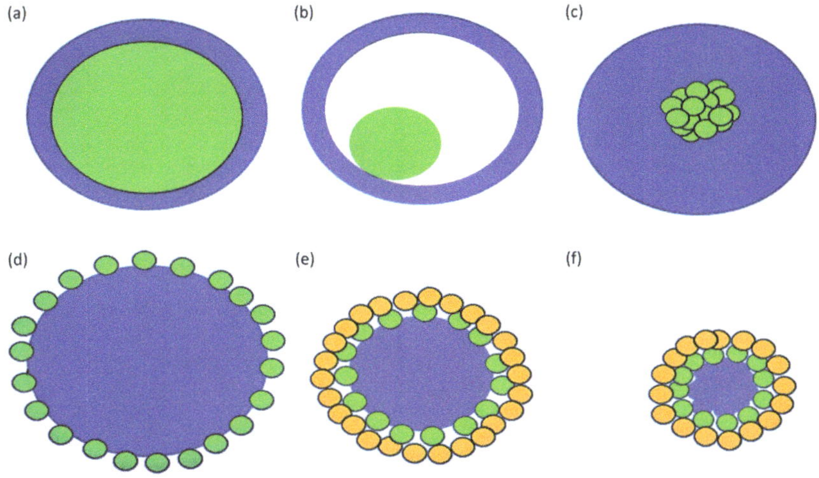

Figure 2.45. The classification of core–shell nanoparticles: (A) a single core integrated with a shell, (B) a hollow shell with a small core, (C) a core consisting of aggregated particles, (D) a big single core covered with a shell of numerous small particles, (E) a big single core covered with double shell layers made from numerous small particles, and (F) an aggregated small-particle core with double shell layers made from numerous small particles. Reproduced from [192] with permission from the Royal Society of Chemistry.

temperature control. Core–shell nanoparticles with temperature-sensitive shell layers can aid in the sequential/controlled delivery of drugs. Sustained sequential release can be designed to release different drugs from different layers using the difference in the biodegradability of the constituent polymer layers. pH-triggered core–shell nanoparticles lose their shell integrity as a result of a change in pH and deliver the therapeutic agent to the surrounding tissue. pH-sensitive core–shell nanoparticles are particularly useful in cancer therapy because cancer tissues have an acidic pH. Therefore, pH-triggered nanoparticles carrying cancer drugs deliver the drug to the target tissue without causing damage to healthy tissues. Figure 2.46 illustrates microfluidic-assisted core–shell biomedical nanoparticle production and its products [193].

In one study, pH-sensitive core–shell nanoparticles were prepared in a cross-junction microfluidic device and developed as a treatment for colorectal cancer [194]. To reduce the off-target toxicity of the chemotherapeutic drugs used, pH-sensitive nanoparticles were prepared for oral delivery. Hydrophobic modified chitosan (HMCS)-based nanoparticles were produced in a microfluidic cross-junction setup so that they could be monodisperse and reproducible and have a high drug loading efficiency. HMCS was chosen to increase the hydrophobic anticancer drug loading capacity. The HMCS core layer was prepared by hydrodynamic flow focusing. The HMCS nanoparticles were coated with a pH-sensitive layer of PMMA by a Tesla micro-mixer microfluidic setup. The PMMA layer was designed to function as a protective layer for the chitosan drug layer on its way from the stomach to the colon (through the gastro-intestinal tract). The upper layer dissolved in the acidic environment encountered in the stomach and caused the

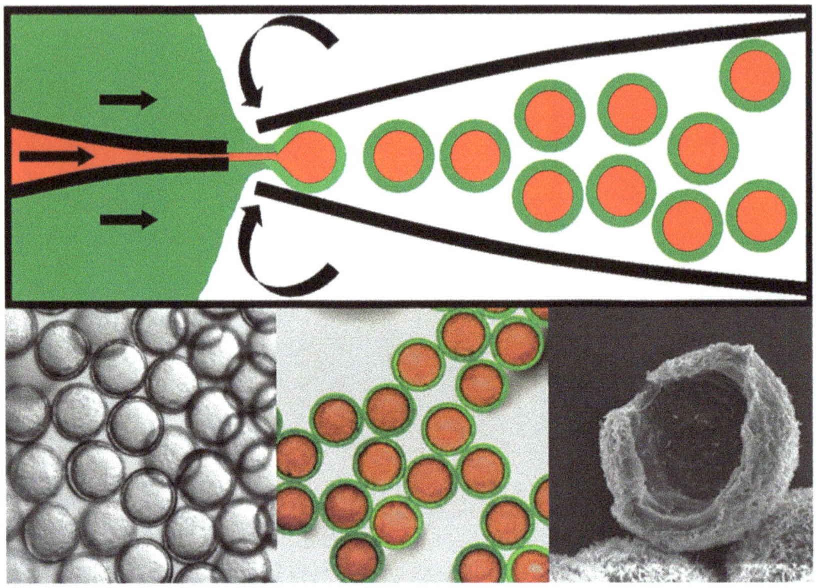

Figure 2.46. Schematic representations and microscopic images of microfluidics-assisted core–shell nanoparticle production and its products. Reprinted with permission from [195]. Copyright (2013) American Chemical Society.

chitosan to swell in the second acid environment in the colon, thereby releasing the drug in a controlled manner. The homogeneity of the prepared double-layer drug delivery system, its high drug loading efficiency, and its adjustable layer thickness and surface load were obtained through the ultra-precise production of low volumes in the microfluidic setup.

2.6 Microfluidics for biological applications

Microfluidic technologies have come to the forefront as an important technical tool with which to determine and define the complex and comprehensive content of biological systems. In addition, microfluidics offers rapid solutions for biological systems such as diagnostic and therapeutic tools.

2.6.1 Microfluidics for omics technologies

All of the technologies that systematically explore and describe biological systems at a large scale, such as the genome, proteome, metabolome, transcriptome, epigenome, lipidome, and microbiome are collectively known as 'omics'. The ability of omics technologies to provide detailed and comprehensive results makes them a key tool in personalised, precision medical applications. In particular, single-cell analysis applications, with the support of omics technologies, offer high sensitivity and accurate results in a wide range of applications from cancers to stem cells and from diagnosis to treatment [196]. The importance of omics technologies and the demand for their widespread use have revealed the need to develop economical, reproducible, sensitive, and accurate systems. As a result of this requirement, microfluidic systems have now attracted a greater focus than the existing conventional methods.

With the increasing importance of omics technologies, microfluidic platforms are becoming a useful and powerful tool for the isolation, processing, and identification of biological sample analytes, as they function in a highly sensitive and high-throughput manner. Microfluidics-assisted omics applications provide a wide range of analytical capabilities from viral to single-cell analysis in automated systems. In addition, single-cell analysis can be carried out at the 'gene to small molecule' level instead of bulk population cell analysis.

The starting point of single-cell studies consists of cell isolation and sorting. The first step in determining spatial features with single-cell resolution is the isolation of a healthy dead cell or a defined cell type from tissue that has a heterogeneous cell source. Cell picking studies started with conventional manual cell picking (mouth pipetting) in the 1970s and has since evolved to use flow cytometric sorters which rely on microfluidic technologies. As a result of microfluidics-based flow cytometry technologies, the adaptation to microfluidic technologies has seen applications with higher efficiency and sensitivity, and lower volumes have been made possible [197]. Microfluidics has become a state-of-the-art tool in the last decade due to the single-cell isolation, manipulation, and identification performed using omics techniques (proteomic, metabolomic, etc).

In microfluidic platforms, single-cell applications are also given multi-dimensional features through the use of chips with different geometries and different flow models (flow focusing, dual flow, etc). It has been reported that ten to thousands of cells can be genomically analysed in less than 24 h as a result of the encapsulation of single cells into individual droplets by microfluidics [198]. Barcoded beads and single cells are encapsulated as separate droplets, enabling genomic analyses to be performed with high reproducibility and sensitivity at the single-cell level in picolitre volume solutions (figure 2.47). In addition to generating labelled cell droplets, microfluidics can also be involved in the cell separation process. Individual cells can easily be isolated by circuit microfluidics. The omics analyses (proteomics, genomics, transcriptomics, etc.) are then completed using mass spectroscopy, which performs cell barcoding and antibody conjugation [198].

Digital microfluidic isolation of single cells for omics (DISCO) is another microfluidics-based single-cell isolation tool for omics analyses. DISCO combines digital microfluidics (DMF), laser cell lysis (LCL) and artificial intelligence (AI) [199]. DISCO-based genomic and/or transcriptomic analyses start with the imaging of a fluorescently labelled target; the resulting images are processed into genomic and/or transcriptomic data with the help of AI. Performing this analysis in a microfluidic system allows separation and omics analyses of single cells to take place with high label selectivity and high-throughput analysis at low volumes.

Microfluidics enables LOC solutions to be produced for omics technologies through integrated combinations of cell isolation, labelling, lysis, and target omics analyses. These omics can be varied from genomics to transcriptomics, epigenomics, proteomics, and metabolomics with single-cell resolution [200].

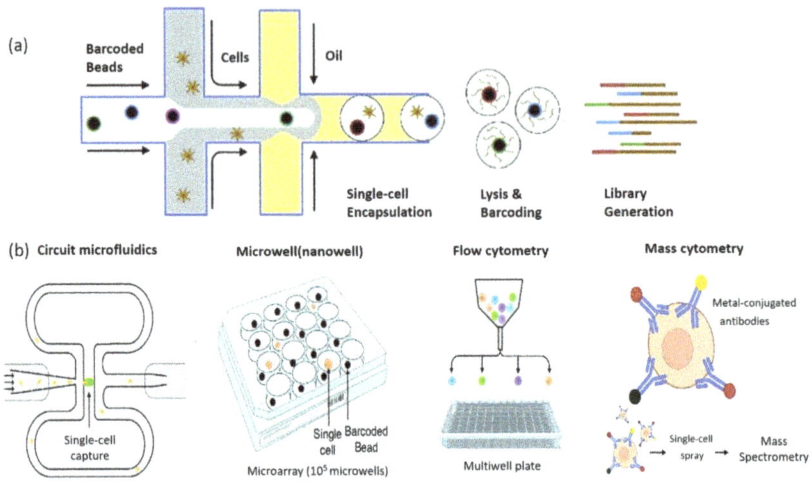

Figure 2.47. Microfluidics for omics technologies. (a) Micro-droplet microfluidics for applications from cell barcoding to single-cell encapsulation and analysis. (b) The pathway from circuit microfluidics to mass spectroscopy analysis for omics. Reproduced with permission from [198]. Copyright (2021) Wolters Kluwer Health, Inc.

2.6.2 Microfluidics in gene therapy

Genetic diseases that negatively affect cellular activity, metabolic activity, and protein synthesis occur due to deficiencies and/or mutations in gene expression. The current path followed in gene therapy is the delivery of genetic material carried as cargo, which passes through the cell membrane to the targeted gene region in the cell. This must be carried out without disturbing the cell integrity. However, the efficient transport of cargo genetic material to the target site without affecting cell viability and without disrupting membrane integrity is a very challenging process. Therefore, effective gene/drug delivery systems are needed. Microfluidic platforms are playing an important role in the development and improvement of gene therapy.

Microfluidic technologies have started to play an active role in gene delivery systems and therapy. Gene studies in which microfluidic systems are integrated offer great advantages compared to traditional methods of gene transfer, gene transfection, and the design and production of carrier systems to perform these functions. Precise production and control, the rapid development of application-specific systems, the ability to work in low volumes, and the ability to develop designs that meet multiple needs are the most important advantages of microfluidics-assisted gene therapy systems. Due to these advantages, it is possible to produce viral and nonviral vectors in closed systems and at low volumes, and optimised production systems can be developed.

Viral vectors such as adenovirus, retrovirus, lentivirus, herpes, etc. are used for gene delivery [201]. However, the most important disadvantage of viral vectors is that they can generate nonspecific immune responses. Nonviral vectors have gained importance because researchers wish to avoid disadvantages associated with of viral vectors. The most widely used nonviral vectors are lipoplex and polyplex structures with cationic charges [202].

In gene therapy, two basic physical methods are used to transport genetic material into the target cell. The first of these is the electroporation technique, which provides transfer by creating pores in the cell membrane through the use of electric pulses. The second is the sonoporation technique, in which acoustic cavitation creates deformation in the cell membrane via the generation of ultrasound waves. The efficiency and effectiveness of the sonoporation technique can be increased using microbubbles. The gas bubbles contained in the microbubbles create local shock waves when ultrasound is applied, inducing the formation of pores in the cell membrane and allowing the genetic material it carries to migrate into the cell. The production and applicability of microbubbles as carrier systems for genetic material is also one step ahead because of the more precise control and rapid production offered by microfluidics-assisted production systems.

Lissandrello *et al* developed a microfluidic device for mRNA delivery to human T-cells [203]. The device was reported to be a next-generation alternative to conventional experimental electroporation setups. The setup was composed of a microfluidic chip, Pt electroporation electrodes, high-conductivity cell media, low-conductivity electroporation media, T-cells, and mRNA transfection agents (figure 2.48). It was determined that the electroporation technique integrated into the microfluidic device exhibited approximately 95% transfection efficiency. It was also reported that in addition to its high transfection efficiency, it was able to detect

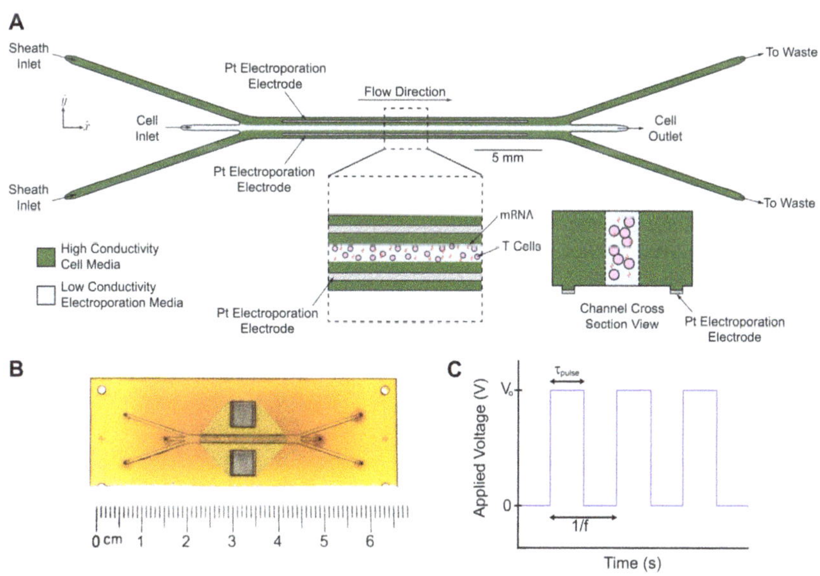

Figure 2.48. A microfluidic electrotransfection device based on continuous flow. (A) A schematic representation of the microfluidic device. The green areas represent high-conductivity cell media and blue areas represent low-conductivity electroporation media. (B) A micrograph of the microfluidic electrotransfection device. (C) A diagram of the voltage waveform applied to the electrodes for transfection. Reprinted by permission from Springer Nature [203], Copyright (2020).

a large number of cells at ultra-fast processing speeds. In the designed microfluidic device, 5 $\times 10^8$ T-cells operated at a reaction rate of 2 $\times 10^7$ cells/min. The results obtained demonstrated that microfluidic electroporation is a promising development for gene therapy applications.

In the microfluidic-assisted electroporation technique, gene transfection can be achieved at very low voltages compared to those of conventional methods. In addition, the low applied voltage benefits the retention of high cell viability. In the design of the microfluidic device, the fluid consists of metal electrodes integrated into the chip, and electrical pulses are transmitted with the help of these electrodes. The metal forming the electrode, the channel design, and the substrate material can be varied for each specific application.

Valero *et al* reported DNA transfection on bone marrow-derived mesenchymal stem cells (MSCs) by electroporation in a microfluidic device at the single-cell level. Their study showed that the limited transfection efficiency of conventional methods (10%) can be successfully increased to more than 75%. In addition, it has been reported that the parallelisation of microfluidic devices has great potential to increase the speed of gene transfer and the number of transfected cells [204].

MHFF was first integrated into flow cytometry and used for particle counting. Combined systems were later developed that contributed to the development of the electroporation technique, which provides high efficiency at low voltages in gene therapy. One of the most important application areas the process has reached today is the microfluidics-assisted confinement (MAC) technique, which allows low-volume, precision production systems to be developed.

Optical transfection is another gene therapy technique used to transport genetic material into living cells. Optical transfection is performed by lasers that transfer the genetic cargo material to the cells. Optical transfection uses continuous-wave and pulsed laser sources to heat local areas in the cell membrane, thereby temporarily forming pores on the cell membrane. These lasers can also provide transfection by creating bubbles and thermoelastic stress, but they are not preferable due to their low transfection efficiency.

Depending on the geometric structure of the surface of microfluidic devices, studies have shown that gene transfection can be achieved through the mechanical deformation of cells. For example, a study by Han *et al* aimed to transport Cas9 ribonucleoproteins into a cell for a genome editing process [205]. Pattern arrays were created on the inner surfaces of microfluidic chips to support the passage of Cas9 molecules, which were intended to be taken into the cell through the cell membrane. The patterns formed on the inner surfaces of the microfluidic channels also preserved the cell viability, even though they created spaces in the membrane that allowed transport. The parallelisation of the created array structures increased the transfection rate (figure 2.49).

Compared with traditional methods, it has been reported that microfluidic-assisted gene therapy applications have succeeded in increasing the ~10% transfection rate to over 50% and the ~50% cell viability rate to over 90% [206]. Considering all these advantages, gene therapy technologies have gained an important place among biomedical applications using microfluidic platforms.

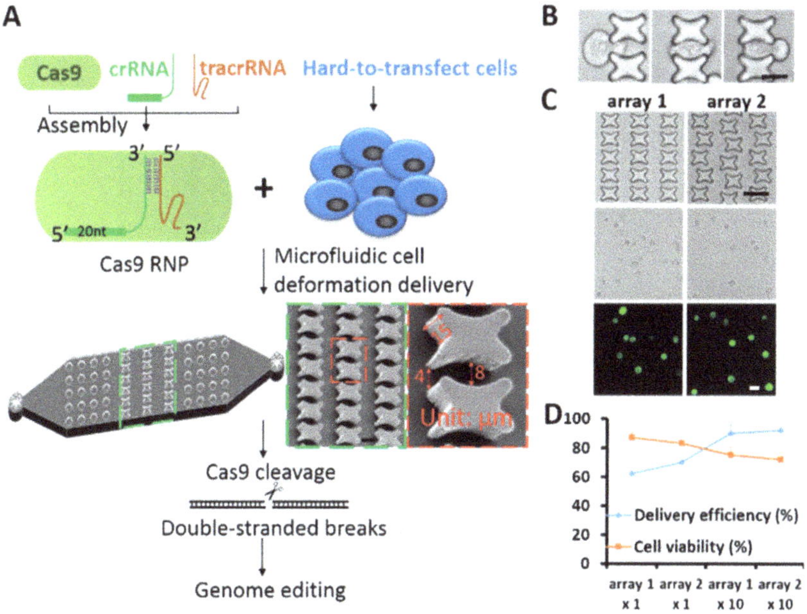

Figure 2.49. A microfluidics-assisted Cas9 RNP delivery strategy with its mechanism and results. (A) A schematic illustration of Cas9/crRNA/tracrRNA ribonucleoprotein (Cas9 RNP) delivery for genome editing in difficult-to-transfect cells via a microfluidic cell deformation chip. SEM micrographs of deformable zones in the microfluidic device (scale bar=10 μm), (B) SEM micrographs of the cell deformation of SK-BR-3 cells (scale bar=10 μm), (C) scanning electron micrographs of SK-BR-3 cells and fluorescein isothiocyanate (FITC)-labelled fluorescence micrographs of arrays 1 and 2 (scale bar=20 μm), (D) delivery efficiency and cell viability diagrams for arrays 1 and 2 at a fluid speed of 150 μl min^{-1}. X10=10 repeats of identical cell deformation zones. (n = 3) [205] John Wiley & Sons. [2017].

2.6.3 Microfluidics in protein separation

Biological applications of microfluidic systems cover a wide area ranging from omics technologies to gene therapies and from drug delivery systems to diagnostic kits. Microfluidic devices provide the potential to mix, concentrate, purify, and separate at low volumes (down to the picolitre level) when working with biological molecules and liquids. Protein purification/separation techniques also offer precise, reproducible, and low-cost operation when integrated into microfluidic devices. In addition to the development of disposable microfluidic chips, the development of integrated systems for complex analytical devices also increases the potential of microfluidic technologies to be used in protein purification/separation applications [207].

Traditional protein separation/purification methods use ultrafiltration, centrifugation, and chromatographic (gel, ion exchange, affinity, hydrophobicity, isoelectric point, high liquid pressure chromatography (HPLC), etc.) techniques. In separation applications tailored to microfluidic devices, complex platforms can be developed using these techniques in which the size distributions can be separated using application-specific channel geometries, charges, and topographies (figure 2.50) [208]. The use of microfluidics as a protein separation technique first began with its

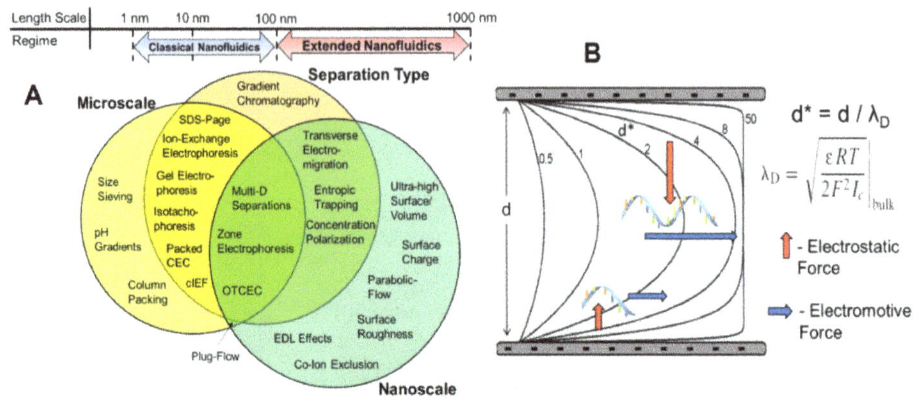

Figure 2.50. (A) A Venn diagram showing microscale (yellow circle) and nanoscale (green circle) phenomena and electrokinetically driven separations (orange circle). KEY–cIEF–capillary isoelectric focusing; multi-D separations–multi-dimensional separations; OTCEC—open tubular capillary electrochromatography; and EDL—electrical double layer. (B) A diagram showing electrokinetically driven transverse electromigration in single-stranded DNAs with different amounts of EDL overlap (d^*), (d is determined using the ratio $d/\lambda d$, where λd is the Debye length). The two major forces acting on the single-stranded DNAs are the electrostatic force and the electromotive force. Reprinted from [208], Copyright (2022), with permission from Elsevier.

integration into chromatography columns. With the development of technology and increased requirements, microfluidic platforms that can operate with high sensitivity and efficiency even at low volumes have started to replace traditional gel electrophoresis (sodium dodecyl sulphate–polyacrylamide gel electrophoresis (SDS-PAGE)) applications [209]. The time saved during analysis is the main reason for the preference for microfluidic platforms. Commercial examples such as the LabChip Protein Characterisation System (PerkinElmer) and the Experion™ Automated Electrophoresis System (Bio-rad) are also prominent examples of commercial products that evolved in line with the need for microfluidic platforms.

Protein separation and detection has become a vital diagnostic tool that is used to maintain patient health and treat patients at an early stage. Microfluidic devices have also gained importance because of the diversity, sensitivity, accuracy, and repeatability they offer. An important example of protein separation from biological fluids is exosome purification and detection. Exosomes are nano-sized vesicles found in biological fluids. They have broad uses ranging from disease detection to cellular therapies, which can be realised by isolating them from their biological environment (figure 2.51) [210]. In another biological application, Wu *et al* developed a prototype of a microfluidic device for the separation of bacteria from human blood cells [211]. Bacteria and blood cells of different sizes are prominent examples of the application of protein separation in the biomedical field. The basis of the developed device was to perform separation through the use of symmetrical and asymmetrical channel geometries in the design of the microfluidic device, which took advantage of the size difference between bacteria and blood cells.

In another microfluidic chip study by Zhao *et al*, exosome detection was developed for ovarian cancer detection in human blood (figure 2.52) [212]. In this

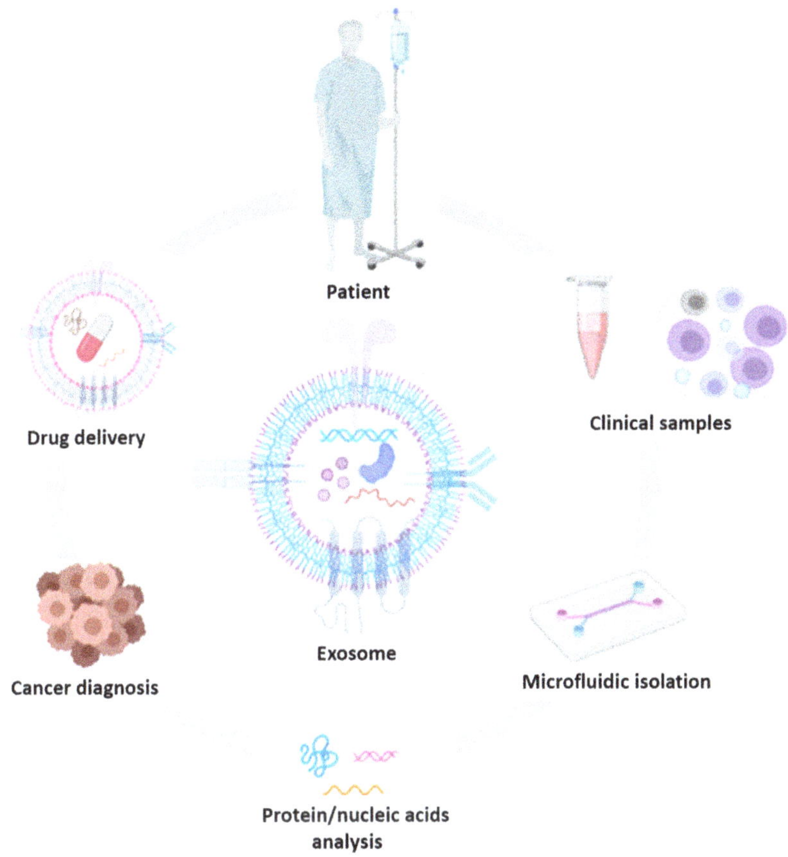

Figure 2.51. A schematic representation of a patient pathway consisting of clinical sample collection, isolation, protein separation, diagnosis, and therapy. Reprinted from [210], Copyright (2021), with permission from Elsevier.

study, which used exosome proteins as biomarkers, a multiplex microfluidic chip called ExoSearch was designed. ExoSearch is a Y-shaped microfluidic chip with a 300 × 500 μm channel size; it has mixing, immunomagnetic bead marking, isolation, and multi-probe compartments and works under continuous flow. A comparison between ExoSearch and the Bradford protein assay showed that the analyte requirement for 1 ml of human plasma decreased to 20 μl and the analysis time decreased from 12 h to 40 min. The detection of exosome proteins (cancer cell fingerprints that freely circulate in blood fluid) using microfluidic chips saved time and analytes. In addition, it created effects that reduced health costs while increasing patient compliance by avoiding the need for invasive procedures. Biomedical applications based on protein separation and purification are not only limited to ovarian cancer and exosome determination but also have wide application potential in the detection of numerous biomarkers.

Microfluidics-assisted protein separation, which started with basic research and the development of automated devices, became complex in line with the needs of the biomedical field and formed the basis of LOC and micro total analysis systems.

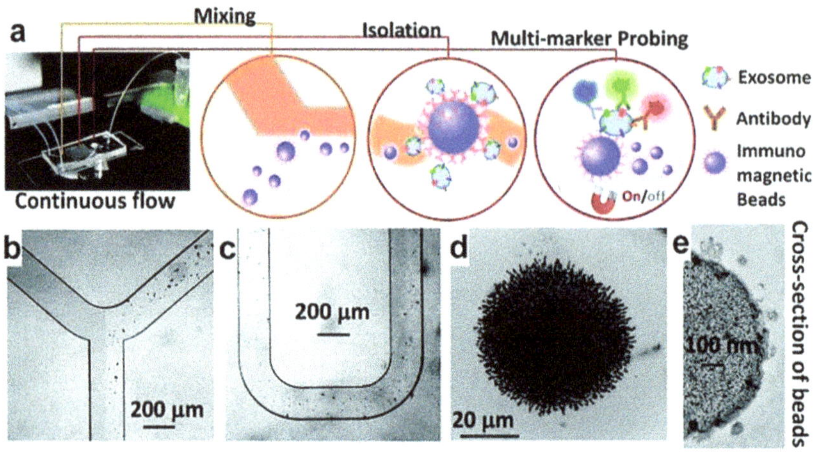

Figure 2.52. (a) The continuous flow scheme of the ExoSearch chip: mixing, isolation, and multi-marker probing. (b) and (c) Bright-field microscope images of immunomagnetic beads manipulated in the microfluidic channel for the mixing and isolation of exosomes. (d) Exosome-bound immunomagnetic beads aggregated in the microchamber with an on/off switchable magnet for the continuous collection and release of exosomes. (e) A cross-sectional transmission electron microscopy (TEM) micrograph of an exosome-bound immunomagnetic bead. Reproduced from [212] with permission from the Royal Society of Chemistry.

Microfluidics-based platforms started with protein purification and integrated the detection and quantity analysis of proteins separated from biological fluids, such as blood, urine, serum, and saliva; microfluidics-based platforms now form the cornerstones of the biomedical kit industry.

2.7 Lab-on-a-chip diagnostic applications

Some of the goals of developing microfluidic systems are to provide a total solution for sample-based applications and to be able to display analytical results. For this reason, microfluidic systems are also called LOCs, biochips, or µTASs. LOC systems allow one or more multi-stage (bio)-chemical processes to be carried out using micro- or nano-sized samples on a single chip. LOC systems range in size from millimetres to several centimetres and are miniaturised microfluidic assemblies.

The main advantages of LOCs are: (1) ease of use, (2) high-speed analysis, (3) small minimum sample amounts, and (4) small reagent volumes. LOCs can perform sequential chemical transformations of the starting sample; these can include steps such as separation, concentration, the mixing of intermediates, transport into different reaction microchambers, and reading the final results.

µTASs are devices that include and automate all the necessary steps for the chemical analysis of a sample, such as sampling, sample handling, chemical reactions, and detection. Due to the unique properties of their microstructures, µTASs can perform complex analyses at a lower cost than conventional systems with reduced consumption of energy and reagents. Thus, µTASs are becoming a valuable alternative in many fields, such as biomedical science, the food sector, chemicals, pharmaceuticals, agriculture, pharmacy, and medicine.

2.7.1 Paper-based microfluidic biosensors

In healthcare applications, the need for cheap and fast solutions for diagnosis and disease follow-up is increasing daily. Whitesides and his group first developed the technology of µPADs in 2007 [41]. Paper, which is cheap, accessible, and recyclable, has become a frequently used material in biomedical applications as a result of these advantages. In addition to being a cheap raw material, its ease of processing is another advantage. µPAD technology, which has grown rapidly to date, has grown in its production techniques and application areas.

Paper-based microfluidic biosensors have been produced using several physical and chemical techniques such as wax patterning, plotting, cutting, inkjet printing, etching, stamping, flexographic printing, laser treatment, photolithography, and plasma and chemical vapour deposition (figure 2.53) [42, 213]. Their advantages and disadvantages are tabulated and classified according to their fabrication techniques in table 2.7.

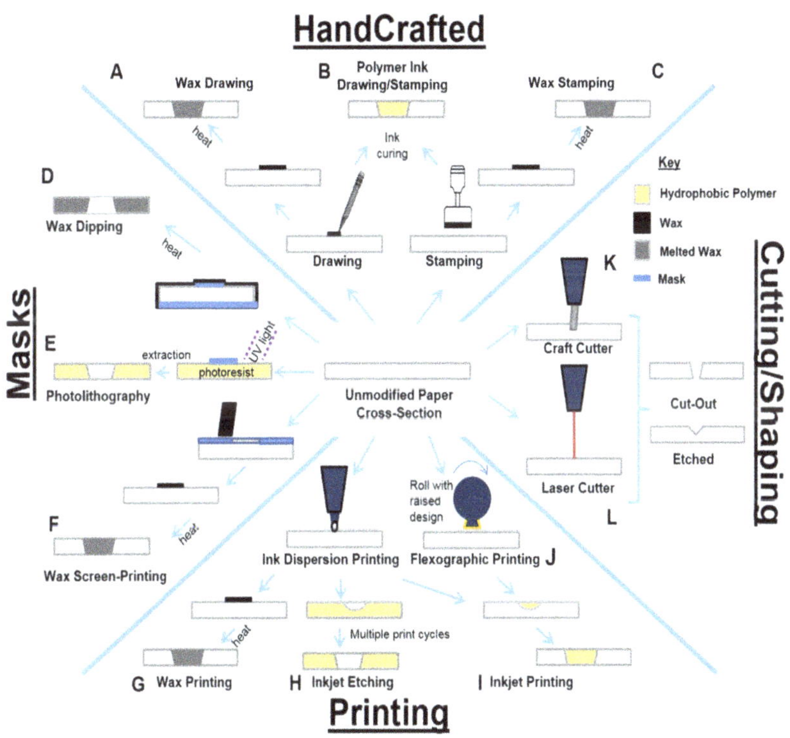

Figure 2.53. Paper-based microfluidic channel production techniques categorised into hand-crafted, mask-based, cutting/shaping, and printing techniques: (a) wax drawing, (b) polymer ink drawing/stamping, (c) wax stamping, (d) wax dipping, (e) photolithography, (f) wax screen printing, (g) wax printing, (h) inkjet etching, (i) inkjet printing, (j) flexographic printing, (k) craft cutter, and (l) laser cutter. Reprinted with permission from [42]. Copyright (2015) American Chemical Society.

Table 2.7. A comparative analysis of the advantages and drawbacks of paper-based microfluidics fabrication techniques. Reprinted with permission from [214]. Copyright (2012) AIP Publishing.

Fabrication techniques	Advantages	Drawbacks
Photolithography	High resolution of microfluidic channels (channel width is as narrow as 200 μm; the barrier is sharp)	Requires expensive equipment; requires an extra washing step to remove non-cross-linked polymer; devices are vulnerable to bending
Plotting	Patterning agent (PDMS) is cheap; devices are flexible	Reduced barrier definition; cannot readily be applied to high-throughput production
Inkjet etching	Requires only a single printing apparatus to create microfluidic channels, which is achieved by etching and printing bio/chemical sensing reagents	The creation of microfluidic channels requires ten printing passes; the printing apparatus must be customised; unsuitable for mass fabrication
Plasma treatment	Uses a very cheap patterning agent (alkyl ketene dimer, AKD), which dramatically reduces the material cost	Requires different masks to create different microfluidic patterns on paper
Wax printing	Produces massive devices using a simple and fast (5–10 min) fabrication process	Requires expensive wax printers; requires an extra heating step after wax deposition
Inkjet printing	Uses very cheap AKD; produces massive devices fast (<10 min) and simply; requires only a desktop printer to produce devices and to print sensing reagents	Requires an extra heating step after AKD deposition; requires modified inkjet printers
Flexography printing	Allows direct roll-to-roll production in existing printing houses; avoids the heat treatment of printed patterns	Requires two prints of polystyrene solution; requires different printing plates; print quality relies on the smoothness of the paper surface
Screen printing	Produces devices via a simple process	The low resolution of microfluidic channels (rough barrier); requires different printing screens to create different patterns
Laser treatment	High resolution (minimum pattern size of about 62 μm)	Microfluidic channels do not allow lateral fluid flows; microfluidic channels require extra coating for liquid flows

The capillary effect provides flow in microfluidic applications without the need for any other equipment. The capillary effect is a key factor, especially in the use of rapid diagnostic kits. μPADs offer economical and practical solutions in diagnostic applications. For this reason, they are preferred as a fast and inexpensive analysis method in food, safety, criminal, and environmental tests, biological diagnosis, and diagnostic kits.

The oldest known paper-based sensor is litmus paper, which provides colorimetric pH analysis. On the other hand, the most frequently used paper-based microfluidic biosensors in daily life are glucometers and pregnancy tests (figure 2.54). During the COVID-19 pandemic, which emerged as a global problem in 2020, the need for disposable biosensors used in virus detection increased day by day. Paper-based biosensors are used in two basic ways: (1) prepared before use by the addition of the reagent and the analyte, and (2) ready to use. The analysis methods used include colorimetric, electrochemical, chemiluminescent, and electrochemiluminescent detection. While the colorimetric method is widely used in pH, protein, and glucose analyses, glucose testing can also be performed using the electrochemical and chemiluminescence methods.

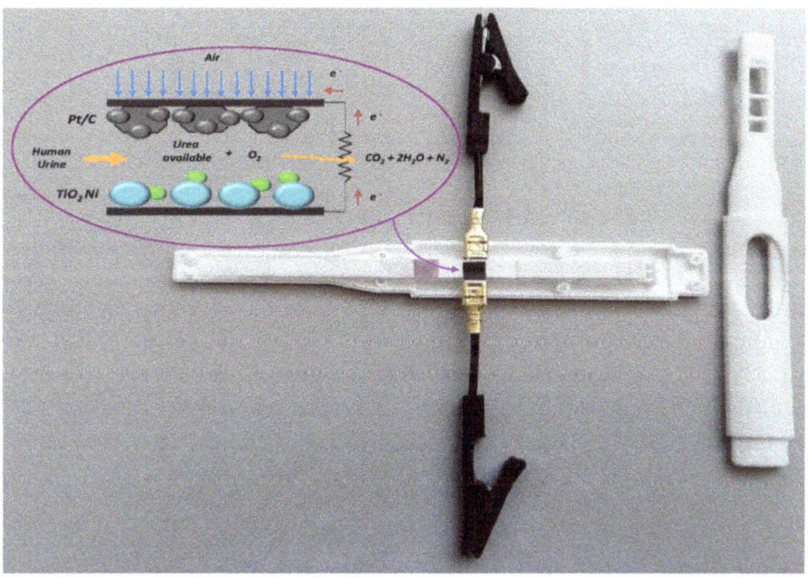

Figure 2.54. μPAD pregnancy test kit and reaction chart. Reproduced from [215]. CC BY 4.0.

Chronic diabetes is a metabolic disease that affects approximately 8.5% of the world's population [216]. The disease is diagnosed and followed up by determining the glucose levels in body fluids (blood, urine, tears). The need for the development of cheap, practical, and patient-friendly analysis methods for blood glucose measurements is very important, as the number of people affected by this disease increases yearly.

Gabriel *et al* designed a μPAD colorimetric biosensor that measures glucose from human tears as an alternative to body fluids such as blood and urine, which are widely used in traditional applications [216] (figure 2.55). Tear glucose level determination is a painless and simple alternative, since it does not require an invasive procedure during the analyte collection stage. The μPAD used in the study was produced by creating hydrophobic channel walls using a wax printing technique. The paper surface was subsequently modified using chitosan. Following the immobilisation of the chromogenic agent and enzyme solutions on the surface, the μPADs were ready to perform lateral flow glucose determination.

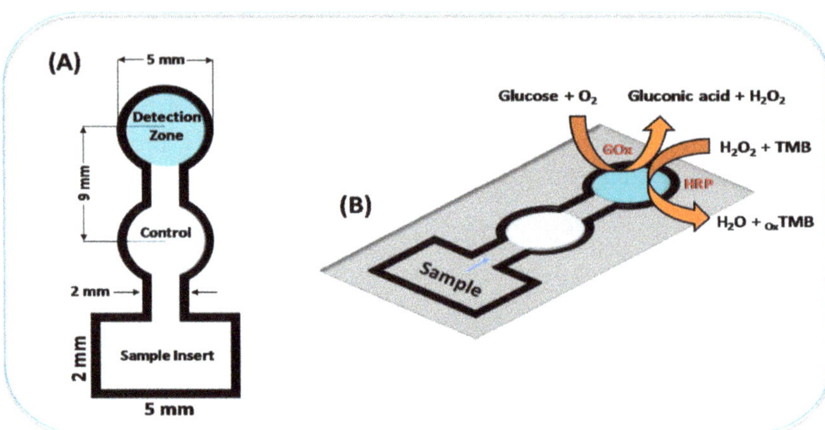

Figure 2.55. Illustrative representations of: (a) the μPAD glucose biosensor, (b) the enzymatic reaction and the glucose detection mechanism of the μPAD. Reproduced from [216]. CC BY 4.0.

Colorimetric analysis of the μPADs was performed by scanning them using an office scanner and then performing calculations using Corel Photo-Paint™ software. As a result of analyses made using tears collected from volunteers, it was determined that the developed biosensor had an analytic sensitivity of 84 AU mM^{-1} and a limit of detection (LOD) of 50 μM. When the measurements were repeated using a commercial glucometer, no statistical difference was observed, and the data fell within the 95% confidence level. High-sensitivity results were obtained using biosensors that could measure the glucose level of patients from tears. This study presented an alternative approach to commercial products that measure blood glucose levels; it thereby offered a way of increasing patient compliance and comfort.

As a result of technological developments, microfluidics-supported biosensors that can make more accurate, easy, and practical measurements are being developed. The increasing usage of smartphones in every field is also shaping paper-based microfluidic biosensor applications. In a recent study by Duan *et al*, a μPAD was used for colorimetric enzyme-linked immunosorbent assay (c-ELISA) and the measurement was made by a smartphone [217]. In addition, smartphone-based measurements have been made with the help of deep learning under different ambient light conditions. Rabbit IgG was used as a reference material. The μPAD was tested using three different light sources (natural light, a table lamp, and fluorescent light) and their combinations (figure 2.56).

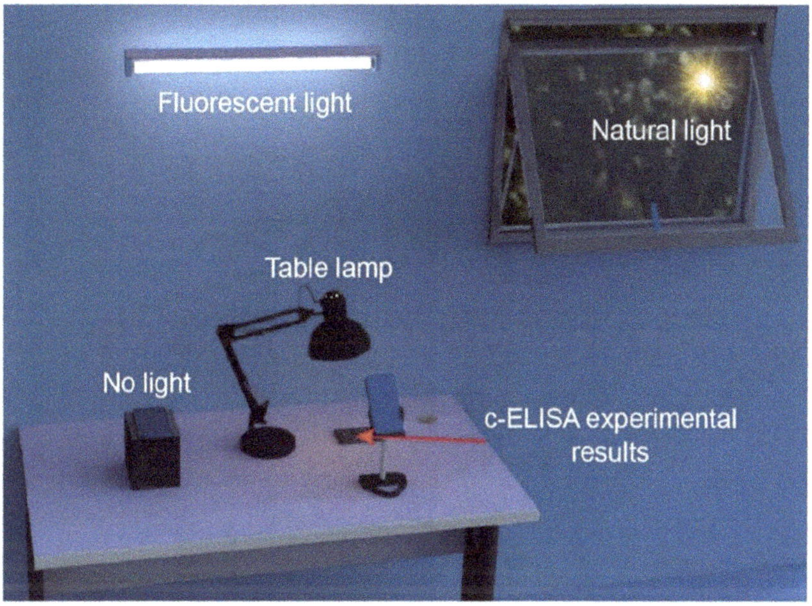

Figure 2.56. Illustrational image of the smartphone-camera-assisted analysis of a paper-based ELISA test in the dark (without light), in fluorescent lighting (F), under a table lamp (L), and under natural lighting (N) conditions. Reprinted from [217], Copyright (2023), with permission from Elsevier.

Whatman chromatography paper was used in the μPADs. Surface-modified paper was produced by a wax printer to obtain multi-well plates. Antigen immobilisation was then performed at different concentrations. After the test samples had interacted with the μPADs, data sets were collected by a smartphone camera under different lighting conditions. The images obtained were simply analysed by the Android system with the help of an image-processing deep learning algorithm (figure 2.57).

The results showed that the designed and tested μPADs exhibited >97% accuracy in determining the rabbit IgG concentration (Picomolar, pM). In addition, three different lights and eight different lighting combinations were tested with different smartphones to prove the accuracy and repeatability of the system. The data obtained revealed that the μPADs developed for integration with mobile devices offered high sensitivity, speed, and accuracy of analysis in qualitative and quantitative settings. In addition, deep learning techniques and image-processing models developed specifically for measurement in mobile devices can support an increasing variety of applications. Adopting the new algorithms and image-processing models

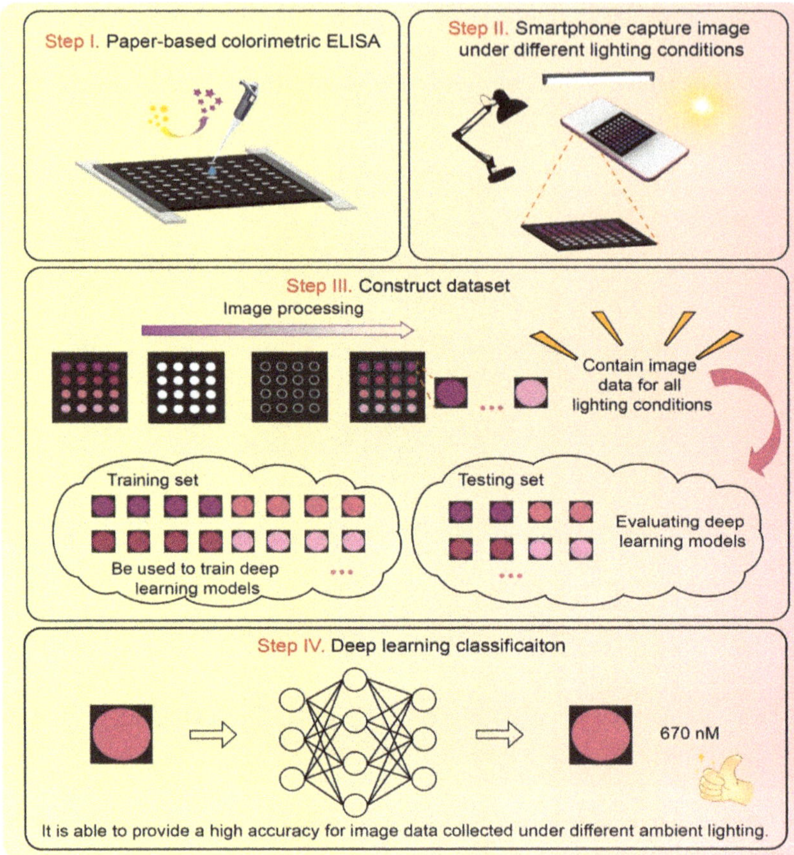

Figure 2.57. A step-by-step schematic representation of the smartphone-assisted testing of µPAD ELISA assays. Reprinted from [217], Copyright (2023), with permission from Elsevier.

for clinical measurements has the potential to strongly impact diversity, speed, and cost reduction in healthcare applications.

2.7.2 Microcirculation-based sensors

As a result of the irregular and aggressive proliferation encountered in primary tumour regions, circulating tumour cells (CTCs) circulate in the blood. These present the risk of seeding cancer tissues into other parts of the body as a result of blood flow through the vascular structure. Therefore, it is vital to remove CTCs that have metastatic potential while they are still in the bloodstream. However, the differentiation and classification of CTCs in the vascular system is a very difficult task due to their low concentration and the heterogeneity of their phenotypes. Over the last two decades, many microfluidics-based approaches have been developed for the successful study and isolation of cells under these challenging situations, which are described in detail below [218]. These separation or isolation methods vary depending on the physical, chemical, or biological properties of the cell type that is intended to be separated from the bloodstream, such as size, membrane composition, or labelling. These studies are based on different mechanisms, including inertial forces, acoustic separation, DEP, and magnetic and optical forces.

Inertial microfluidics is a promising approach for the separation and sorting of CTCs from blood cells based on differences in cell size and deformability [219]. The general principle of inert microfluidics is based on the use of hydrodynamic forces to push cells towards specific positions in a microchannel, depending on their size and shape. This approach separates cells based on their size and deformability using hydrodynamic forces. An important element that distinguishes inert microfluidic systems from other microfluidic systems is that they operate at relatively higher Reynolds numbers. Although the first inert microfluidic systems were developed to concentrate particles, devices that can differentiate cells according to their size and elasticity have been developed using geometric designs such as multi-orifice straight, spiral, and serpentine designs (figure 2.58). Inert microfluidics can isolate CTCs with high efficiency and purity and have been used for CTC isolation in a variety of cancers, including lung, breast, and prostate cancers [220–222].

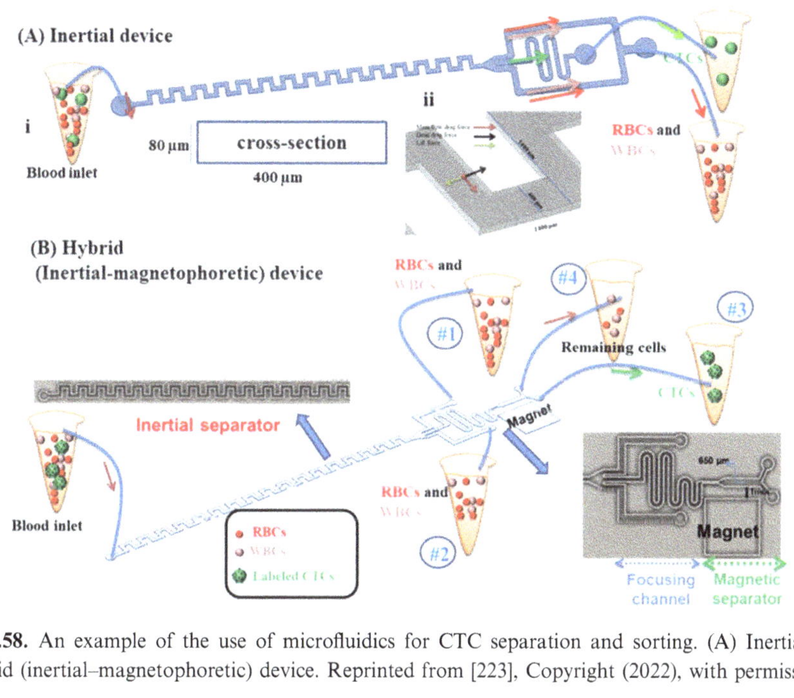

Figure 2.58. An example of the use of microfluidics for CTC separation and sorting. (A) Inertial device, (B) hybrid (inertial–magnetophoretic) device. Reprinted from [223], Copyright (2022), with permission from Elsevier.

Acoustic-based microfluidics, also called 'acoustophoresis', offers a label-free and noninvasive approach for separating and sorting CTCs from blood cells based on differences in physical properties. This noninvasive approach uses sound waves to separate cells based on their size, density, and compressibility. High precision and purity are also possible using this approach. Ultrasonic standing waves controlled by a piezoelectric transducer are applied to the system, and low-pressure nodes occur along the separation channel. The amplitude of the wave is adjusted to push particles larger than the target size towards the centre of the channel, while the smaller ones remain at the edges of the channel (figure 2.59) [224]. The amplitude can be changed, and separation by size can be made possible by gradually classifying the cells by adjusting the voltage applied to the piezoelectric transducer.

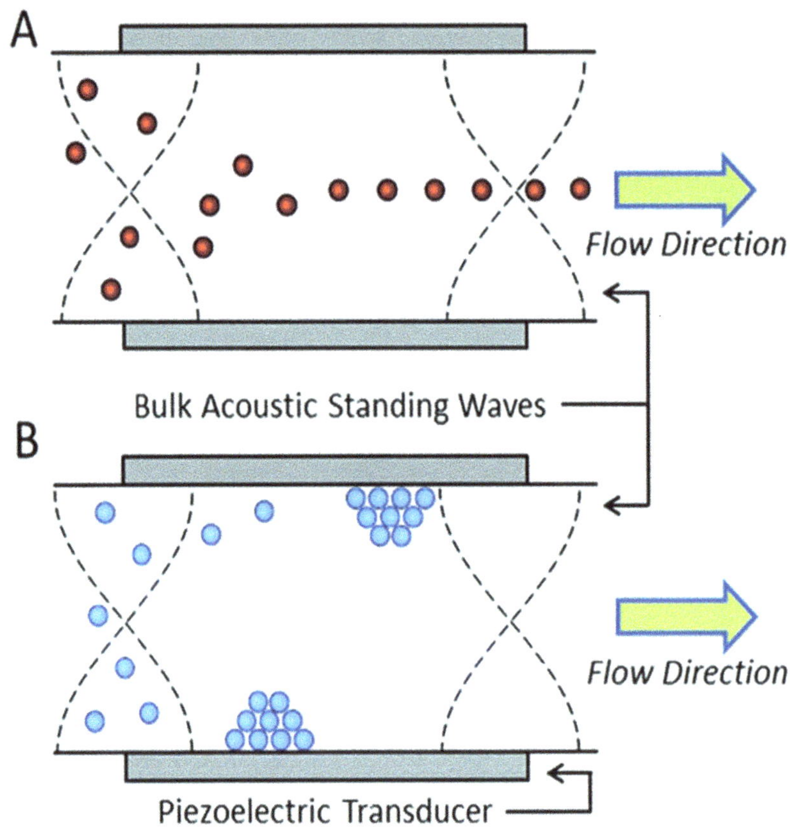

Figure 2.59. Acoustophoretic cell manipulation. Objects migrate to the pressure node(s) and antinodes, depending on their acoustic contrast characters. Reproduced from [224] with permission from the Royal Society of Chemistry.

Another approach used to separate CTCs from other cells in the bloodstream is DEP. Using DEP, cells can be classified according to their particle size and polarizability. After an electric field is applied to the microfluidic channel, the polarised cells interact with the applied field and encounter a net electric force. Cells have different dielectric properties, according to their polarizability and factors such as membrane composition and size. When normal blood cells and CTCs with different polarisation potentials are exposed to a non-uniform electric field, they move in different directions according to the force they are affected by. This method has many advantages; for example, there is no need to mark or label the cells before they acquire an electrical charge. This is because the dipoles induced when the cells are exposed to an uneven electric field align the cells within that electric field (figure 2.60) [225].

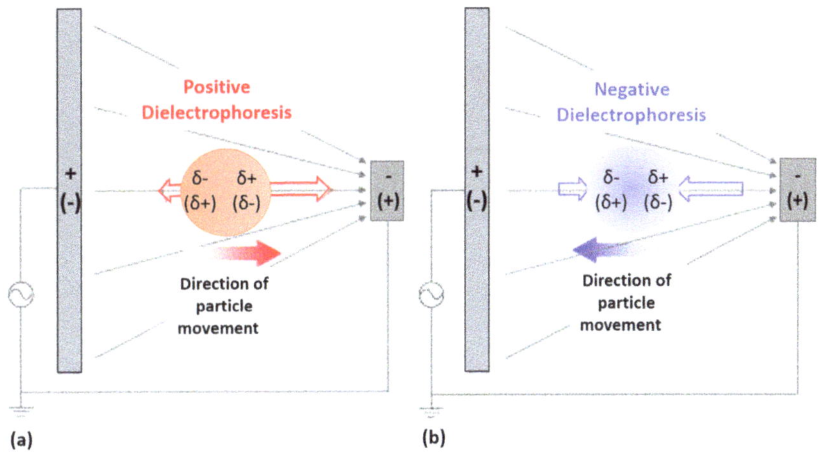

Figure 2.60. The direction of cell movement depends on the dielectrophoretic response: (a) positive dielectrophoretic cells and (b) negative dielectrophoretic cells. Reprinted from [225], Copyright (2005), with permission from Elsevier.

Magnetophoresis is defined as 'the movement of particles under the influence of a magnetic field' and is similar to the abovementioned dielectrophoretic approach. Magnetophoresis is a high-throughput, powerful approach for isolating CTCs from blood cells using magnetic nanoparticles that are functionalized with specific antibodies or aptamers that bind to the specific surface markers on CTCs. The sample interacts with magnetic nanoparticles functionalized with specific antibodies or aptamers that target CTCs before the magnetic field is applied. The mixture of magnetised CTCs and blood is then passed through a microfluidic channel that has a magnetic field gradient. As a result of this gradient, the CTCs are attracted towards the magnet and can be separated from the rest of the blood (figure 2.61) [226]. The remaining blood components are either removed from the microfluidics or transferred to the bloodstream, leaving behind the CTCs bound to the magnetic nanoparticles in the collecting zone. The concentrated analyte can be further analysed for possible early detection or metastatic circulation.

Microfluidic devices in which cells are separated and classified using their refractive index and size in a mixture also have significant usage areas and examples. These optical systems utilise light that can provide high-purity CTC separation, but their effectiveness may vary depending on the type of cancer. In optofluidic systems for CTC detection, a fluid or blood sample containing CTCs is passed through a microfluidic channel designed to interact with light in a specific way. This interaction

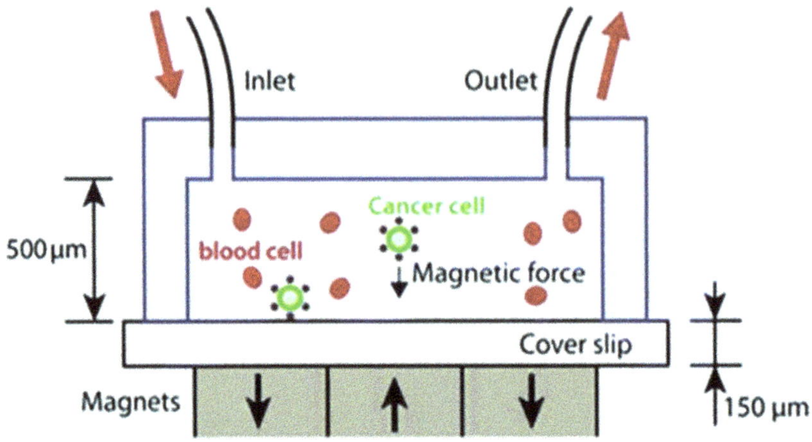

Figure 2.61. A schematic illustration of a microfluidic design for the immunomagnetic detection of cancer cells, showing the principle of operation. Reproduced from [226] with permission from the Royal Society of Chemistry.

can be achieved if the channel has a surface pattern that scatters light in a specific direction or by covering it with a material that enhances the interaction between light and CTCs. These interactions cause light to be scattered or refracted in a way that can be detected by a camera or other optical sensor. The captured images can then be analysed to identify and count CTCs. Because the optical properties of CTCs resulting from their size, shape, and refractive index differ from those of other blood cells, this approach has the potential to be highly sensitive and specific.

2.8 The future scope of microfluidic technology

The technology of microfluidics was founded on fluid dynamics and then continued its development via lithography, MEMs, and LOC applications. However, microfluidic technologies experienced their biggest revolution with the discovery of PDMS. The main advantage of microfluidics is that it provides fast, economical, and reproducible solutions in the biomedical field. The biotechnological and biomedical applications of microfluidics have expanded as a result of the discovery of PDMS.

Microfluidics is used in a wide range of applications ranging from drug delivery systems to imaging agents, tissue scaffolds, cell culture reactors, organ-on-a-chip applications, separation, diagnosis, detection, and biosensor applications. Microfluidics provide primary benefits such as automation, integration, and miniaturisation. The ability to develop inexpensive, tailor-made, and fast microfluidics platforms is also the cornerstone of state-of-the-art microfluidics (figure 2.62).

The COVID-19 pandemic, a global health problem that emerged in 2019, has also hinted at the fact that microfluidics will gain greater importance and development in the coming years. Examples such as the production of COVID-19 mRNA vaccines in microfluidic reactors and rapid diagnostic kits such as paper-based microfluidic

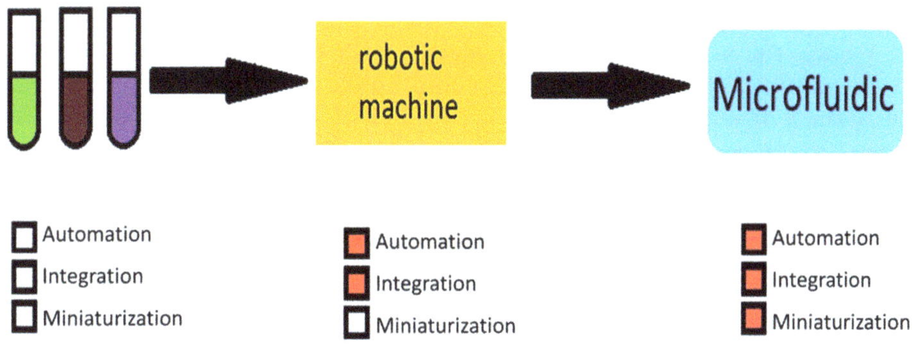

Figure 2.62. The development process and advantages of microfluidics. Reproduced from [192] with permission from the Royal Society of Chemistry.

chips and PCR tests demonstrate the need for microfluidics on a global scale. Considering the developments reported in the scientific literature, it can be predicted that developments in microfluidics-assisted diagnostics and treatment and the use of FDA-approved microfluidic products will increase in the coming years. In view of the miniaturisation capabilities of microfluidic devices, it is highly feasible that they will be used to provide fast and economical solutions to wider diagnostic applications. In addition, the inability of laboratory studies to simulate the 3D and dynamic human body in 2D cell culture vessels under static conditions has revealed the importance of microfluidic devices once again. The development of microfluidic tissue models that imitate the human body in dynamic conditions instead of animal experiments shows great promise in preclinical applications as an economical solution that is friendly to the environment, nature, and other living things. The most important area in which microfluidic platforms are developing is undoubtedly human-on-a-chip applications.

References and further reading

[1] Castillo-León J 2015 Microfluidics and lab-on-a-chip devices: history and challenges *Lab-on-a-Chip Devices and Micro-Total Analysis Systems* (Berlin: Springer) pp 1–15

[2] Delaquilla A 2021 Five Short Stories on The History of Microfluidics https://www.elveflow.com/microfluidic-reviews/general-microfluidics/history-of-microfluidics/

[3] Janna W S 2020 *Introduction to Fluid Mechanics* (Boca Raton, FL: CRC Press) 6th edn

[4] Young D F, Munson B R, Okiishi T H and Huebsch W W 2010 *A Brief Introduction to Fluid Mechanics* (New York: Wiley)

[5] Prakash S, Karacor M and Banerjee S 2009 Surface modification in microsystems and nanosystems *Surf. Sci. Rep.* **64** 233–54

[6] Venkateshwarlu A and Bharti R P 2021 Effects of capillary number and flow rates on the hydrodynamics of droplet generation in two-phase cross-flow microfluidic systems *J. Taiwan Inst. Chem. Eng.* **129** 64–79

[7] Kleinstreuer C 2013 *Microfluidics and Nanofluidics: Theory and Selected Applications* (New York: Wiley)

[8] Cheri M S, Shahraki H, Sadeghi J, Moghaddam M S and Latifi H 2014 Measurement and control of pressure driven flows in microfluidic devices using an optofluidic flow sensor *Biomicrofluidics* **8** 054123
[9] Ajdari A 2004 Steady flows in networks of microfluidic channels: building on the analogy with electrical circuits *C.R. Phys.* **5** 539–46
[10] Bier M 2013 *Electrophoresis: Theory, Methods, and Applications* (Amsterdam: Elsevier)
[11] McCallum C and Pennathur S 2016 Accounting for electric double layer and pressure gradient-induced dispersion effects in microfluidic current monitoring *Microfluid. Nanofluid.* **20** 1–9
[12] Kirby B J and Hasselbrink Jr E F 2004 Zeta potential of microfluidic substrates: 2. Data for polymers *Electrophoresis* **25** 203–13
[13] Sprague I B and Dutta P 2011 Modeling of diffuse charge effects in a microfluidic based laminar flow fuel cell *Numer. Heat Transf.* A **59** 1–27
[14] Prakash S and Yeom J 2014 *Nanofluidics and Microfluidics: Systems and Applications* (William Andrew)
[15] Yadavali S, Jeong H-H, Lee D and Issadore D 2018 Silicon and glass very large scale microfluidic droplet integration for terascale generation of polymer microparticles *Nat. Commun.* **9** 1–9
[16] Iliescu C, Taylor H, Avram M, Miao J and Franssila S 2012 A practical guide for the fabrication of microfluidic devices using glass and silicon *Biomicrofluidics* **6** 016505
[17] Wen J, Legendre L A, Bienvenue J M and Landers J P 2008 Purification of nucleic acids in microfluidic devices *Anal. Chem.* **80** 6472–9
[18] Lapierre F, Piret G, Drobecq H, Melnyk O, Coffinier Y, Thomy V and Boukherroub R 2011 High sensitive matrix-free mass spectrometry analysis of peptides using silicon nanowires-based digital microfluidic device *Lab Chip* **11** 1620–8
[19] Qi Z, Xu L, Xu Y, Zhong J, Abedini A, Cheng X and Sinton D 2018 Disposable silicon-glass microfluidic devices: precise, robust and cheap *Lab Chip* **18** 3872–80
[20] Terry S C, Jerman J H and Angell J B 1979 A gas chromatographic air analyzer fabricated on a silicon wafer *IEEE Trans. Electron Devices* **26** 1880–6
[21] Tian W-C and Finehout E 2009 *Microfluidics for Biological Applications* (Berlin: Springer Science & Business Media)
[22] Hwang J, Cho Y H, Park M S and Kim B H 2019 Microchannel fabrication on glass materials for microfluidic devices *Int. J. Precis. Eng. Manuf.* **20** 479–95
[23] Attia U M, Marson S and Alcock J R 2009 Micro-injection moulding of polymer microfluidic devices *Microfluid. Nanofluid.* **7** 1–28
[24] Liga A, Morton J A and Kersaudy-Kerhoas M 2016 Safe and cost-effective rapid-prototyping of multilayer PMMA microfluidic devices *Microfluid. Nanofluid.* **20** 1–12
[25] Chen Y, Zhang L and Chen G 2008 Fabrication, modification, and application of poly (methyl methacrylate) microfluidic chips *Electrophoresis* **29** 1801–14
[26] Ma X, Li R, Jin Z, Fan Y, Zhou X and Zhang Y 2020 Injection molding and characterization of PMMA-based microfluidic devices *Microsyst. Technol.* **26** 1317–24
[27] Chen X, Shen J and Zhou M 2016 Rapid fabrication of a four-layer PMMA-based microfluidic chip using CO_2-laser micromachining and thermal bonding *J. Micromech. Microeng.* **26** 107001

[28] Li J, Liu C, Dai X, Chen H, Liang Y, Sun H, Tian H and Ding X 2008 PMMA microfluidic devices with three-dimensional features for blood cell filtration *J. Micromech. Microeng.* **18** 095021

[29] Kim E, Xia Y and Whitesides G M 1995 Polymer microstructures formed by moulding in capillaries *Nature* **376** 581–4

[30] Xia Y, Mrksich M, Kim E and Whitesides G M 1995 Microcontact printing of octadecylsiloxane on the surface of silicon dioxide and its application in microfabrication *J. Am. Chem. Soc.* **117** 9576–7

[31] Wilbur J L, Kim E, Xia Y and Whitesides G M 1995 Lithographic molding: a convenient route to structures with sub-micrometer dimensions *Adv. Mater.* **7** 649–52

[32] McDonald J C and Whitesides G M 2002 Poly (dimethylsiloxane) as a material for fabricating microfluidic devices *Acc. Chem. Res.* **35** 491–9

[33] Tang S K and Whitesides G M 2010 *Basic Microfluidic and Soft Lithographic Techniques* (New York: McGraw-Hill)

[34] Becker H and Locascio L E 2002 Polymer microfluidic devices *Talanta* **56** 267–87

[35] Fujii T 2002 PDMS-based microfluidic devices for biomedical applications *Microelectron. Eng.* **61** 907–14

[36] Tsao C-W 2016 Polymer microfluidics: simple, low-cost fabrication process bridging academic lab research to commercialized production *Micromachines* **7** 225

[37] Guan Y, Xu F, Wang X, Hui Y, Sha J, Tian Y, Wang Z, Zhang S, Chen D and Yang L 2021 Implementation of hybrid PDMS-graphite/Ag conductive material for flexible electronic devices and microfluidic applications *Microelectron. Eng.* **235** 111455

[38] Mehling M and Tay S 2014 Microfluidic cell culture *Curr. Opin. Biotechnol.* **25** 95–102

[39] Halldorsson S, Lucumi E, Gómez-Sjöberg R and Fleming R M 2015 Advantages and challenges of microfluidic cell culture in polydimethylsiloxane devices *Biosens. Bioelectron.* **63** 218–31

[40] Davy J 1812 VI. On a gaseous compound of carbonic oxide and chlorine *Philos. Trans. Royal Soc. London* **102** 144–51

[41] Martinez A W, Phillips S T, Butte M J and Whitesides G M 2007 Patterned paper as a platform for inexpensive, low-volume, portable bioassays *Angew. Chem.* **119** 1340–2

[42] Cate D M, Adkins J A, Mettakoonpitak J and Henry C S 2015 Recent developments in paper-based microfluidic devices *Anal. Chem.* **87** 19–41

[43] Osborn J L, Lutz B, Fu E, Kauffman P, Stevens D Y and Yager P 2010 Microfluidics without pumps: reinventing the T-sensor and H-filter in paper networks *Lab Chip* **10** 2659–65

[44] Lisowski P and Zarzycki P K 2013 Microfluidic paper-based analytical devices (μPADs) and micro total analysis systems (μTAS): development, applications and future trends *Chromatographia* **76** 1201–14

[45] Chung B G, Lee K-H, Khademhosseini A and Lee S-H 2012 Microfluidic fabrication of microengineered hydrogels and their application in tissue engineering *Lab Chip* **12** 45–59

[46] Choi N W, Cabodi M, Held B, Gleghorn J P, Bonassar L J and Stroock A D 2007 Microfluidic scaffolds for tissue engineering *Nat. Mater.* **6** 908–15

[47] Mu X, Zheng W, Sun J, Zhang W and Jiang X 2013 Microfluidics for manipulating cells *Small* **9** 9–21

[48] Nie J, Gao Q, Wang Y, Zeng J, Zhao H, Sun Y, Shen J, Ramezani H, Fu Z and Liu Z 2018 Vessel-on-a-chip with hydrogel-based microfluidics *Small* **14** 1802368

[49] Meng Q, Wang Y, Li Y and Shen C 2021 Hydrogel microfluidic-based liver-on-a-chip: mimicking the mass transfer and structural features of liver, *Biotechnol. Bioeng.* **118** 612–21

[50] Burdick J A, Khademhosseini A and Langer R 2004 Fabrication of gradient hydrogels using a microfluidics/photopolymerization process *Langmuir* **20** 5153–6

[51] Lee U N, Day J H, Haack A J, Bretherton R C, Lu W, DeForest C A, Theberge A B and Berthier E 2020 Layer-by-layer fabrication of 3D hydrogel structures using open microfluidics *Lab Chip* **20** 525–36

[52] Hou X, Zhang Y S, Santiago G T D, Alvarez M M, Ribas J, Jonas S J, Weiss P S, Andrews A M, Aizenberg J and Khademhosseini A 2017 Interplay between materials and microfluidics *Nat. Rev. Mater.* **2** 1–15

[53] Ren K, Chen Y and Wu H 2014 New materials for microfluidics in biology *Curr. Opin. Biotechnol.* **25** 78–85

[54] Plecis A and Chen Y 2007 Fabrication of microfluidic devices based on glass–PDMS–glass technology *Microelectron. Eng.* **84** 1265–9

[55] Abdelgawad M, Watson M W and Wheeler A R 2009 Hybrid microfluidics: a digital-to-channel interface for in-line sample processing and chemical separations *Lab Chip* **9** 1046–51

[56] Hou X, Hu Y, Grinthal A, Khan M and Aizenberg J 2015 Liquid-based gating mechanism with tunable multiphase selectivity and antifouling behaviour *Nature* **519** 70–3

[57] Zhou W, Dou M, Timilsina S S, Xu F and Li X 2021 Recent innovations in cost-effective polymer and paper hybrid microfluidic devices *Lab Chip* **21** 2658–83

[58] Dou M, Sanjay S T, Benhabib M, Xu F and Li X 2015 Low-cost bioanalysis on paper-based and its hybrid microfluidic platforms *Talanta* **145** 43–54

[59] Giri B 2017 *Laboratory Methods in Microfluidics* (Amsterdam: Elsevier)

[60] Mailly D and Vieu C 2007 Lithography and etching processes *Nanoscience* (Berlin: Springer) pp 3–40

[61] Ferry M S, Razinkov I A and Hasty J 2011 Microfluidics for synthetic biology: from design to execution *Methods in Enzymology* (Amsterdam: Elsevier) 295–372

[62] Lin Y, Gao C, Gritsenko D, Zhou R and Xu J 2018 Soft lithography based on photolithography and two-photon polymerization *Microfluid. Nanofluid.* **22** 1–11

[63] Zhao X-M, Xia Y and Whitesides G M 1997 Soft lithographic methods for nano-fabrication *J. Mater. Chem.* **7** 1069–74

[64] Sia S K and Whitesides G M 2003 Microfluidic devices fabricated in poly (dimethylsiloxane) for biological studies *Electrophoresis* **24** 3563–76

[65] Stephan K, Pittet P, Renaud L, Kleimann P, Morin P, Ouaini N and Ferrigno R 2007 Fast prototyping using a dry film photoresist: microfabrication of soft-lithography masters for microfluidic structures *J. Micromech. Microeng.* **17** N69

[66] Abdelgawad M, Watson M W, Young E W, Mudrik J M, Ungrin M D and Wheeler A R 2008 Soft lithography: masters on demand *Lab Chip* **8** 1379–85

[67] Han X, Zhang Y, Tian J, Wu T, Li Z, Xing F and Fu S 2022 Polymer-based microfluidic devices: a comprehensive review on preparation and applications, *Polym. Eng. Sci.* **62** 3–24

[68] Ng J M, Gitlin I, Stroock A D and Whitesides G M 2002 Components for integrated poly (dimethylsiloxane) microfluidic systems *Electrophoresis* **23** 3461–73

[69] Yazdi A A, Popma A, Wong W, Nguyen T, Pan Y and Xu J 2016 3D printing: an emerging tool for novel microfluidics and lab-on-a-chip applications *Microfluid. Nanofluid.* **20** 1–18

[70] Huang S H, Liu P, Mokasdar A and Hou L 2013 Additive manufacturing and its societal impact: a literature review *Int. J. Adv. Manuf. Technol.* **67** 1191–203
[71] Gibson I, Rosen D W, Stucker B and Khorasani M 2021 *Additive Manufacturing Technologies* (Berlin: Springer)
[72] Zhang X, Jiang X and Sun C 1999 Micro-stereolithography of polymeric and ceramic microstructures *Sensors Actuators* A **77** 149–56
[73] Weisgrab G, Ovsianikov A and Costa P F 2019 Functional 3D printing for microfluidic chips *Adv. Mater. Technol.* **4** 1900275
[74] Van den Driesche S, Lucklum F, Bunge F and Vellekoop M J 2018 3D printing solutions for microfluidic chip-to-world connections *Micromachines* **9** 71
[75] He Y, Wu Y, Fu J Z, Gao Q and Qiu J J 2016 Developments of 3D printing microfluidics and applications in chemistry and biology: a review *Electroanalysis* **28** 1658–78
[76] Waldbaur A, Rapp H, Länge K and Rapp B E 2011 Let there be chip—towards rapid prototyping of microfluidic devices: one-step manufacturing processes, *Anal. Methods* **3** 2681–716
[77] Sood A K, Ohdar R and Mahapatra S S 2009 Improving dimensional accuracy of fused deposition modelling processed part using grey Taguchi method *Mater. Des.* **30** 4243–52
[78] Sochol R, Sweet E, Glick C, Venkatesh S, Avetisyan A, Ekman K, Raulinaitis A, Tsai A, Wienkers A and Korner K 2016 3D printed microfluidic circuitry via multijet-based additive manufacturing *Lab Chip* **16** 668–78
[79] Costa P F, Albers H J, Linssen J E, Middelkamp H H, Van Der Hout L, Passier R, Van Den Berg A, Malda J and Van Der Meer A D 2017 Mimicking arterial thrombosis in a 3D-printed microfluidic *in vitro* vascular model based on computed tomography angiography data *Lab Chip* **17** 2785–92
[80] Bhusal A, Dogan E, Nieto D, Mousavi Shaegh S A, Cecen B and Miri A K 2022 3D Bioprinted hydrogel microfluidic devices for parallel drug screening *ACS Appl. Bio Mater.* **5** 4480–92
[81] Knowlton S, Yu C H, Ersoy F, Emadi S, Khademhosseini A and Tasoglu S 2016 3D-printed microfluidic chips with patterned, cell-laden hydrogel constructs *Biofabrication* **8** 025019
[82] Ku X, Zhang Z, Liu X, Chen L and Li G 2018 Low-cost rapid prototyping of glass microfluidic devices using a micromilling technique *Microfluid. Nanofluid.* **22** 1–8
[83] Guckenberger D J, De Groot T E, Wan A M, Beebe D J and Young E W 2015 Micromilling: a method for ultra-rapid prototyping of plastic microfluidic devices *Lab Chip* **15** 2364–78
[84] Aurich J C, Reichenbach I G and Schüler G M 2012 Manufacture and application of ultra-small micro end mills *CIRP Ann.* **61** 83–6
[85] Aramcharoen A, Mativenga P, Yang S, Cooke K and Teer D 2008 Evaluation and selection of hard coatings for micro milling of hardened tool steel *Int. J. Mach. Tools Manuf* **48** 1578–84
[86] Lopes R, Rodrigues R O, Pinho D, Garcia V, Schütte H, Lima R and Gassmann S 2015 Low cost microfluidic device for partial cell separation: micromilling approach *IEEE Int. Conf. on Industrial Technology (ICIT)* (Piscataway, NJ: IEEE) pp 3347–50
[87] Kosoff D, Yu J, Suresh V, Beebe D J and Lang J M 2018 Surface topography and hydrophilicity regulate macrophage phenotype in milled microfluidic systems *Lab Chip* **18** 3011–7

[88] Lin Y-S, Yang C-H, Wang C-Y, Chang F-R, Huang K-S and Hsieh W-C 2012 An aluminum microfluidic chip fabrication using a convenient micromilling process for fluorescent poly (DL-lactide-co-glycolide) microparticle generation *Sensors* **12** 1455–67
[89] Singhal J, Pinho D, Lopes R, Sousa P C, Garcia V, Schütte H, Lima R and Gassmann S 2015 Blood flow visualization and measurements in microfluidic devices fabricated by a micromilling technique *Micro Nanosyst.* **7** 148–53
[90] Wan L, Skoko J, Yu J, Ozdoganlar O, LeDuc P and Neumann C 2017 Mimicking embedded vasculature structure for 3D cancer on a chip approaches through micromilling *Sci. Rep.* **7** 1–8
[91] Chien R-D 2006 Hot embossing of microfluidic platform *Int. Commun. Heat Mass Transfer* **33** 645–53
[92] Mathur A, Roy S, Tweedie M, Mukhopadhyay S, Mitra S and McLaughlin J 2009 Characterisation of PMMA microfluidic channels and devices fabricated by hot embossing and sealed by direct bonding *Curr. Appl Phys.* **9** 1199–202
[93] Yang S and DeVoe D L 2013 Microfluidic device fabrication by thermoplastic hot-embossing *Microfluidic Diagnostics: Methods and Protocols* (Totowa, NJ: Humana Press) pp 115–23
[94] Jeon J S, Chung S, Kamm R D and Charest J L 2011 Hot embossing for fabrication of a microfluidic 3D cell culture platform *Biomed. Microdevices* **13** 325–33
[95] Giboz J, Copponnex T and Mélé P 2007 Microinjection molding of thermoplastic polymers: a review *J. Micromech. Microeng.* **17** R96
[96] Heckele M and Schomburg W 2003 Review on micro molding of thermoplastic polymers *J. Micromech. Microeng.* **14** R1
[97] Scott S M and Ali Z 2021 Fabrication methods for microfluidic devices: an overview *Micromachines* **12** 319
[98] Lee C-Y, Chang C-L, Wang Y-N and Fu L-M 2011 Microfluidic mixing: a review *Int. J. Mol. Sci.* **12** 3263–87
[99] Shi H, Nie K, Dong B, Long M, Xu H and Liu Z 2019 Recent progress of microfluidic reactors for biomedical applications *Chem. Eng. J.* **361** 635–50
[100] Kardous F, Rouleau A, Simon B, Yahiaoui R, Manceau J-F and Boireau W 2010 Improving immunosensor performances using an acoustic mixer on droplet microarray *Biosens. Bioelectron.* **26** 1666–71
[101] Buchegger W, Haller A, van den Driesche S, Kraft M, Lendl B and Vellekoop M 2012 Studying enzymatic bioreactions in a millisecond microfluidic flow mixer *Biomicrofluidics* **6** 012803
[102] Lee H-B, Oh K, Yeo W-H, Lee T-R, Chang Y-S, Choi J-B, Lee K-H, Kramlich J, Riley J J and Kim Y-J 2012 Enhanced bioreaction efficiency of a microfluidic mixer toward high-throughput and low-cost bioassays *Microfluid. Nanofluid.* **12** 143–56
[103] Li Y, Xu Y, Feng X and Liu B-F 2012 A rapid microfluidic mixer for high-viscosity fluids to track ultrafast early folding kinetics of G-quadruplex under molecular crowding conditions *Anal. Chem.* **84** 9025–32
[104] Li Y, Liu C, Feng X, Xu Y and Liu B-F 2014 Ultrafast microfluidic mixer for tracking the early folding kinetics of human telomere G-quadruplex *Anal. Chem.* **86** 4333–9
[105] Li Y, Zhang D, Feng X, Xu Y and Liu B-F 2012 A microsecond microfluidic mixer for characterizing fast biochemical reactions *Talanta* **88** 175–80

[106] Burke K S, Parul D, Reddish M J and Dyer R B 2013 A simple three-dimensional-focusing, continuous-flow mixer for the study of fast protein dynamics *Lab Chip* **13** 2912–21

[107] Jiang L, Zeng Y, Sun Q, Sun Y, Guo Z, Qu J Y and Yao S 2015 Microsecond protein folding events revealed by time-resolved fluorescence resonance energy transfer in a microfluidic mixer *Anal. Chem.* **87** 5589–95

[108] Kennedy M J, Ladouceur H D, Moeller T, Kirui D and Batt C A 2012 Analysis of a laminar-flow diffusional mixer for directed self-assembly of liposomes *Biomicrofluidics* **6** 044119

[109] Lim J-M, Swami A, Gilson L M, Chopra S, Choi S, Wu J, Langer R, Karnik R and Farokhzad O C 2014 Ultra-high throughput synthesis of nanoparticles with homogeneous size distribution using a coaxial turbulent jet mixer *ACS Nano* **8** 6056–65

[110] Maeki M, Saito T, Sato Y, Yasui T, Kaji N, Ishida A, Tani H, Baba Y, Harashima H and Tokeshi M 2015 A strategy for synthesis of lipid nanoparticles using microfluidic devices with a mixer structure *RSC Adv.* **5** 46181–5

[111] Lin Y-H, Wang C-C and Lei K F 2014 Bubble-driven mixer integrated with a microfluidic bead-based ELISA for rapid bladder cancer biomarker detection *Biomed. Microdevices* **16** 199–207

[112] Aeinehvand M M, Ibrahim F, Harun S W, Djordjevic I, Hosseini S, Rothan H A, Yusof R and Madou M J 2015 Biosensing enhancement of dengue virus using microballoon mixers on centrifugal microfluidic platforms *Biosens. Bioelectron.* **67** 424–30

[113] Tian F, Cai L, Liu C and Sun J 2022 Microfluidic technologies for nanoparticle formation *Lab Chip* **22** 512–29

[114] Rhee M, Valencia P M, Rodriguez M I, Langer R, Farokhzad O C and Karnik R 2011 Synthesis of size-tunable polymeric nanoparticles enabled by 3D hydrodynamic flow focusing in single-layer microchannels *Adv. Mater.* **23** H79–83

[115] Stroock A D, Dertinger S K, Ajdari A, Mezic I, Stone H A and Whitesides G M 2002 Chaotic mixer for microchannels *Science* **295** 647–51

[116] Jahn A, Stavis S M, Hong J S, Vreeland W N, DeVoe D L and Gaitan M 2010 Microfluidic mixing and the formation of nanoscale lipid vesicles *ACS Nano* **4** 2077–87

[117] Liu D, Cito S, Zhang Y, Wang C F, Sikanen T M and Santos H A 2015 A versatile and robust microfluidic platform toward high throughput synthesis of homogeneous nanoparticles with tunable properties *Adv. Mater.* **27** 2298–304

[118] Zhigaltsev I V, Belliveau N, Hafez I, Leung A K K, Huft J, Hansen C and Cullis P R 2012 Bottom-up design and synthesis of limit size lipid nanoparticle systems with aqueous and triglyceride cores using millisecond microfluidic mixing *Langmuir* **28** 3633–40

[119] Kim Y, Lee Chung B, Ma M, Mulder W J M, Fayad Z A, Farokhzad O C and Langer R 2012 Mass production and size control of lipid–polymer hybrid nanoparticles through controlled microvortices *Nano Lett.* **12** 3587–91

[120] Therriault D, White S R and Lewis J A 2003 Chaotic mixing in three-dimensional microvascular networks fabricated by direct-write assembly *Nat. Mater.* **2** 265–71

[121] Squires T M and Quake S R 2005 Microfluidics: fluid physics at the nanoliter scale *Rev. Mod. Phys.* **77** 977

[122] Sun J *et al* 2018 Control over the emerging chirality in supramolecular gels and solutions by chiral microvortices in milliseconds *Nat. Commun.* **9** 2599

[123] Ahmed H, Ramesan S, Lee L, Rezk A R and Yeo L Y 2020 On-chip generation of vortical flows for microfluidic centrifugation *Small* **16** 1903605

[124] Javadi A, Eggers J, Bonn D, Habibi M and Ribe N 2013 Delayed capillary breakup of falling viscous jets *Phys. Rev. Lett.* **110** 144501

[125] Dewandre A, Rivero-Rodriguez J, Vitry Y, Sobac B and Scheid B 2020 Microfluidic droplet generation based on non-embedded co-flow-focusing using 3D printed nozzle *Sci. Rep.* **10** 21616

[126] Guerrero J, Chang Y W, Fragkopoulos A A and Fernandez-Nieves A 2020 Capillary-based microfluidics—coflow, flow-focusing, electro-coflow, drops, jets, and instabilities *Small* **16** 1904344

[127] Utada A S, Fernandez-Nieves A, Gordillo J M and Weitz D A 2008 Absolute instability of a liquid jet in a coflowing stream *Phys. Rev. Lett.* **100** 014502

[128] Gultekinoglu M, Jiang X, Bayram C, Ulubayram K and Edirisinghe M 2018 Honeycomb-like PLGA-b-PEG structure creation with T-Junction microdroplets *Langmuir* **34** 7989–97

[129] Duraiswamy S and Khan S A 2009 Droplet-based microfluidic synthesis of anisotropic metal nanocrystals *Small* **5** 2828–34

[130] Niculescu A-G, Mihaiescu D E and Grumezescu A M 2022 A review of microfluidic experimental designs for nanoparticle synthesis *Int. J. Mol. Sci.* **23** 8293

[131] Christopher G F and Anna S L 2007 Microfluidic methods for generating continuous droplet streams *J. Phys.* D **40** R319

[132] Hung L-H, Teh S-Y, Jester J and Lee A P 2010 PLGA micro/nanosphere synthesis by droplet microfluidic solvent evaporation and extraction approaches *Lab Chip* **10** 1820–5

[133] Shang L, Cheng Y and Zhao Y 2017 Emerging droplet microfluidics *Chem. Rev.* **117** 7964–8040

[134] Xuan X, Zhu J and Church C 2010 Particle focusing in microfluidic devices *Microfluid. Nanofluid.* **9** 1–16

[135] Rajawat A and Tripathi S 2020 Disease diagnostics using hydrodynamic flow focusing in microfluidic devices: beyond flow cytometry *Biomed. Eng. Lett.* **10** 241–57

[136] Lu M, Ozcelik A, Grigsby C L, Zhao Y, Guo F, Leong K W and Huang T J 2016 Microfluidic hydrodynamic focusing for synthesis of nanomaterials *Nano Today* **11** 778–92

[137] Gañán-Calvo A, Montanero J, Martín-Banderas L and Flores-Mosquera M 2013 Building functional materials for health care and pharmacy from microfluidic principles and flow focusing *Adv. Drug Delivery Rev.* **65** 1447–69

[138] Yang R-J, Fu L-M and Hou H-H 2018 Review and perspectives on microfluidic flow cytometers *Sensors Actuators* B **266** 26–45

[139] Wang H, Liu H, Liu H, Su W, Chen W and Qin J 2019 One-step generation of core–shell gelatin methacrylate (GelMA) microgels using a droplet microfluidic system *Adv. Mater. Technol.* **4** 1800632

[140] Koryakina I G, Afonicheva P K, Arabuli K V, Evstrapov A A, Timin A S and Zyuzin M V 2021 Microfluidic synthesis of optically responsive materials for nano-and biophotonics *Adv. Colloid Interface Sci.* **298** 102548

[141] Mogensen K B and Kutter J P 2009 Optical detection in microfluidic systems *Electrophoresis* **30** S92–S100

[142] Myers F B and Lee L P 2008 Innovations in optical microfluidic technologies for point-of-care diagnostics *Lab Chip* **8** 2015–31

[143] Fan X and White I M 2011 Optofluidic microsystems for chemical and biological analysis *Nat. Photonics* **5** 591–7

[144] Gao Y, Wu M, Lin Y and Xu J 2020 Acoustic microfluidic separation techniques and bioapplications: a review *Micromachines* **11** 921
[145] Wang S, Huang X and Yang C 2012 Microfluidic bubble generation by acoustic field for mixing enhancement *J. Heat Transfer* **134** 051014
[146] Wiklund M 2012 Acoustofluidics 12: biocompatibility and cell viability in microfluidic acoustic resonators *Lab Chip* **12** 2018–28
[147] Reboud J, Bourquin Y, Wilson R, Pall G S, Jiwaji M, Pitt A R, Graham A, Waters A P and Cooper J M 2012 Shaping acoustic fields as a toolset for microfluidic manipulations in diagnostic technologies *Proc. Natl Acad. Sci.* **109** 15162–7
[148] Lenshof A, Evander M, Laurell T and Nilsson J 2012 Acoustofluidics 5: building microfluidic acoustic resonators *Lab Chip* **12** 684–95
[149] Wu J, Cao W, Wen W, Chang D C and Sheng P 2009 Polydimethylsiloxane microfluidic chip with integrated microheater and thermal sensor *Biomicrofluidics* **3** 012005
[150] Kopparthy V L, Tangutooru S M, Nestorova G G and Guilbeau E J 2012 Thermoelectric microfluidic sensor for bio-chemical applications *Sensors Actuators* B **166** 608–15
[151] Nestorova G G, Kopparthy V L, Crews N D and Guilbeau E J 2015 Thermoelectric lab-on-a-chip ELISA *Anal. Methods* **7** 2055–63
[152] Shin J H, Seo J, Hong J and Chung S K 2017 Hybrid optothermal and acoustic manipulations of microbubbles for precise and on-demand handling of micro-objects *Sensors Actuators* B **246** 415–20
[153] Kopparthy V L, Tangutooru S M and Guilbeau E J 2015 Label free detection of L-glutamate using microfluidic based thermal biosensor *Bioengineering* **2** 2–14
[154] Hossan M R, Dutta D, Islam N and Dutta P 2018 Electric field driven pumping in microfluidic device *Electrophoresis* **39** 702–31
[155] Link D R, Grasland-Mongrain E, Duri A, Sarrazin F, Cheng Z, Cristobal G, Marquez M and Weitz D A 2006 Electric control of droplets in microfluidic devices *Angew. Chem. Int. Ed.* **45** 2556–60
[156] Grant K M, Hemmert J W and White H S 2002 Magnetic field-controlled microfluidic transport *J. Am. Chem. Soc.* **124** 462–7
[157] Cao Q, Han X and Li L 2014 Configurations and control of magnetic fields for manipulating magnetic particles in microfluidic applications: magnet systems and manipulation mechanisms *Lab Chip* **14** 2762–77
[158] Keller M W, Glasheen W and Kaul S 1989 Albunex: a safe and effective commercially produced agent for myocardial contrast echocardiography *J. Am. Soc. Echocardiogr.* **2** 48–52
[159] Stride E and Edirisinghe M 2008 Novel microbubble preparation technologies *Soft Matter* **4** 2350–9
[160] Li Y, Liu X, Huang Q, Ohta A T and Arai T 2021 Bubbles in microfluidics: an all-purpose tool for micromanipulation *Lab Chip* **21** 1016–35
[161] Zhou Y, Kang P, Huang Z, Yan P, Sun J, Wang J and Yang Y 2020 Experimental measurement and theoretical analysis on bubble dynamic behaviors in a gas-liquid bubble column *Chem. Eng. Sci.* **211** 115295
[162] Whitesides G M 2006 The origins and the future of microfluidics *Nature* **442** 368–73
[163] Lin H, Chen J and Chen C 2016 A novel technology: microfluidic devices for microbubble ultrasound contrast agent generation *Med. Biol. Eng. Comput.* **54** 1317–30

[164] Bayram C, Jiang X, Gultekinoglu M, Ozturk S, Ulubayram K and Edirisinghe M 2019 Biofabrication of gelatin tissue scaffolds with uniform pore size via microbubble assembly *Macromol. Mater. Eng.* **304** 1900394
[165] Huang D, Zhang X, Zhao C, Fu X, Zhang W, Kong W, Zhang B and Zhao Y 2021 Ultrasound-responsive microfluidic microbubbles for combination tumor treatment *Adv. Therap.* **4** 2100050
[166] Gartshore A, Kidd M and Joshi L T 2021 Applications of microwave energy in medicine *Biosensors* **11** 96
[167] Decadt B and Siriwardena A K 2004 Radiofrequency ablation of liver tumours: systematic review *Lancet Oncol.* **5** 550–60
[168] Elsayed M, Kothandaraman A, Edirisinghe M and Huang J 2016 Porous polymeric films from microbubbles generated using a T-junction microfluidic device *Langmuir* **32** 13377–85
[169] Parhizkar M, Edirisinghe M and Stride E 2013 Effect of operating conditions and liquid physical properties on the size of monodisperse microbubbles produced in a capillary embedded T-junction device *Microfluid. Nanofluid.* **14** 797–808
[170] Elsayed M, Huang J and Edirisinghe M 2015 Bioinspired preparation of alginate nanoparticles using microbubble bursting *Mater. Sci. Eng.* C **46** 132–9
[171] Reinke N, Vossnacke A, Schütz W, Koch M and Unger H 2001 Aerosol generation by bubble collapse at ocean surfaces *Water Air Soil Pollut: Focus* **1** 333–40
[172] Cesur S, Cam M E, Sayın F S, Su S, Harker A, Edirisinghe M and Gunduz O 2021 Metformin-loaded polymer-based microbubbles/nanoparticles generated for the treatment of type 2 diabetes mellitus *Langmuir* **38** 5040–51
[173] Gnyawali V, Moon B-U, Kieda J, Karshafian R, Kolios M C, Tsai S S and Honey 2017 I shrunk the bubbles: microfluidic vacuum shrinkage of lipid-stabilized microbubbles *Soft Matter* **13** 4011–6
[174] Zalloum I O, Paknahad A A, Kolios M C, Karshafian R and Tsai S S 2022 Controlled shrinkage of microfluidically generated microbubbles by tuning lipid concentration *Langmuir* **38** 13021–9
[175] Hettiarachchi K, Talu E, Longo M L, Dayton P A and Lee A P 2007 On-chip generation of microbubbles as a practical technology for manufacturing contrast agents for ultrasonic imaging *Lab Chip* **7** 463–8
[176] Khan A H *et al* 2020 Effectiveness of oil-layered albumin microbubbles produced using microfluidic t-junctions in series for *in vitro* inhibition of tumor cells *Langmuir* **36** 11429–41
[177] Wu B *et al* 2022 Generating lifetime-enhanced microbubbles by decorating shells with silicon quantum nano-dots using a 3-series t-junction microfluidic device *Langmuir* **38** 10917–33
[178] Ghamkhari A, Tafti H A, Rabbani S, Ghorbani M, Ghiass M A, Akbarzadeh F and Abbasi F 2023 Ultrasound-triggered microbubbles: novel targeted core–shell for the treatment of myocardial infarction disease *ACS Omega* **8** 11335–50
[179] Valencia P M, Farokhzad O C, Karnik R and Langer R 2012 Microfluidic technologies for accelerating the clinical translation of nanoparticles *Nat. Nanotechnol.* **7** 623–9
[180] Xu S, Nie Z, Seo M, Lewis P, Kumacheva E, Stone H A, Garstecki P, Weibel D B, Gitlin I and Whitesides G M 2005 Generation of monodisperse particles by using microfluidics: control over size, shape, and composition *Angew. Chem.* **117** 734–8
[181] Shepherd S J, Issadore D and Mitchell M J 2021 Microfluidic formulation of nanoparticles for biomedical applications *Biomaterials* **274** 120826

[182] Karnik R, Gu F, Basto P, Cannizzaro C, Dean L, Kyei-Manu W, Langer R and Farokhzad O C 2008 Microfluidic platform for controlled synthesis of polymeric nanoparticles *Nano Lett.* **8** 2906–12
[183] Gultekinoglu M, Jiang X, Bayram C, Wu H, Ulubayram K and Edirisinghe M 2020 Self-assembled micro-stripe patterning of sessile polymeric nanofluid droplets *J. Colloid Interface Sci.* **561** 470–80
[184] Känkänen V, Fernandes M, Liu Z, Seitsonen J, Hirvonen S-P, Ruokolainen J, Pinto J F, Hirvonen J, Balasubramanian V and Santos H A 2023 Microfluidic preparation and optimization of sorafenib-loaded poly (ethylene glycol-block-caprolactone) nanoparticles for cancer therapy applications *J. Colloid Interface Sci.* **633** 383–95
[185] Satta S, Shahabipour F, Gao W, Lentz S R, Perlman S, Ashammakhi N and Hsiai T 2022 Engineering viral genomics and nano-liposomes in microfluidic platforms for patient-specific analysis of SARS-CoV-2 variants *Theranostics* **12** 4779
[186] Gregoriadis G 2021 Liposomes and mRNA: two technologies together create a COVID-19 vaccine *Med. Drug Discov.* **12** 100104
[187] Wilson B and Geetha K M 2022 Lipid nanoparticles in the development of mRNA vaccines for COVID-19 *J. Drug Deliv. Sci. Technol.* **74** 103553
[188] Khorshid S, Montanari M, Benedetti S, Moroni S, Aluigi A, Canonico B, Papa S, Tiboni M and Casettari L 2022 A microfluidic approach to fabricate sucrose decorated liposomes with increased uptake in breast cancer cells *Eur. J. Pharm. Biopharm.* **178** 53–64
[189] Jaradat E, Weaver E, Meziane A and Lamprou D A 2022 Microfluidic paclitaxel-loaded lipid nanoparticle formulations for chemotherapy *Int. J. Pharm.* **628** 122320
[190] Bressan L P, Robles-Najar J, Adamo C B, Quero R F, Costa B M, de Jesus D P and da Silva J A 2019 3D-printed microfluidic device for the synthesis of silver and gold nanoparticles *Microchem. J.* **146** 1083–9
[191] Mahdavi Z, Rezvani H and Moraveji M K 2020 Core–shell nanoparticles used in drug delivery-microfluidics: a review, *RSC Adv.* **10** 18280–95
[192] Kashani S Y, Afzalian A, Shirinichi F and Moraveji M K 2021 Microfluidics for core–shell drug carrier particles–a review *RSC Adv.* **11** 229–49
[193] Liu D, Zhang H, Fontana F, Hirvonen J T and Santos H A 2017 Microfluidic-assisted fabrication of carriers for controlled drug delivery *Lab Chip* **17** 1856–83
[194] Hasani-Sadrabadi M M, Taranejoo S, Dashtimoghadam E, Bahlakeh G, Majedi F S, VanDersarl J J, Janmaleki M, Sharifi F, Bertsch A and Hourigan K 2016 Microfluidic manipulation of core/shell nanoparticles for oral delivery of chemotherapeutics: a new treatment approach for colorectal cancer *Adv. Mater.* **28** 4134–41
[195] Windbergs M, Zhao Y, Heyman J and Weitz D A 2013 Biodegradable core–shell carriers for simultaneous encapsulation of synergistic actives *J. Am. Chem. Soc.* **135** 7933–7
[196] Caen O, Lu H, Nizard P and Taly V 2017 Microfluidics as a strategic player to decipher single-cell omics? *Trends Biotechnol.* **35** 713–27
[197] Geng S and Huang Y 2018 From mouth pipetting to microfluidics: the evolution of technologies for picking healthy single cells *Adv. Biosyst.* **2** 1800099
[198] Li H and Humphreys B D 2021 Single cell technologies: beyond microfluidics *Kidney 360* **7** 1196–204
[199] Lamanna J *et al* 2020 Digital microfluidic isolation of single cells for-omics *Nat. Commun.* **11** 5632

[200] Xu X, Wang J, Wu L, Guo J, Song Y, Tian T, Wang W, Zhu Z and Yang C 2020 Microfluidic single-cell omics analysis *Small* **16** e1903905

[201] Robbins P D and Ghivizzani S C 1998 Viral vectors for gene therapy *Pharmacol. Therap.* **80** 35–47

[202] Yin H, Kanasty R L, Eltoukhy A A, Vegas A J, Dorkin J R and Anderson D G 2014 Non-viral vectors for gene-based therapy *Nat. Rev. Genet.* **15** 541–55

[203] Lissandrello C A, Santos J A, Hsi P, Welch M, Mott V L, Kim E S, Chesin J, Haroutunian N J, Stoddard A G and Czarnecki A 2020 High-throughput continuous-flow microfluidic electroporation of mRNA into primary human T cells for applications in cellular therapy manufacturing *Sci. Rep.* **10** 18045

[204] Valero A, Post J N, van Nieuwkasteele J W, ter Braak P M, Kruijer W and van den Berg A 2008 Gene transfer and protein dynamics in stem cells using single cell electroporation in a microfluidic device *Lab Chip* **8** 62–7

[205] Han X, Liu Z, Ma Y, Zhang K and Qin L 2017 Cas9 ribonucleoprotein delivery via microfluidic cell-deformation chip for human T-cell genome editing and immunotherapy *Adv. Biosyst.* **1** 1600007

[206] Kim J, Hwang I, Britain D, Chung T D, Sun Y and Kim D-H 2011 Microfluidic approaches for gene delivery and gene therapy *Lab Chip* **11** 3941–8

[207] Vicente F A, Plazl I, Ventura S P and Žnidaršič-Plazl P 2020 Separation and purification of biomacromolecules based on microfluidics *Green Chem.* **22** 4391–410

[208] Rathnayaka C, Amarasekara C A, Akabirov K, Murphy M C, Park S, Witek M A and Soper S A 2022 Nanofluidic devices for the separation of biomolecules *J. Chromatogr.* A **1683** 463539

[209] Rodríguez-Ruiz I, Babenko V, Martínez-Rodríguez S and Gavira J 2018 Protein separation under a microfluidic regime *Analyst* **143** 606–19

[210] Wang J, Ma P, Kim D H, Liu B-F and Demirci U 2021 Towards microfluidic-based exosome isolation and detection for tumor therapy *Nano Today* **37** 101066

[211] Wu Z, Willing B, Bjerketorp J, Jansson J K and Hjort K 2009 Soft inertial microfluidics for high throughput separation of bacteria from human blood cells *Lab Chip* **9** 1193–9

[212] Zhao Z, Yang Y, Zeng Y and He M 2016 A microfluidic ExoSearch chip for multiplexed exosome detection towards blood-based ovarian cancer diagnosis *Lab Chip* **16** 489–96

[213] He Y, Wu Y, Fu J-Z and Wu W-B 2015 Fabrication of paper-based microfluidic analysis devices: a review *RSC Adv.* **5** 78109–27

[214] Li X, Ballerini D R and Shen W 2012 A perspective on paper-based microfluidics: current status and future trends *Biomicrofluidics* **6** 011301

[215] Vera-Estrada I L *et al* 2022 Digital pregnancy test powered by an air-breathing paper-based microfluidic fuel cell stack using human urine as fuel *Sensors* **22** 6641

[216] Gabriel E F M, Garcia P T, Lopes F M and Coltro W K T 2017 Paper-based colorimetric biosensor for tear glucose measurements *Micromachines* **8** 104

[217] Duan S *et al* 2023 Deep learning-assisted ultra-accurate smartphone testing of paper-based colorimetric ELISA assays *Anal. Chim. Acta* **1248** 340868

[218] Farahinia A, Zhang W and Badea I 2021 Novel microfluidic approaches to circulating tumor cell separation and sorting of blood cells: A review *J. Sci.: Adv. Mater. Devices* **6** 303–20

[219] Huang D, Man J, Jiang D, Zhao J and Xiang N 2020 Inertial microfluidics: recent advances *Electrophoresis* **41** 2166–87

[220] Wang J, Lu W, Tang C, Liu Y, Sun J, Mu X, Zhang L, Dai B, Li X and Zhuo H 2015 Label-free isolation and mRNA detection of circulating tumor cells from patients with metastatic lung cancer for disease diagnosis and monitoring therapeutic efficacy *Anal. Chem.* **87** 11893–900

[221] Lee M G, Shin J H, Bae C Y, Choi S and Park J-K 2013 Label-free cancer cell separation from human whole blood using inertial microfluidics at low shear stress *Anal. Chem.* **85** 6213–8

[222] Zhou J, Giridhar P V, Kasper S and Papautsky I 2013 Modulation of aspect ratio for complete separation in an inertial microfluidic channel *Lab Chip* **13** 1919–29

[223] Nasiri R, Shamloo A and Akbari J 2022 Design of two inertial-based microfluidic devices for cancer cell separation from blood: a serpentine inertial device and an integrated inertial and magnetophoretic device *Chem. Eng. Sci.* **252** 117283

[224] Shields IV C W, Reyes C D and López G P 2015 Microfluidic cell sorting: a review of the advances in the separation of cells from debulking to rare cell isolation *Lab Chip* **15** 1230–49

[225] Doh I and Cho Y-H 2005 A continuous cell separation chip using hydrodynamic dielectrophoresis (DEP) process *Sensors Actuators* A **121** 59–65

[226] Hoshino K, Huang Y-Y, Lane N, Huebschman M, Uhr J W, Frenkel E P and Zhang X 2011 Microchip-based immunomagnetic detection of circulating tumor cells *Lab Chip* **11** 3449–57

Chapter 3

Electrohydrodynamic manufacturing

Electrohydrodynamic systems are an important method for producing fibres and particles using the combination of an electric field with a fluid flow. The applied electric field, flow rate, solution–collector distance, and solution properties allow fibres and particles to be produced from the microscale to the nanoscale. The produced particles and fibres have a wide range of applications. Particles are frequently used as drug delivery vehicles, while fibres have a wide application potential ranging from filtration materials to wound dressings and scaffolds. This chapter discusses electrohydrodynamics (EHD) thoroughly and describes how its products are being used to create the next generation of biomaterials.

3.1 The principles of electrohydrodynamics

EHD is a field of physics and engineering that examines the behaviour of electrically charged fluids under the influence of electric fields (figure 3.1) [1–3]. EHD has been used in many studies across a range of fields, including materials science, biology, and engineering, for several years. This technology, which has been used in many state-of-the-art studies in recent years, has received significant attention due to its ability to control fluid motion using electric fields, which provides new possibilities for the fabrication of advanced materials and devices.

The history of EHD technology began when researchers first observed the effects of electric fields on fluid motion. In the early 20th century, Lord Rayleigh [4, 5] and Sir Geoffrey Ingram Taylor [6, 7], who were the pioneers in this field, first described the instability of a charged liquid jet and studied the behaviour of charged droplets. These pioneers paved the way for different types of research into EHD, which led to significant advances in our understanding of fluid behaviour under electric fields.

Taylor first described the Taylor Cone in 1964, which is a very important principle in EHD. The Taylor cone can be characterised as a cone-shaped projection formed at the tip of a liquid droplet or jet when a high electric field is applied [8, 9].

doi:10.1088/978-0-7503-5187-4ch3

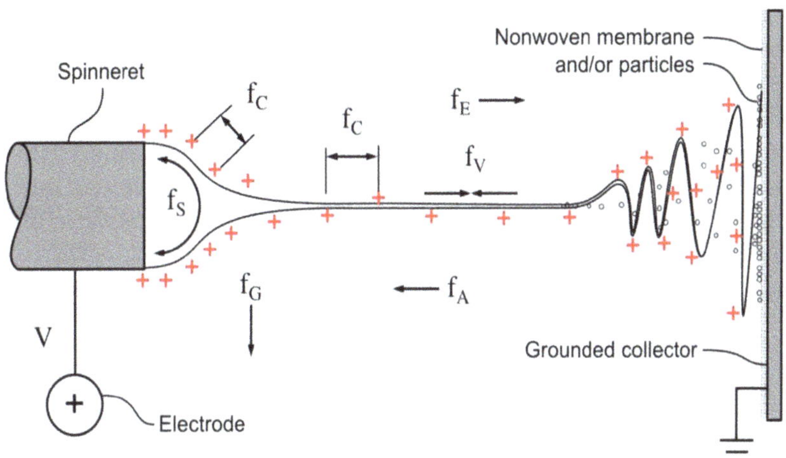

Figure 3.1. A schematic illustration of the electrospinning setup and the mechanism of reaction between the electrode-connected spinneret and the grounded collector. The abbreviations are defined as follows: coulombic (f_C), electric field (f_E), viscoelastic (f_V), surface tension (f_S), air drag (f_A), and gravitational (f_G) forces. Reprinted from [3], Copyright (2019), with permission from Elsevier.

According to EHD, applying a potential difference between the surface of the liquid and an electrode creates an electric field that can cause a cone-shaped protrusion at the apex of the liquid. If this electric field is strong enough, the liquid can be drawn out of the cone in the form of a fine jet or a series of droplets. The shape and stability of the Taylor cone are affected by various factors, such as the properties of the liquid or solution, solution flow rate, the electric field strength, and the environment. The Taylor cone is used in many applications such as electrospinning and electrospraying.

Over the years, EHD has expanded to include a spectrum of applications in the manufacture of nanomaterials, drug delivery systems [10, 11], flexible sensors [12–15], and in many fields of biomedical engineering research. EHD technology depends on principles such as fluid dynamics and electric fields. These principles of EHD are summarised in the following sections.

3.1.1 Fluid dynamics in EHD

Fluid dynamics plays an important role in EHD principles, as it describes the behaviour of fluids in the presence of an electric field. The Reynolds number is a key concept in fluid dynamics; it is a dimensionless parameter that characterises the relative importance of inertial forces (associated with the fluid's mass and velocity) versus viscous forces (associated with the fluid's resistance to deformation) [16, 17].

The influence of fluid dynamics on EHD is evident in the behaviour of fluids under electric fields, which can cause changes in fluid velocity and viscosity [18]. By understanding the Reynolds number and other principles of fluid dynamics, engineers can design optimised EHD systems for specific applications. In comparison to microfluidic devices, in which fluid volumes are small and the Reynolds number is low, laminar flow is often preferred because it allows for precise control of fluid motion [19, 20].

Electrostatics, which involves the study of stationary electric fields, is also a crucial aspect of fluid dynamics in EHD. Managing fluid behaviour using EHD involves understanding how electrostatics can be used to move a fluid in a certain direction [21, 22]. Electrostatics can also be used to produce electrohydrodynamic flow, in which an electric field is applied to a fluid (figure 3.2) [3]. These flows are characterised by small length scales, high velocities, and low Reynolds numbers [23].

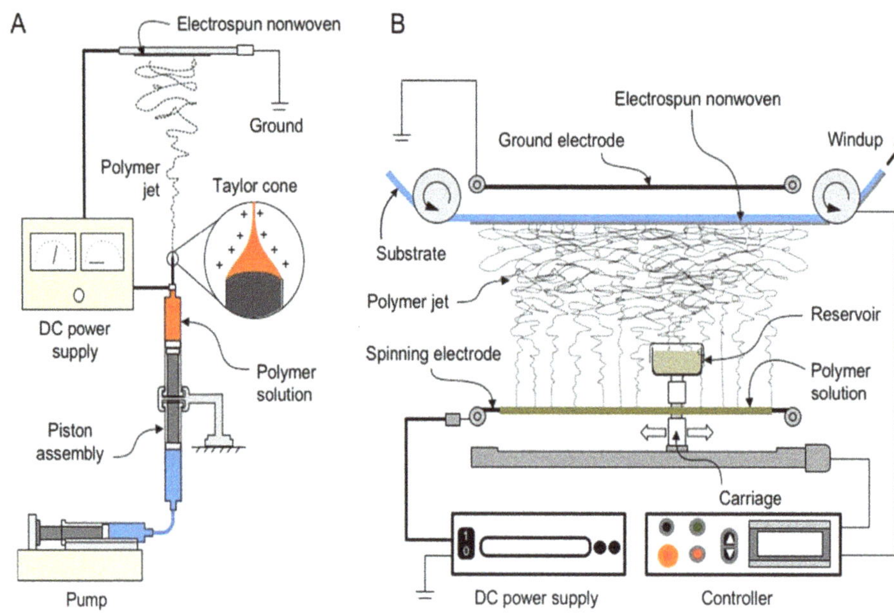

Figure 3.2. A representative illustration of an electrospinning setup: (A) Taylor cone and nonwoven fibre formation, (B) complex setup and nonwoven fibre formation. Reprinted from [3], Copyright (2019), with permission from Elsevier.

Magnetohydrodynamics is a part of fluid dynamics in EHD. It is the study of the behaviour of electrically conducting fluids in the presence of magnetic fields [24–26]. In EHD, magnetohydrodynamics can be used to control fluid flow accurately. Flow regulation can be achieved by placing a fluid in a magnetic field. This technique has applications in microfluidic mixers and fluid pumps [24]. These pumps have no moving parts, making them perfect for use in lab-on-a-chip and microfluidic systems. They are suitable for a variety of applications due to their simple integration into micro-electromechanical systems (MEMs) [27].

3.1.2 Electric field in EHD systems

Electric fields play a vital role in EHD systems; the movement of fluids can be regulated by changing the intensity and distribution of the electric field.

Understanding electric field dynamics in EHD systems is essential for designing and improving EHD devices and processes.

Surface charges are one of the key elements of the dynamics of an electric field. When a liquid is exposed to an electric field, charges may accumulate on its surface. These charges then interact with the electric field, causing the liquid to flow. The distribution of surface charges can impact the intensity and direction of fluid flow. In addition, fluid polarisation resulting from the electric field can affect both the electric field strength and the fluid's response to it.

In the context of EHD, the Navier–Stokes equations (equation (3.1)) are used to model the behaviour of a fluids under the influence of electric fields [28, 29].

In their most general form, the Navier–Stokes equations are expressed as:

$$\rho(\partial v/\partial t + (v.\ \nabla)v) = -\nabla p + \mu\nabla\hat{}2v\ +\ f \tag{3.1}$$

Here, ρ is the density of the fluid, v is the velocity vector, p is the pressure, μ is the dynamic viscosity of the fluid, and f represents the electric fields. The term $(\partial v/\partial t + (v.\nabla)\ v)$ represents the acceleration of the fluid, which is a function of both the velocity and the rate of change of the velocity.

In EHD, the Navier–Stokes equations are commonly used together with the Maxwell equations that describe the behaviour of electric fields [25, 29, 30]. The two sets of equations are coupled through the use of the Lorentz force, which represents the force exerted on the fluid by the electric field (equation (3.2)). The Lorentz force is defined by:

$$f = \rho E + J \times B \tag{3.2}$$

where E is the electric field, J is the current density, B is the magnetic field, and X represents the cross product.

Engineers can develop mathematical models that predict the behaviour of fluids under the influence of electric fields by combining the Navier–Stokes equations with the Maxwell equations and the Lorentz force. These models can be used to design and optimise electrohydrodynamic systems for a wide range of applications, from microfluidic devices to industrial-scale electrostatic precipitators [23].

3.2 Material properties used in EHD

EHD is a field of study that investigates the interactions between electric fields and fluid flow. The material properties of a fluid can significantly impact its behaviour under these conditions, making it essential to understand the properties of fluids used in EHD applications.

3.2.1 Viscosity

In EHD experiments, viscosity is an important material property, as it affects the flow behaviour of the fluid when affected by an electric field.

The electric field in EHD exerts a force on charged particles within the solution, causing them to move and create a flow. This flow can be either a jet or a spray, depending on the experimental setup. The viscosity of the solution affects the magnitude of the forces acting on the charged particles, ultimately influencing fluid motion.

Usually, a higher solution viscosity leads to slower fluid motion, requiring additional force to move the fluid [31]. As a result, higher viscosity can lead to a thicker and more stable jet, as the fluid is less prone to breaking up into smaller droplets. However, higher-viscosity solutions may cause increased clogging and blockages in the experimental setup, negatively impacting the overall performance of the EHD system [32]. Therefore, when designing an EHD experiment, it is critical to consider the viscosity of the solution being used and the potential effects on the resulting fluid motion and system performance.

The formation of a stable Taylor cone during electrospraying is heavily influenced by the viscosity of the solution used. If the viscosity is too low, the surface tension and viscoelasticity are not strong enough to counteract the forces of gravity and electrostatic attraction, leading to dripping instead of the formation of a cone jet [33]. Conversely, high-viscosity solutions are unable to facilitate a stable Taylor cone, as the drying of polymeric particles through solvent evaporation blocks the capillary tip. Therefore, it is necessary to use solutions with a specific range of viscosity values (typically from 1.5 to 5500 mPa·s) to achieve a cone jet during electrospraying [34].

Ku *et al* presented their experimental findings on the electrospraying parameters of highly viscous solutions [35]. The behaviour of NaI-doped glycerol solutions was investigated under varying electrical fields, with a particular focus on the size distributions of droplets emitted by the Taylor cone. The study found that due to the low volatility of the glycerol solutions, the size distribution of unnaturalised glycerol electrosprayed products ranged between 0.3 and 1.2 μm. In addition, the study found that manipulation of the liquid flow rate could lead highly viscous liquids to produce monodisperse droplets that ranged between 0.3 and 0.44 μm in diameter. These findings have significant implications for the development of precise and controlled electrospraying techniques, particularly in the fields of materials science and drug delivery systems.

3.2.2 Dielectric properties

The dielectric properties of a fluid are critical in EHD, as they determine how the fluid responds to an applied electric field. The dielectric properties of a material describe its ability to store and transmit electrical charge and energy; they include parameters such as permittivity and conductivity [36, 37].

One of the most important effects of dielectric properties on EHD is the strength of the electric field [38, 39]. The strength of the electric field depends on the permittivity of the medium surrounding the charged particles, which affects the extent to which the electric field is distorted or screened by the surrounding material [40]. Higher-permittivity materials (i.e. those that can store more electric charge) cause the electric field to be screened more effectively, which reduces the strength of the electric field and can result in weaker EHD effects [41].

In addition, the conductivity of the material can also affect its electrohydrodynamic behaviour. Conductive materials can transfer electrical charge more easily, which can lead to increased current flow and more pronounced EHD effects. However, high conductivity can also lead to undesired effects such as Joule heating, which can heat the fluid and cause it to break down or evaporate [42].

Another important factor to consider is the dielectric breakdown strength, which is the maximum electric field that a material can withstand before breaking down and becoming conductive itself [43]. This can be an important consideration in EHD systems, particularly those that involve high electric fields or high voltages.

3.2.3 Solvent evaporation kinetics

In EHD, it is important to consider the evaporation kinetics of solvents, as they can significantly impact the properties of the fluid and the resulting EHD behaviour. Solvent evaporation kinetics refers to the rate at which the solvent in a solution evaporates; it can be influenced by factors such as temperature, humidity, and the properties of the solvent itself.

The rate of solvent evaporation can affect the size and morphology of the resulting droplets or particles in an EHD system. If the solvent evaporates too quickly, droplets or particles may not have enough time to fully form and solidify, leading to smaller or more irregular particles. On the other hand, if the solvent evaporates too slowly, the droplets or particles may become too large or coalesce, leading to a less uniform particle size distribution.

The solvent vapour pressure is a key factor in determining the rate of evaporation and drying time [44]. By influencing the phase separation process, solvent volatility plays a significant role in the development of nanostructures [41]. Decreases in jet width and velocity may be caused when high-vapour-pressure solvents start to evaporate [45]. For instance, tetrahydrofuran/dimethylformamide/polystyrene (PS) fibres spun using various solvent combinations produced micro- and nanostructure morphologies at higher solvent volatilities and a greatly increased size at lower solvent volatilities [41].

In addition to affecting the particle size and morphology, solvent evaporation kinetics can also affect the overall stability of the EHD system. Rapid solvent evaporation can lead to instabilities in the electric field or the fluid flow, which can result in less stable and more variable system performance. This can be particularly problematic in EHD systems that require a high degree of precision or control.

3.2.4 Shear stress

Shear stress is a crucial factor in EHD, as it can affect the stability and flow behaviour of the fluid as well as the resulting patterns and structures formed under the influence of the electric field [46]. Shear stress refers to the force exerted on a fluid by parallel or tangential flow and is typically quantified by the viscosity of the fluid [47].

One of the key effects of shear stress on EHD is the deformation and stretching of the charged fluid or particles [48]. Shear force can cause the particles to elongate or align in the direction of flow, which can affect their motion in the electric field. This can be particularly important in applications such as electrospraying or electrospinning, in which the size and morphology of the resulting droplets or fibres can be influenced by the shear stress [49]. In addition to affecting particle morphology, shear stress can also affect the stability of the EHD system [50, 51]. High shear forces can lead to instabilities in the electric field or the fluid flow, which can result in less stability and more variability in product formation [52]. This can be particularly problematic in EHD systems that require a high degree of precision or control.

The effect of shear stress on EHD can be quantified using various theoretical and experimental techniques [53, 54], including rheological measurements and particle tracking methods. By understanding the influence of shear stress on EHD, it is possible to optimise the design and operation of EHD systems for a variety of applications. In table 3.1, the parameter-dependent effects for electrospinning are examined in detail [55].

Table 3.1. Parameter-dependent effects in the electrospinning technique [55]. John Wiley & Sons. [2020].

Parameter	Effect
Working distance	Decreasing the distance beyond a critical point → thicker fibres and morphological defects. Increasing the distance → thinner fibres; but may lead to increased coronal discharge and Rayleigh instability, resulting in beaded or fused fibre defects beyond a critical distance.
Voltage	Must exceed critical voltage, V_K, to overcome the surface tension of the polymer solution and maintain a jet. Increased voltage → decreased flight time, increased fibre diameter; above a critical point, increased voltage induces erratic jets and bead formation, and vice versa.
Flow rate	Increasing flow rate (above the critical flow rate) → low stretching, larger pore size and fibre diameter.
Spinneret orifice	Smaller spinneret orifice diameter → narrower fibres and reduces morphological defects; also increases the probability of nozzle clogging. Hollow or blended fibre morphology possible.
Collector geometry	Different fibre arrangements can be obtained using different collector shapes. Aligned, crossed array, braided, nanoweb, or coiled fibres can be obtained using geometries such as rotating drum, plate, disc, etc.

(Continued)

Table 3.1. (*Continued*)

Parameter	Effect
Polymer concentration, viscosity, and surface tension	• Sufficient polymer concentration → molecular chain entanglements → surface tension overcome without fragmentation of the jet → uniform continuous fibres. • Molecular chain entanglement increases → viscosity increases → decreases electrospinnability, increases fibre thickness. • Low viscosity → electrospraying, bead defects, requires a higher voltage field or higher solution viscosity for electrospinnability.
Electrical conductivity	• Appropriate conductivity → improved charge accumulation → the jet eruption requires less voltage. • High conductivity has been reported to cause unstable multi-jetting likely due to electrical discharge to the surrounding air.
Dielectric constant	• A solvent's higher capability to retain electric charge in a solution helps to distribute the surface charge of a jet uniformly, and leads to better fibre electrospinnability with smaller diameters.
Solvent volatility	• Sufficiently volatile solutions → prevention of wet fusion of fibres at the collector. • Highly volatile solutions → premature solidification without sufficient elongation → morphological defects, hinders thin fibre production, increases the risk of blockage at the spinneret.
Relative humidity	• Increased humidity → delay in solidification before deposition → increases elongation time → thinner fibres • High humidity (>60%) has been known to produce non-uniform fused fibres for especially hygroscopic polymers such as poly(vinylpyrrolidone) (PVP). • If the polymer is insoluble in water, precipitation of polymer may cause spinneret blockage, thicker diameters, morphological defects, and other issues attributed to phase separation.
Temperature	Temperature affects most of the parameters listed above. For example: temperature increase → decrease in solution viscosity, increase in electrical conductivity → thin uniform fibres with greater polymer chain alignment. Temperature increase → decrease in evaporation and elongation time before solidification → counteracts the formation of finer fibres. An operating temperature of 10 °C has been shown to decrease fibre diameter due to increased elongation time.

3.3 Electrohydrodynamic fabrication techniques

Electrohydrodynamic techniques are a family of methods that use electric fields to manipulate the behaviour of fluids and suspensions to create functional materials and structures [56, 57]. These techniques are based on the principles of EHD, which involves the interaction between electric fields and fluids or charged particles.

Electrohydrodynamic techniques can be used to produce a wide range of functional materials and structures, including thin films, coatings, fibres, particles, and complex 3D structures. These materials can have a variety of properties, such as high surface area, high conductivity, high strength and can be used in a range of applications, such as in energy generation and storage, biomedical devices, sensors, and electronics [15, 58–61].

Some common electrohydrodynamic fabrication techniques include electrospraying, electrospinning, electrohydrodynamic atomisation, and direct writing. These techniques have unique advantages and limitations, and the choice of technique depends on the specific application and the desired material properties.

3.3.1 Electrohydrodynamic atomisation

Electrohydrodynamic atomisation (EHDA) is a technique that utilises an electric field to generate a high-intensity electric charge on the surface of a liquid [62]. This electric charge produces a series of complex fluid instabilities that ultimately result in the formation of a highly charged meniscus or a cone-shaped droplet known as the Taylor cone. EHDA includes two main sub-techniques, electrospraying and electrospinning, which differ mainly in the size and shape of the resulting droplets or fibres. Electrospraying produces submicrometre- to micrometre-sized droplets, while electrospinning produces nanometre- to micrometre-sized fibres [63]. EHDA has several advantages over traditional atomisation methods, including the ability to produce smaller droplets or fibres, narrow size distributions, the ability to precisely control the size and shape of the resulting particles. EHDA has been applied in various fields, including drug delivery, tissue engineering, and energy storage devices [63, 64].

In electrospraying, a liquid solution is introduced into a capillary or needle, which is connected to a high-voltage power supply. As the voltage is applied, an electric field is created between the needle and a grounded or oppositely charged electrode. This electric field causes the liquid to become charged and form a cone-shaped meniscus at the tip of the needle. As the voltage is increased, the meniscus becomes unstable and breaks up into fine droplets, which are then ejected from the needle and carried by a gas flow towards the opposite electrode. The size of the droplets produced by electrospraying depends on several factors, such as the properties of the liquid, the voltage applied, and the distance between the needle and the electrode (figure 3.3) [65–67]. Generally, smaller droplets can be produced by increasing the voltage, reducing the distance between the needle and the electrode, or using liquids with lower viscosity or surface tension.

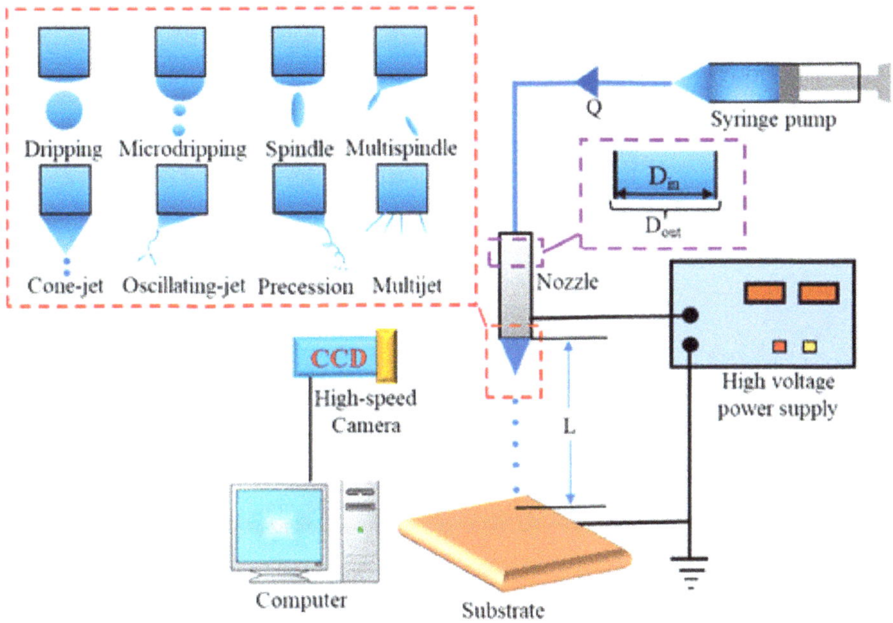

Figure 3.3. EHDA setup. Reprinted with permission from [68]. Copyright (2022) American Chemical Society.

Electrospinning is a process that involves the creation of fibres using an electrostatic force to draw a polymer solution or melt through a small nozzle. In this process, a high voltage is applied to a syringe containing the polymer solution, which forms a droplet at the tip of the metallic nozzle. The electrostatic force causes the droplet to elongate into a fine jet, and the solvent evaporates as the jet moves towards the collector. As a result, a thin and continuous fibre is formed and collected on a grounded surface. The process can be used with a variety of polymers, allowing for the creation of fibres with different physical and chemical properties. Electrospinning also has a wide range of applications, including tissue engineering, drug delivery, and antimicrobial filtration [69, 70].

3.3.1.1 Electrospraying

Electrospraying (electrohydrodynamic spraying) is an EHD fabrication technique that uses an electric field to produce fine droplets or particles from a liquid solution, which can then also be deposited onto a substrate to create various types of thin films or coatings [66, 71]. Electrospraying encompasses a range of bulk and surface forces, such as electrodynamic, gravity, inertia, and drag forces, as well as electrodynamic stress, pressure differential, and liquid dynamic viscosity. A scaling correlation has been established to determine the size of droplets emitted by a Taylor cone jet. The correlation depends on various factors, including flow rate, surface tension, solution conductivity, and a coefficient related to solution permittivity [72–74]. In addition, the nozzle apparatus design varies the product size and shape. Figure 3.4 shows micrographs of single-nozzle apparatuses [62].

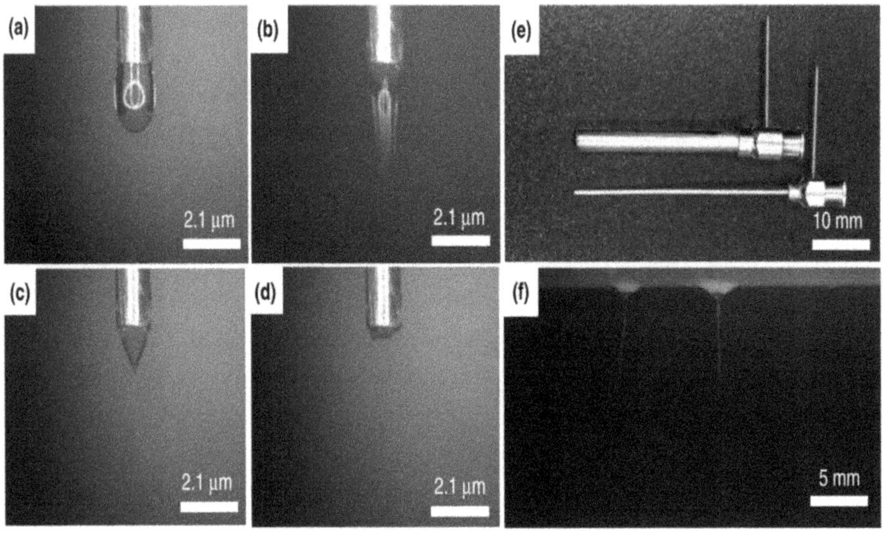

Figure 3.4. Micrographs of single-nozzle apparatus used for EHDA jetting: (a) dripping regime (no applied voltage), (b) unstable jetting regime, (c) Taylor cone stable jetting regime, (d) single-nozzle multiple jet formation, (e) coaxial nozzle examples showing the inner and outer layers of the system, and (f) a nozzle-less approach, namely the formation of jets by pores. Reprinted from [62], Copyright (2017), with permission from Elsevier.

The electrospraying method has some advantages. One advantage is that it is sustainable under ambient temperature and pressure conditions, making it ideal for producing certain biomolecules and living cells. In addition, the width of the surface area and the uniform distribution of the droplets have shown promise in many biomedical studies. This has made it an increasingly valuable tool for pharmaceutical and multidisciplinary applications [75].

Electrospraying is a state-of-the-art technology used in the fabrication of novel dual-adhesive hydrogel particles for bone regeneration [76]. It is a microfluidic technique that uses a high voltage to generate a fine, charged spray of liquid droplets. The technology offers precise control over the size, morphology, and composition of the resulting particles. In this study, electrospraying was used to fabricate hydrogel particles with a hierarchical porous morphology similar to that of pollen particles. The particles were rapidly solidified via liquid nitrogen-assisted cryoablation, resulting in structure-related adhesion. Electrospraying is a promising technology for the fabrication of various types of particles for different applications, including drug delivery, tissue engineering, and nanotechnology.

The majority of microfluidic systems for the manufacture of microcapsules work by solidifying many layers of emulsion droplets. To create hydrogel microcapsules, Wang *et al* [77] created a co-flow capillary microfluidic synthesis chip with three-bore microchannel injectors and an electrospray collection device. The target enzyme was initially immobilised in inverse opal particles during the production process and then enclosed in hollow alginate hydrogel utilising microfluidic electrospray. Through the immobilisation of various inverse opal particles in a single capsule, the electrospray approach made it possible to achieve multi-enzyme cascades. The viability of the proposed device was demonstrated through the development of a multi-enzyme system to lower the alcohol content in aqueous solutions.

Enzyme immobilisation represents a crucial challenge in standardising biosensors and obtaining the right analytical performance in terms of sensitivity, selectivity, and stability. In research conducted by Castrovilli *et al* [60], electrospray deposition (ESD) was used as a cutting-edge method to immobilise laccase enzyme on electrodes modified by screen printing with carbon black. The goal of this study was the creation of an amperometric biosensor for the detection of phenolic compounds. Scanning electron microscopy analysis and electrochemical characterisation of the electrodes produced using ESD demonstrated that this immobilisation method is appropriate for the production of high-performance biosensors. The findings demonstrated that the laccase enzyme maintains its activity during electrospray ionisation and deposition and that the constructed biosensor had increased storage performance.

Researchers have developed three-dimensional porous graphene electrodes using an electrostatic spray deposition technique for supercapacitor applications [78]. The electrode structure had superior characteristics compared to previous graphene-based supercapacitors, with open-pore structures that allowed for ion diffusion and electron transport. This technique eliminated the need for conductive binders or additives, making it a simple approach to electrode production. The technology has potential for use in small energy storage systems.

3.3.1.2 Electrospinning

Electrospinning is a versatile technique that is used to produce nanofibres with diameters ranging from nanometres to micrometres [79]. The technique involves the use of an electric field to draw a polymer solution or melt from a nozzle, resulting in the formation of nanofibres that are collected on a substrate [80].

Recent advances in electrospinning have focused on improving the processing parameters to produce fibres with more uniform morphologies and narrower size distributions [81, 82]. For example, researchers have investigated the effects of solution properties, such as viscosity and electrical conductivity, on fibre formation. They have also studied the effects of processing parameters such as the applied voltage, the nozzle-to-collector distance, and the solution flow rate on fibre morphology and size.

Another area of research has been the development of electrospinning for specific applications. For example, researchers have used electrospinning to produce nanofibres for tissue engineering, drug delivery, and wound healing. In tissue engineering, electrospinning has been used to produce scaffolds with tailored mechanical and biological properties that can support cell growth and tissue regeneration [83]. In drug delivery, electrospun fibres can be used to encapsulate drugs and release them in a controlled manner. Electrospun fibres have also been used for wound healing applications, in which they can provide a scaffold for cell growth and promote tissue regeneration. Several EHDA-induced polymer-based products are shown in figure 3.5, from core–shell microcapsules to microparticles, nanofibres, patterns, and bubbles [62].

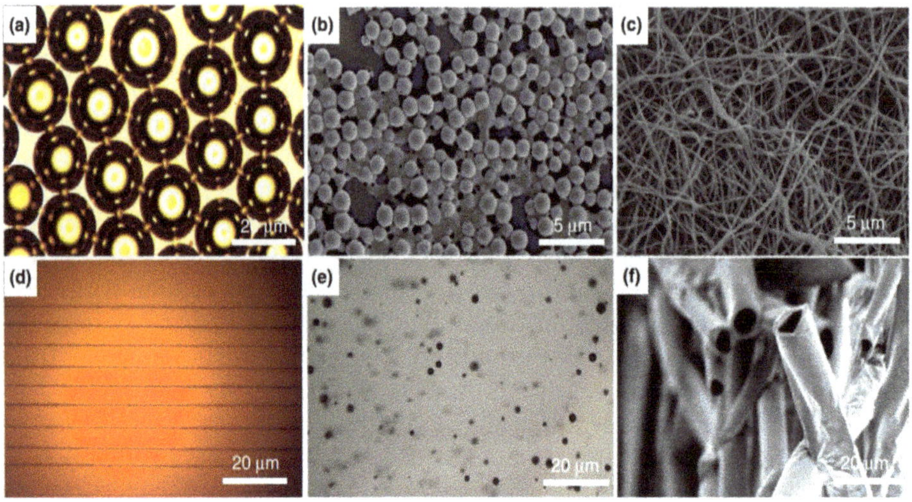

Figure 3.5. EHDA-induced polymer products: (a) core–shell microcapsules (coaxial electrospraying), (b) microparticles (single-nozzle electrospraying), (c) nanofibres (single-nozzle electrospraying), (d) linear patterns (direct writing), (e) microbubbles (micro bubbling), and (f) microtube bundles (coaxial electrospinning). Reprinted from [62], Copyright (2017), with permission from Elsevier.

Furthermore, researchers have explored the use of electrospinning for the production of hybrid materials, such as nanofibre-reinforced composites [84–86]. By incorporating different materials into the fibres, researchers have been able to enhance their mechanical and functional properties [87].

Multijet electrospinning is a technique used to produce nanofibres with controlled morphology and composition. It uses multiple nozzles to simultaneously extrude different polymer solutions or suspensions [88, 89]. The use of multiple jets allows for the production of more complex structures, including core–shell and hollow fibres, and enables the incorporation of different materials into the nanofibres [90–92].

Recent advances in multijet electrospinning have focused on improving the processing parameters to produce fibres with more uniform morphologies and size distributions [88, 89]. For example, researchers have investigated the effects of different electric field configurations, nozzle spacings, and solution properties on fibre formation.

The development of multijet electrospinning is important for biomedical applications. For example, researchers have used this technique to produce nanofibres for tissue engineering, drug delivery, and water filtration [88, 93]. In tissue engineering, multijet electrospinning has been used to produce scaffolds with tailored mechanical and biological properties, while in drug delivery, it has been used to produce fibres that release drugs at controlled rates. In addition, researchers have also explored the use of multijet electrospinning for the production of hybrid materials, such as nanofibre-reinforced composites. By incorporating different materials into the fibres, researchers have been able to enhance their mechanical and functional properties.

As a state-of-the-art technology for nanofibre production, the electrohydrodynamic gun has gained significant attention in recent years due to its ability to produce high-quality nanofibres with precise control over their diameter, morphology, and orientation. A study was conducted on the potential use of nanofibres for wound healing in diabetic patients [94]. The study utilised a portable electrohydrodynamic gun to produce the nanofibres, and several tests were performed to assess their safety and effectiveness. Drug release studies were also conducted to determine the rate at which drugs such as Metformin and *Ginkgo biloba* were released from the nanofibres over time.

Nanofibre-based biosensors have emerged as another state-of-the-art technology in the field of electrospinning, offering high sensitivity, selectivity, and stability in the detection of a wide range of analytes. They are being extensively researched due to their potential use in various applications, including disease diagnosis, drug screening, and environmental monitoring [15]. This study demonstrated that electrospun porous copper oxide (CuO)/cadmium oxide (CdO) composite nanofibres represent a promising platform for the development of non-enzymatic glucose sensors, and their high sensitivity and selectivity make them a potential candidate for use in various other biomedical applications [95].

3.3.2 Direct writing

Direct writing is an EHD technique that enables the precise deposition of functional materials, such as polymers or metals, onto a substrate using a fine nozzle and an electric field to control the flow of the material [96–98]. This technique can be used to create complex structures and patterns with high resolution and accuracy. Direct writing can deposit or pattern materials onto a substrate in a controlled manner, usually in a layer-by-layer fashion [99].

Direct writing and EHDA are two distinct techniques that share similarities in their ability to create complex and precise structures [62, 99]. Direct writing utilises a printing-like process controlled by a computer system to deposit materials in a precise pattern or shape. EHDA, on the other hand, involves the atomisation and spraying of a solution or suspension through an electric field.

In direct writing, a material in the form of a solution or paste is dispensed from a nozzle or pen tip, which is connected to a high-voltage power supply [100]. As the material is extruded from the nozzle, an electric field is applied, which causes the material to become charged and form a jet. The trajectory of the jet is then controlled by the electric field, which can be adjusted by changing the voltage, the distance between the nozzle and the substrate, and other parameters.

The deposited material can be either solidified immediately upon deposition or left to dry and solidify at a later time. This process can be repeated layer by layer to create complex 3D structures.

Direct writing has many applications in various fields, such as in the production of electronic devices, sensors, and biomedical implants [96, 98, 100, 101]. It allows for precise patterning and the deposition of materials with high spatial resolution and control, making it a promising technique for the fabrication of structures with unique properties and functions.

There are several variations of direct writing, such as electrohydrodynamic lithography, which uses a photomask to pattern the electric field and create more complex structures, and electrohydrodynamic jet printing, which uses multiple nozzles to print multiple materials simultaneously [102–104].

Some recent advances in direct writing have focused on improving the resolution, speed, and versatility of the technique. For example, researchers have developed new nozzle designs and ink formulations to enable the deposition of a wider range of materials, including conductive, semiconducting, and biological materials. In the development of this method, researchers have used direct writing to produce electronic devices, such as sensors and transistors, by depositing conductive materials in precise patterns [105, 106]. They have also used direct writing to produce tissue engineering scaffolds by depositing biological materials in three-dimensional patterns that can support cell growth and tissue regeneration [107, 108].

Moreover, researchers have explored the use of direct writing for the fabrication of complex structures, such as microfluidic devices, by using multiple nozzles or pens to deposit different materials in precise patterns [102, 109]. Table 3.2 gives brief information about nozzle characteristics and their relationship to the end product [98]. By combining multiple materials and deposition techniques, researchers have been able to create complex, multi-functional structures with high resolution.

Table 3.2. Nozzle structure characteristics and related applications. Reproduced from [98] with permission from the Royal Society of Chemistry.

Nozzles	Structures	Applications
Multi-nozzle	• Parallel nozzles	• Printing solar cell electrodes with high manufacturing efficiency
	• Addressable nozzles	• Printing transistors using different materials in the corresponding nozzles
	• Revolver nozzles	
Tip-in-nozzle	• Non-conductive tip-in-nozzle	• Reducing the applied voltage
	• Conductive tip-in-nozzle	• Adjusting the diameter of the fibre
		• Control the deposition frequency

(*Continued*)

Table 3.2. (*Continued*)

Nozzles	Structures	Applications
Coaxial nozzle	• Two coaxially arranged needles	• Coaxial fibres
	• Three coaxially arranged needles	• Core–shell fibres
		• Nanowire-in-microtube structure
		• Single Microchannel
		• OLED
Multi-hole nozzle	• Two parallel holes in the needle	• Multi-channel fibre
	• Multiple parallel holes in the needle	• Materials and structures for biomimicry

Direct writing, which allows for the precise deposition of materials at the micrometre or nanometre scale, has emerged as a state-of-the-art technology with a wide range of applications in various fields such as electronics, medicine, and materials science. Shen *et al* presented a study on the fabrication of 3D microstructures for flexible pressure sensors based on direct writing printing [110]. This work demonstrated the potential of direct writing technologies using a state-of-the-art example of 3D microstructure fabrication. Two forms of direct writing, namely the EHD and aerosol jet (AJ) printing methods, were used to create highly controllable 3D microstructures with different shapes and sizes. Because the printing processes were programmable, both methods were able to control the shape of the fabricated microstructures, and the height and shape of the 3D microstructure could be effectively controlled by changing the number of printing layers and the printing speed. The EHD printing method was found to have higher manufacturing precision, while the AJ printing method had higher stacking efficiency. The ability to precisely fabricate 3D microstructures using direct writing technology has significant potential for various applications, including the development of flexible sensors, MEMs, and biomedical devices with the aid of EHD (figure 3.6) [98].

3.4 Electrohydrodynamic fabrication products

EHDA has a simple physical process which includes a combination of electrospraying and electrospinning. The EHDA setup consists of a high-voltage source and a conductive collector. The applied voltage, flow rate, capillary nozzle–conductive collector distance, ambient temperature, humidity, and the physicochemical characteristics of the solution are the main operational parameters of EHDA. Electrospraying is a useful technique for the manufacture of micro/nanoparticles and microbubble suspensions. On the other hand, micro/nanofibres can also be produced by electrospinning. In

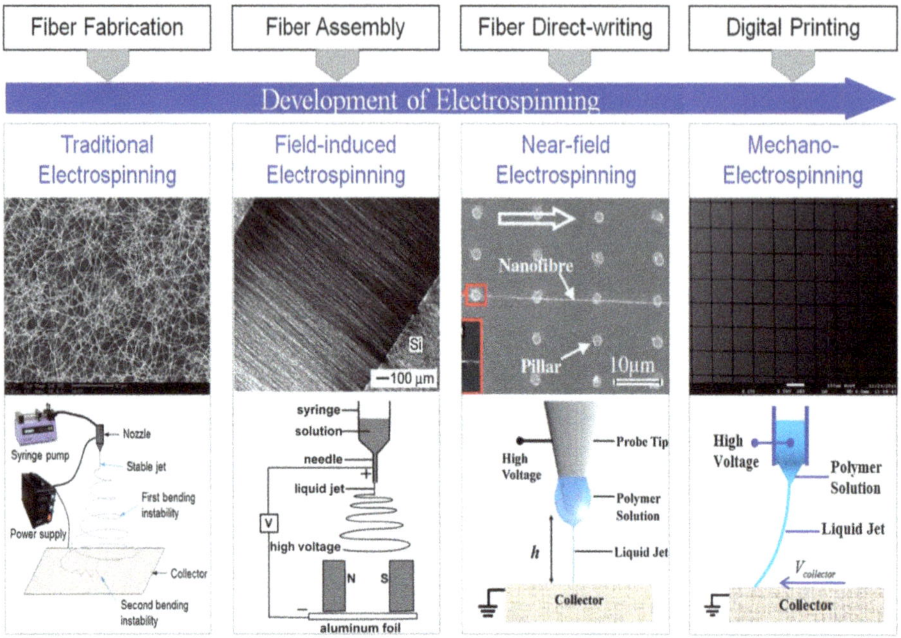

Figure 3.6. A timeline showing the development of EHD fibre production from traditional electrospinning to mechano-electrospinning. Reproduced from [98] with permission from the Royal Society of Chemistry.

addition, more complex, multilayer particle and fibre applications can also be generated.

In a study by Husain and co-workers, a particle-to-fibre transition phenomenon was investigated [111]. A polymer, polylactic-co-glycolic acid (PLGA), was used in the study at different concentrations (2 wt%, 4 wt%, 10 wt%, 15 wt%, 20 wt%, and 25 wt%). When the flow rate, applied voltage, and working distance tested were kept constant (50 μL min^{-1}, 15 kV, and 200 mm, respectively), the particle-to-fibre transition was induced by increasing the polymer concentration (figure 3.7). Low PLGA concentrations (2 wt% and 4 wt%) resulted in electrospraying, and particle formation occurred. At moderate PLGA concentrations (10 wt% and 15 wt%), products were obtained in the intermediate phase of transition from particle to fibre, these were called 'tailed particles'. When PLGA was used at a 20 wt% concentration, fibre formation was the dominant process, although a few beads were produced. At the highest concentration of 25 wt% of PLGA solution, smooth, non-beaded, homogeneous fibre formation was established.

3.4.1 Particles

Natural and synthetic polymers can be used in studies that produce particles using EDHA. In addition to the concentration of the polymer used, the flow rate, collector distance, and even the solvent used have an effect on the size and

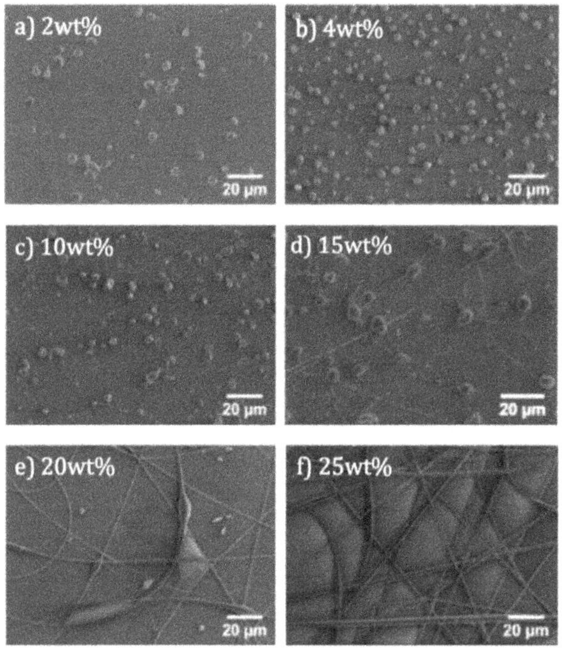

Figure 3.7. SEM micrographs of PLGA particles and fibre products at a constant flow rate, applied voltage, and working distance (50 μL min^{-1}, 15 kV, and 200 mm, respectively) and at different polymer concentrations: (a) 2 wt%, (b) 4 wt%, (c) 10 wt%, (d) 15 wt%, (e) 20 wt%, and (f) 25 wt% (scale bar = 20 μm). Reprinted from [111], Copyright (2016), with permission from Elsevier.

morphology of the produced particles. The increase in flow rate also causes an increase in particle size. The solvent is not only important in the preparation of a homogeneous mixture of the polymer to be used but also affects the evaporation rate after jet formation. While rapid evaporation induces the formation of irregular particle shapes with pores that appear on the particle surface, slow evaporation leads to the production of homogeneous spherical particles with smooth surfaces (figure 3.8) [64].

In a study by C J Hogan Jr *et al*, hydrophilic and hydrophobic single-layer particles and core–shell structures were produced by EHDA. Water-soluble polyethylene glycol (PEG), polyvinylpyrrolidone (PVP) and water-insoluble poly-methylmethacrylate (PMMA) particles were produced using EHDA (figures 3.9–3.11) [67]. The parametric effects of the surface tension, viscosity, electrical conductivity, and dielectric constant of the polymer solutions on the particle size distribution were investigated. In addition, the particle sizes were evaluated to determine the effect of the polymer's molecular weight on the physicochemical parameters of the polymer solution. It was concluded that controllable particle formation could occur at sizes between 0.35 and 2.71 μm. The EHDA technique is a simple, versatile, and robust way to produce particles from polymer solutions that vary widely in terms of solubility, electrical conductivity, viscosity, etc. Moreover,

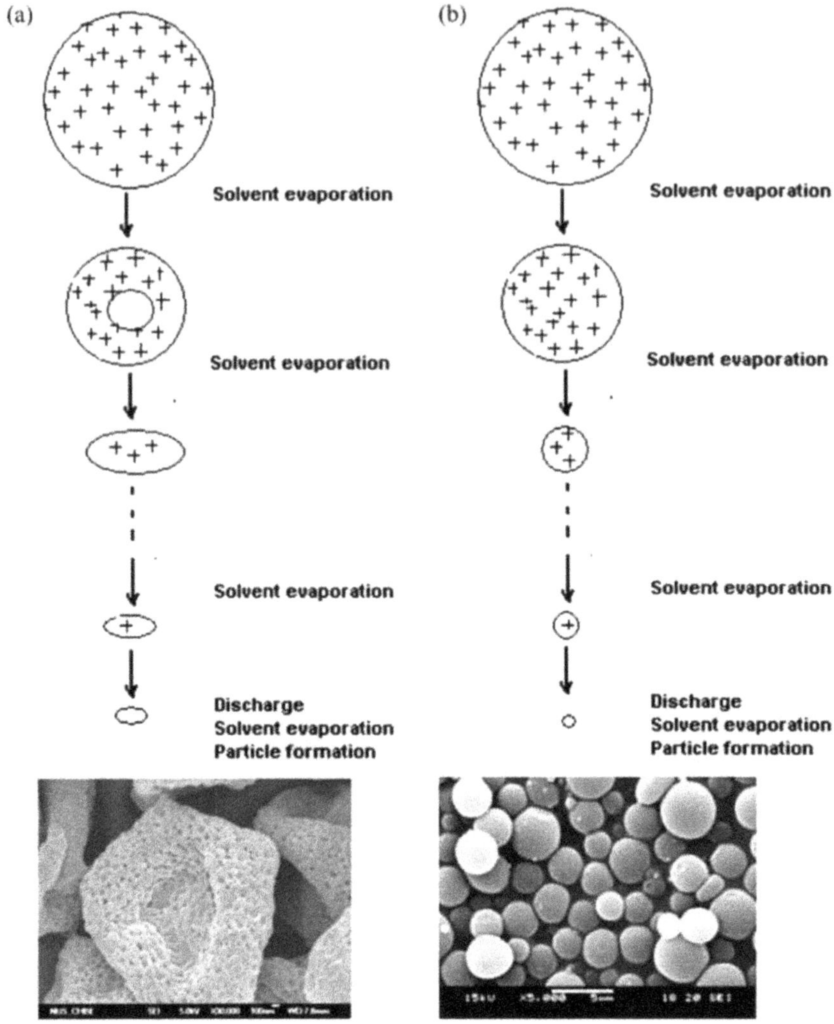

Figure 3.8. Strategies for the production of PLGA nanoparticles via EHDA and SEM micrographs of the resulting nanoparticles for: (a) rapid and (b) slow solvent evaporation. Reprinted from [64], Copyright (2006), with permission from Elsevier.

particle formation is not only limited to a monolayer but is also conducive to producing core–shell structures [112].

3.4.2 Fibres

Fibre production using EHDA is commonly referred to as the electrospinning technique. Through the use of this technique, synthetic and natural polymers can be produced separately, by blending, or according to a core–shell model. In addition, the polymer types used are classified not only as natural versus synthetic but also according to their solubility properties. The relationship between solvents and

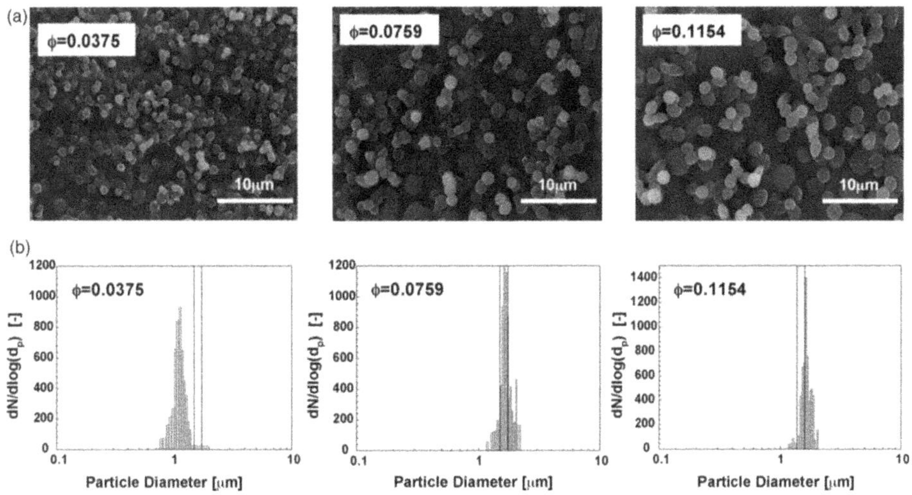

Figure 3.9. (a) SEM micrographs and (b) size distribution graphs of PEG particles. Reprinted from [67], Copyright (2007), with permission from Elsevier.

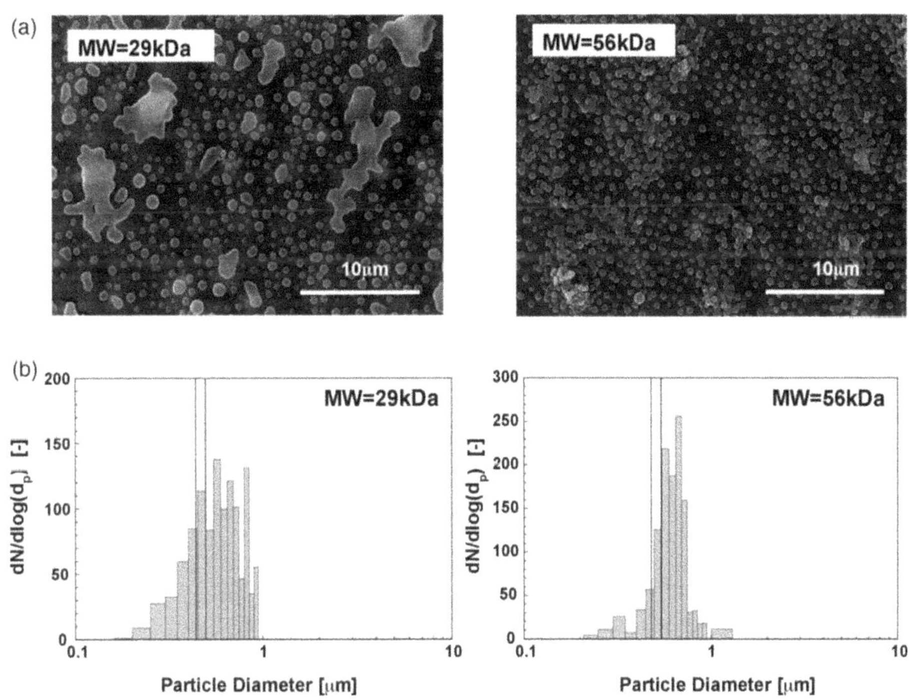

Figure 3.10. (a) SEM micrographs and (b) size distribution graphs of PVP particles. Reprinted from [67], Copyright (2007), with permission from Elsevier.

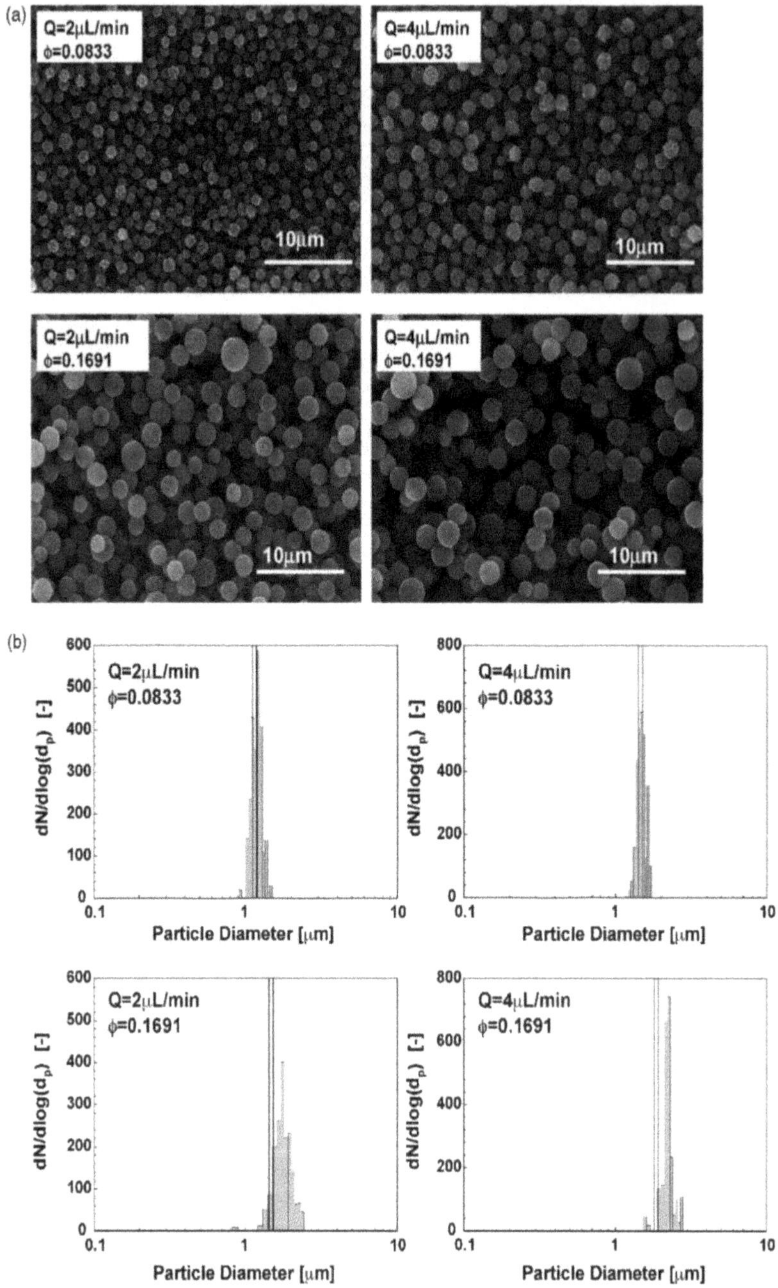

Figure 3.11. (a) SEM micrographs and (b) size distribution graphs of PMMA particles. Reprinted from [67], Copyright (2007), with permission from Elsevier.

polymers affects the production control through the parameters of concentration, electrical conductivity, viscosity, surface tension. EHD-induced fibre production techniques can also take the form of direct writing. The direct writing device is a sister device of the electrospinning device. The main difference between them is that the direct printing assembly has a collector with the ability to move in the *x–y–z* axes. The motion sensitivity of the movable printer and the diameter of the printed fibres have an effect on the resolution of the resulting pattern.

In a study, Ahmad and co-workers produced polyurethane (PU) and poly(methylsilsesquioxane) (PMSQ) particles, fibres, and patterned structures by electrospraying, electrospinning, and direct writing techniques (figures 3.12–3.14) [113]. In addition, the voltage and collection-distance parameters were evaluated. This study showed that

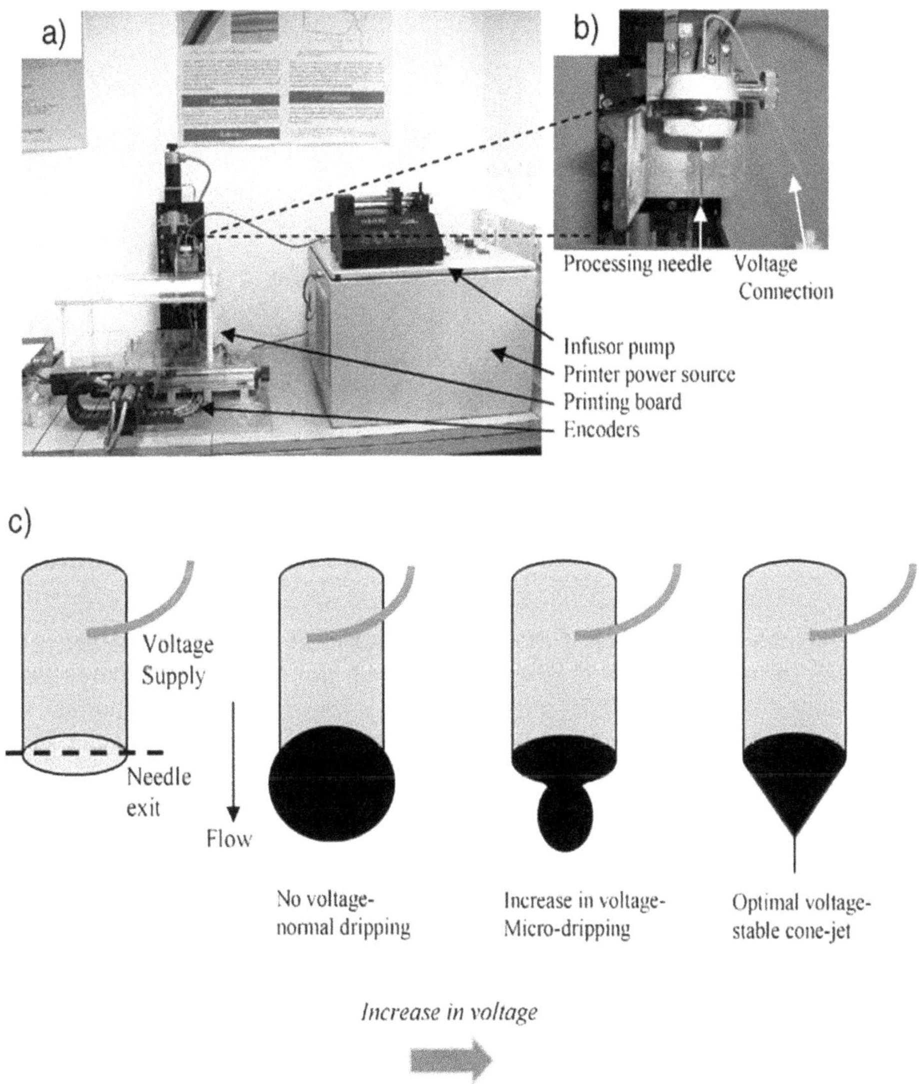

Figure 3.12. Optical images of: (a) an EHD setup, (b) processing needle and voltage connector on a printing head. (c) An illustrative image of voltage-induced stable cone jet formation [113]. John Wiley & Sons. [2010].

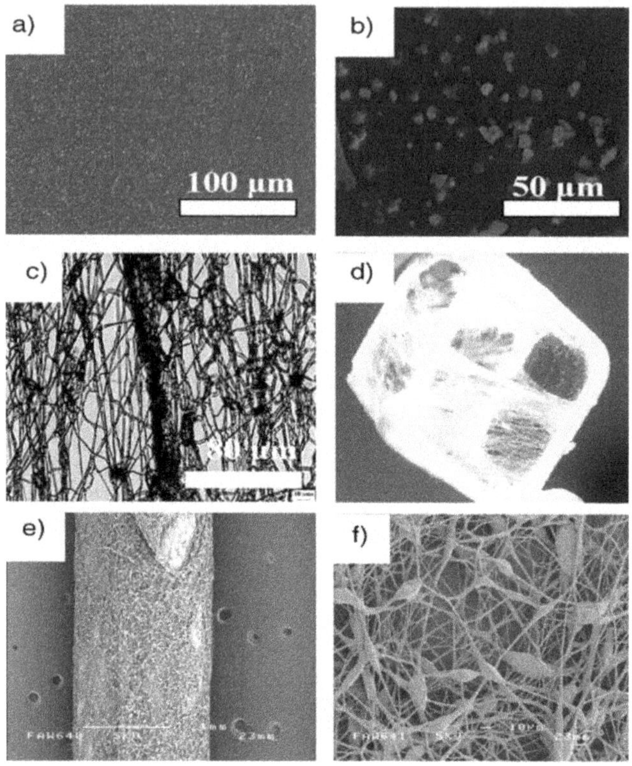

Figure 3.13. SEM micrographs of (a) PMSQ particles (scale bar=100 µm) produced by electrospraying, (b) PMSQ particles (scale bar=50 µm) produced by electrospraying, (c) PU fibres produced by electrospinning, (d) nHA–PU fibres spun directly onto a stainless steel hollow cube and (e) a stainless steel rod. (f) A high-magnification view of stainless steel with a nano-hydroxyapatite (nHA)–PU fibre coating [113]. John Wiley & Sons. [2010].

EHD techniques can be extended to derive fibre applications for biomedical applications; these are not only bulk fibre applications but also layered fibres patterned by direct printing techniques. The importance and usage of EHD-supported fibre production methods in biomedical applications will be examined in detail in the following section.

3.5 Electrohydrodynamic technology-based biomedical engineering

3.5.1 Tissue engineering

Electrospun nanofibres have a wide range of uses from military applications to sensors and biomedicine, in which they are particularly used as tissue engineering constructs (figure 3.15) [114]. Biodegradable and biocompatible tissue scaffolds are the most important component in tissue engineering, which is a research area that utilises multidisciplinary approaches at the intersection of medicine and engineering sciences with the aim of restoring the function of damaged tissues or those with lost functionality [115]. Studies in which synthetic or natural biopolymers are used in

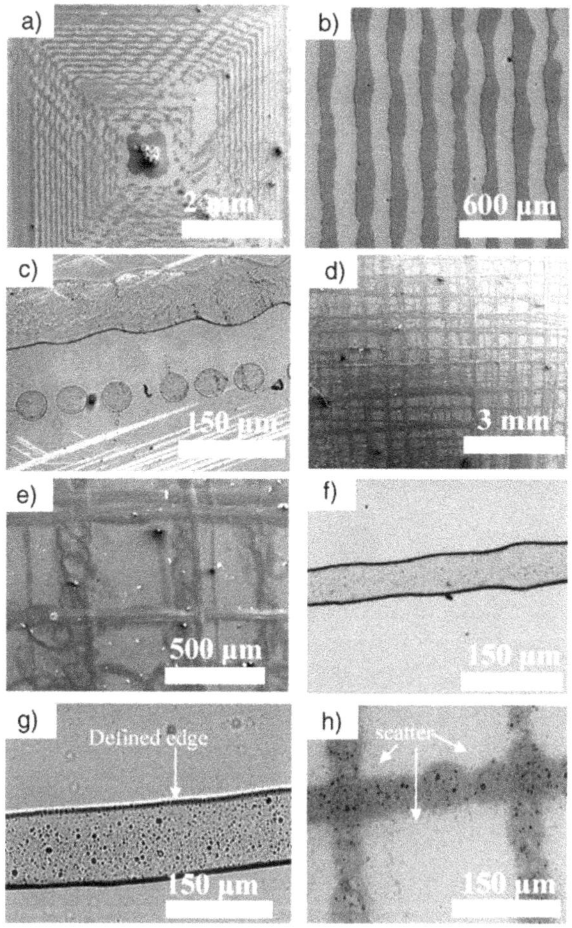

Figure 3.14. SEM micrographs of PMSQ written using EHD: (a) scale bar=2 mm, (b) scale bar=600 μm, (c) patterns printed by dripping and stable jets, (d) PU produced by direct writing with multiple layers produced by overwriting, (e) higher-magnification view of PU produced by direct writing with multiple layers produced by overwriting, (f) a single line of PU created by direct writing, (g) a PU-nHA composite produced by direct writing on a glass surface, and (h) direct writing of an nHA pattern showing scatter [113] John Wiley & Sons. [2010].

tissue engineering applications have increased greatly since the very first years of the tissue scaffold concept. Many examples of these wide-ranging biocompatible and degradable polymers are of synthetic, bacterial, vegetable, or animal origin, such as poly (alpha hydroxy acids), polylactic, and glycolic acids, polycaprolactone (PCL), chitosan, and silk fibroin (SF) [114, 116–118].

To successfully imitate native three-dimensional tissues, the produced biodegradable structures must allow the movement of nutrients, growth hormones, and even cells into the depths of the scaffold; therefore they must have a porous nature. Along with these properties, the cells of the relevant tissue must attach, proliferate,

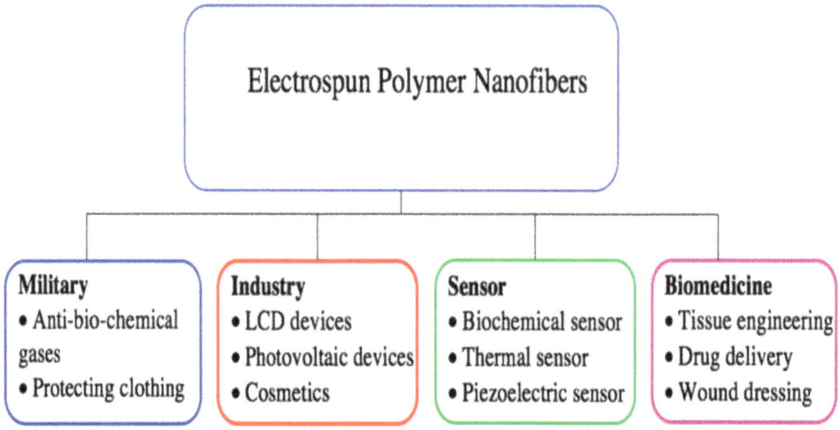

Figure 3.15. Uses of electrospun nanofibres, from military applications to biomedicine. Reproduced from [114]. CC BY 4.0.

and spread onto scaffolds. The structural fibrous proteins, linear glycosaminoglycans, and glycoproteins that make up the natural tissues of the extracellular matrix (ECM) work together to provide structural support to the tissue, regulation of cell behaviour, and differentiation. From this point of view, we can conclude that electrospinning is a very suitable manufacturing method for the production of scaffolds used for the imitation of these ECM structures, which are largely composed of linear macromolecular chains and voids; numerous examples and sub-techniques of such production have been described in research literature [55, 119].

The electrospinning technique is extensively utilised for the fabrication of tissue engineering scaffolds for several reasons. First and foremost, the electrospinning technique allows for the fabrication of scaffolds with a high surface-to-volume ratio and a porous structure, resembling the ECM of native tissues. In addition, mimicry of the ECM promotes cell attachment, migration, and proliferation. Furthermore, electrospun scaffolds offer tunable properties such as fibre diameter, alignment, and porosity, which can be tailored to mimic specific tissue characteristics and requirements. This versatility enables scaffolds to be designed that closely resemble the architecture of the target tissue, thereby facilitating cell integration and tissue regeneration.

The use of electrospinning is a highly preferable and feasible approach for the preparation of scaffolds for bone tissue regeneration [120–122]. Successful imitation of the porous and matrix components of the scaffold (which are used as a filler materials, especially in critical size defects) can be simply achieved using electrospun fibres [123]. Collagen fibres are the most important and largest organic component of bone tissue. In studies of synthetic and natural polymers such as PCL, PLGA, gelatine, chitosan, and SF, collagen structures have been imitated in terms of both size and mechanical characteristics [124, 125].

Bone tissue also contains hydroxyapatite (HA), one of its most important inorganic components, and it is possible to add this to the porous scaffold by dispersing nanosized calcium phosphate minerals into the electrospinning solution or by soaking the resulting fibres in simulated body fluid, where nucleation occurs. The versatility of electrospinning in utilising various materials and its ability to produce biomimetic scaffolds have made it an established choice in bone tissue engineering (figure 3.16) [124].

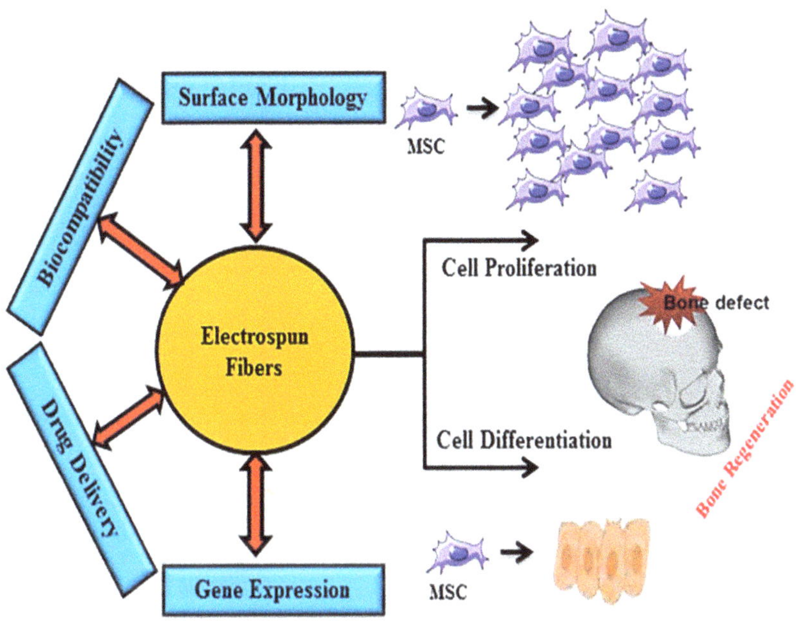

Figure 3.16. A schematic illustration of the effect of electrospun fibre scaffolds on cell proliferation and differentiation for bone regeneration. Reprinted from [124], Copyright (2019), with permission from Elsevier.

In addition to basic tissue regeneration issues such as viability, proliferation, and motility, it has been shown that cell phenotype characteristics strictly depend on the spatial organisation of the scaffold material. Better chondrocyte differentiation results were achieved using three-dimensional cultures that imitated the natural cartilage ECM structures. The use of layered scaffolds in the treatment of defects in articular cartilage, subchondral bone, and the overall osteochondral region has aroused interest in recent studies [126–128]. In the osteochondral region, the matrix components and the mechanical properties of layers change vertically. This is why the ECM density and the orientation of collagen fibres in articular cartilage tissue differ. This is one of the major challenges that faces *in vitro* cartilage tissue engineering in recreating the hierarchical orientation of the collagen network of native tissue [129]. Currently, scientists are showing significant interest in electrospinning that can imitate the pattern characteristics of the articular cartilage ECM. This technique has garnered attention for its potential applications in the field of cartilage regeneration. The use of oriented nanofibres in varying concentrations is important for the parameters of overall cartilage regeneration. Reboredo *et al* proposed a multilayered collagen-based porous scaffold for total cartilage replacement material. The scaffold they fabricated consisted of five layers and allows for the differentiation of human mesenchymal stem cells from chondrocytes. The layers consisted of two collagen types with both random and aligned oriented fibres; these were electrospun step by step to achieve the final five-layered structure that mimicked the native tissue hierarchy from the top to the bottom (figure 3.17) [130]. Wise *et al* developed nano- and microfibre PCL scaffolds with controlled orientation and tested these scaffolds using human mesenchymal stem cells [131]. The results of their study demonstrated that the creation of an organised ECM environment to control tissue alignment can be enhanced through the utilisation of aligned electrospun nanofibres. Furthermore, the combination of stem cells and

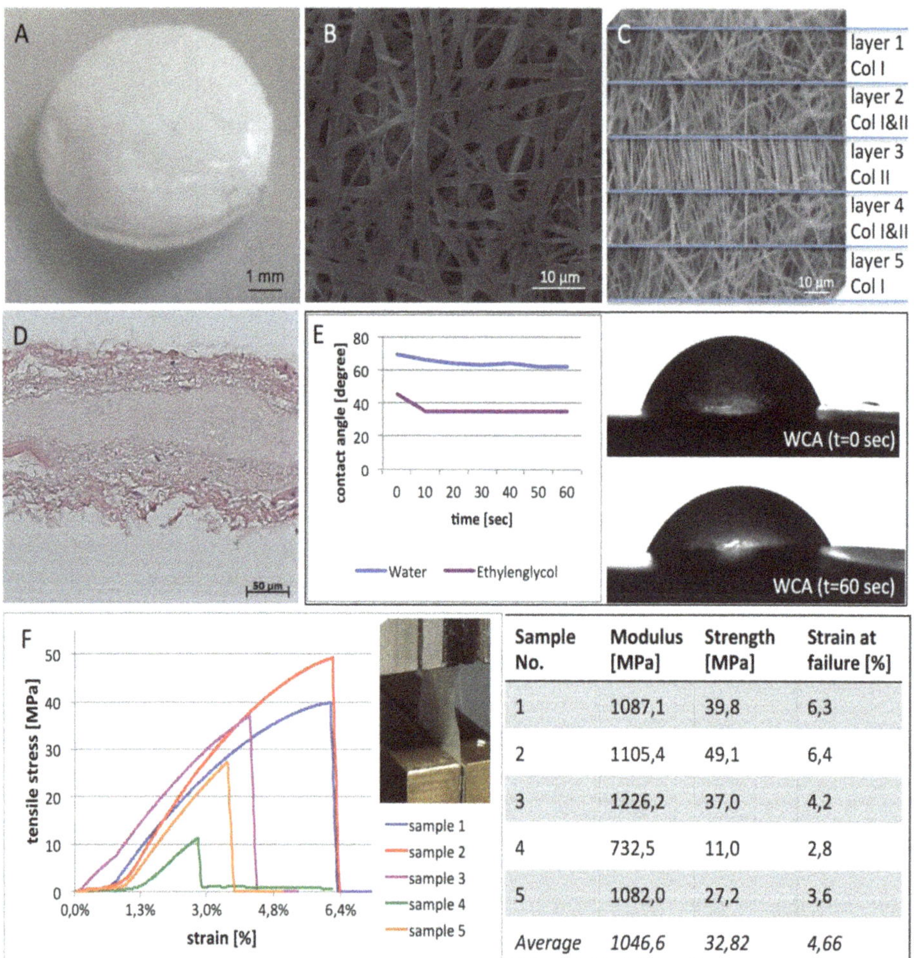

Sample No.	Modulus [MPa]	Strength [MPa]	Strain at failure [%]
1	1087,1	39,8	6,3
2	1105,4	49,1	6,4
3	1226,2	37,0	4,2
4	732,5	11,0	2,8
5	1082,0	27,2	3,6
Average	*1046,6*	*32,82*	*4,66*

Figure 3.17. Multilayered collagen-based scaffold fibres: (a) a micrograph of collagen-based scaffold fibres (scale bar = 1 mm), (b) an SEM micrograph of collagen fibres (scale bar = 10 µm), (c) SEM micrographs of the collagen fibre scaffold cross-sections (scale bar = 10 µm), (d) haematoxylin and eosin (H&E) staining of the collagen fibre scaffold (scale bar = 50 µm), (e) contact angles of collagen fibre scaffolds, and (f) tensile stress–strain curves (left) and modulus, strength, and strain at failure results (right) of fibre samples (n = 5) [130] John Wiley & Sons. [2016].

nanofibre scaffolds can lead to notable improvements in specific tissue engineering applications, particularly in the construction of the surface layer of articular cartilage. Aligned electrospun PCL scaffolds with nano- and microscale fibres appeared to promote the growth of mesenchymal stem cells, while nanofibre scaffolds enhanced chondrogenic activity. This resulted in higher sulphated glycosaminoglycan (sGAG) production and increased collagen type II synthesis, which indicated that nano-fibrous scaffolds may be particularly suitable for the development of the superficial region.

In recognition of the importance of blood vessels in the human body and their widespread network, tissue engineering studies have also been carried out to create a blood vessel using electrohydrodynamic systems. In a study by Stankus *et al*, small-diameter elastomeric poly(ester urethane) urea (PEUU) conduits were produced using the electrospinning method. During fibre production, smooth muscle cells (SMCs) were simultaneously electrosprayed to overcome the cell penetration difficulties encountered by 3D structures (figure 3.18) [132]. In this study, electro-spinning and electrohydrodynamic atomisation (electrospraying) techniques were used in an integrated manner. This approach confirmed the synergistic effect that occurs when these techniques are used together as well as the benefit of using these techniques in tissue engineering applications.

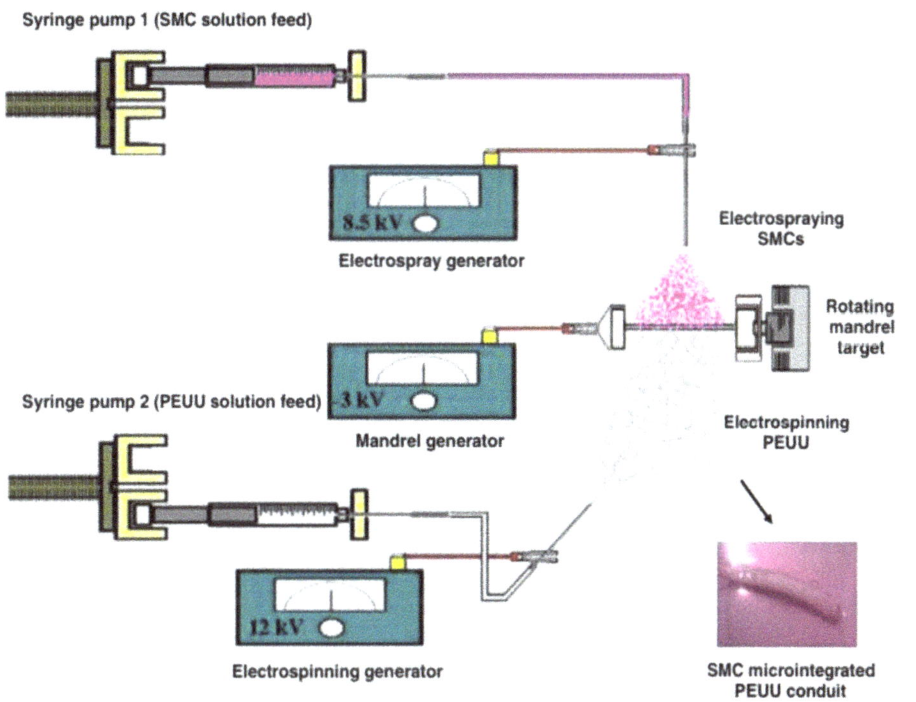

Figure 3.18. A schematic representation of the use of integrated electrospinning and electrospraying techniques to produce SMCs microintegrated into PEUU conduits. The inset shows an optical image of the SMC microintegrated into the PEUU conduit product. Reprinted from [132], Copyright (2007), with permission from Elsevier.

Heart tissue may be damaged as a result of ischaemia or infarction and may experience loss of function. At this point, artificial tissue materials and scaffolds can be used to support regeneration. In addition for basic requirements such as cell compatibility and cell adhesion, it is important that biomimetic materials used to mimic heart tissue are suitable for electrical conduction in order to permit the spontaneous and simultaneous contraction of cardiac cells. Therefore, scaffold materials adopted should contain materials with high electrical conductivity, such as conductive polymers or carbon nanotubes, to facilitate communication and electrical signal transmission. In their recently published work, Gil-Castell *et al* proposed a nanofibre scaffold structure that contained PCL, gelatine, and polyaniline (PANI) as a suitable material for cardiac tissue engineering. In scaffold structures in which PANI microparticles acted as cellular centres for cardiomyocyte proliferation, electrical conduction was provided by nanofibres with diameters of 300 nm or less. Testing was carried out using HL-1 cardiac muscle cells (figure 3.19) [133].

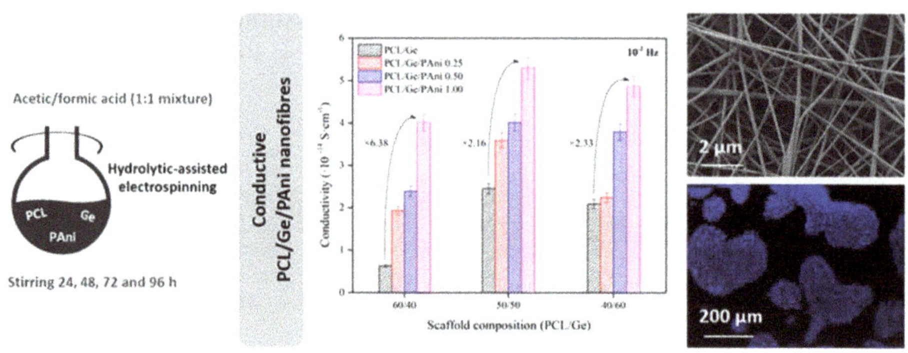

Figure 3.19. The preparation of conductive polycaprolactone/gelatine/polyaniline fibres via hydrolysis-assisted electrospinning (left), their conductivity/scaffold properties (centre), SEM micrograph (upper right; scale bar = 2μm), and DAPI staining (lower right, HL-1 cardiac muscle cell line; scale bar = 200 μm). Reprinted from [133], Copyright (2022), with permission from Elsevier.

In a study in which electrical conduction was facilitated by the use of carbon nanotubes (CNTs), nanofibre scaffolds with random and aligned orientations were tested with H9C2 (rat cardiac myoblasts) and human umbilical vessel endothelial cells (HUVECs). Electrical conduction was observed to be greater in the aligned nanofibre structures in which polyurethane and chitosan were used, compared to a random fibre structure [134]. In a study published in 2020, Flaig *et al* pointed out that many scaffolds produced for use in cardiac tissue engineering cannot support the necessary biological activity because they contain only hydrophobic polymers. To reinforce this argument, researchers who added 30% polyglycerol sebacate (PGS) to poly(lactic acid) (PLA) solutions stated that cell–material interactions increased with increasing wettability. In addition, it was reported that the inflammatory response was decreased compared to that of the control group and the cardiomyocyte cell morphology in the PGS-doped fibre scaffolds was closer to that found in natural tissue (figures 3.20–3.21) [135].

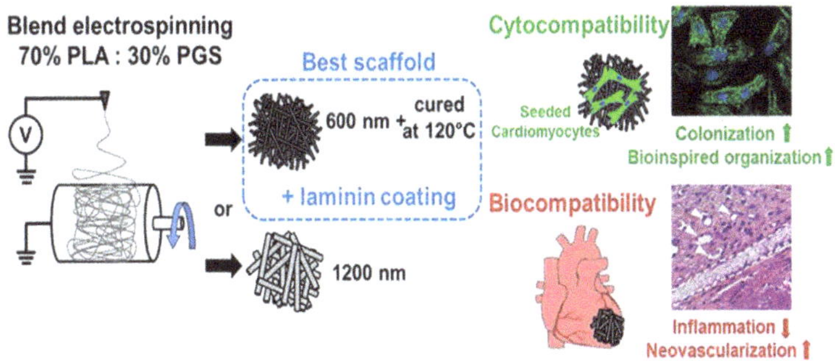

Figure 3.20. A schematic representation of the production of PLA:PGS polymer blend fibre scaffolds and their effect on inflammation, colonisation, bioinspired organisation, and neovascularization for cardiac regeneration. Reprinted with permission from [135]. Copyright (2020) American Chemical Society.

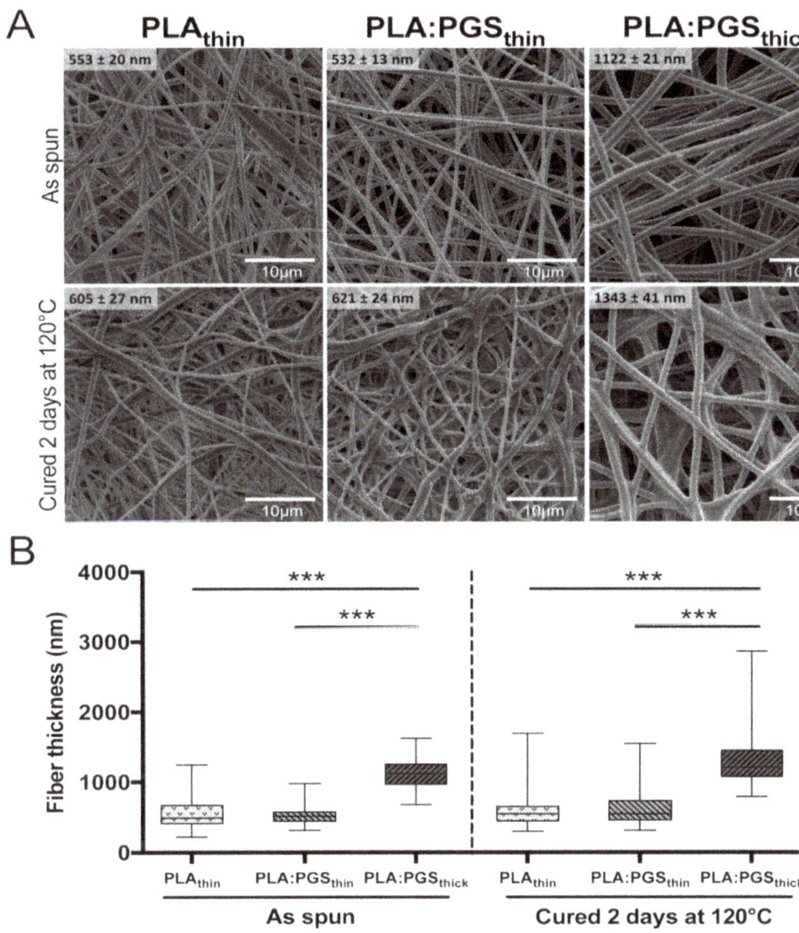

Figure 3.21. PLA and PLA:PGS electrospun nanofibres as spun and after thermal curing. (A) SEM micrographs (scale bar=10μm), (B) fibre thickness (nm). Reprinted with permission from [135]. Copyright (2020) American Chemical Society.

Another scenario in which electrical conduction is important is the materials used in neural tissue engineering. In nerve conduction, the structure must be able to transmit the stimulus created by the action potential to the tissue scaffold. An important indicator of whether tissue regeneration will be successful is neurite outgrowth. A suitable approach would encourage the orientation of cells through aligned nanofibres to obtain synaptic conductivity between axons and dendrites in a regular and unidirectional manner and form a structure in which interneuron communication can take place during nerve transmission. The structural alignment of nanofibre scaffolds serves as a physical guide for nerve cells, allowing them to extend their neurites in the desired direction. This alignment creates a surface with a specific topography that enables cells to grow in a unidirectional manner as they align. Nanofibres have a small diameter and a high aspect ratio, similar to the fibres of the ECM of natural tissue. As nerve cells contact these nanofibres, they adhere to the surface and orient themselves in the direction of the fibres. Consequently, this alignment facilitates the elongation of neurites along the scaffold. In addition, if the nanofibres are conductive, they can provide electrical stimulation to the nerve cells, supporting their growth, differentiation, and directional guidance. This electrical stimulation further enhances the alignment and elongation of neurites along the scaffold. Studies showing that electrically conductive scaffolds encourage stem cells to adopt the neural differentiation pathway are quite abundant in the research literature. Carbon nanomaterials such as CNTs and mixtures of conductive polymers such as PANI, polypyrrole (Ppy) and poly(3,4-ethylenedioxythiophene) (PEDOT) have been used as electrically conductive elements in cardiac tissue engineering. In the study by Babaie *et al* in which PEDOT was added to PVA (as indicated by the numbers following the PEDOT in figure 3.22), it was shown that mesenchymal stem cells cultured in tissue scaffolds containing 1% PEDOT showed higher metabolic activity compared with other sample groups and that electrical stimulation increased neural differentiation markers (figure 3.22) [136].

Another study showed that linearly aligned PLA nanofibres with various nanoporous surface structures can be used as a promising material approach in tissue engineering, especially for neuro-regeneration; such fibres also inhibit bacterial colonisation. It has been reported that neural stem cells are more prone to migrate onto aligned fibres with small ellipsoid roughness, but increases in proliferation and differentiation develop as the pore size increases, which has been induced by the ambient humidity ratio (figure 3.23) [137].

3.5.2 Drug delivery

Electrohydrodynamic production methods are preferred because of their fast, easy, economical, and adjustable properties in fibre and particle production. Due to their advantageous features and their ability to produce at the microscale and the nanoscale, EHD systems have the potential to achieve widespread use. Their low sizes, high surface areas, and layered structures also allow the fibre and particle structures produced by EHD to be used as drug delivery systems. The fact that the EHD technique offers the opportunity to work with numerous polymers also allows for the diversification of the drugs or active substances used in drug delivery systems.

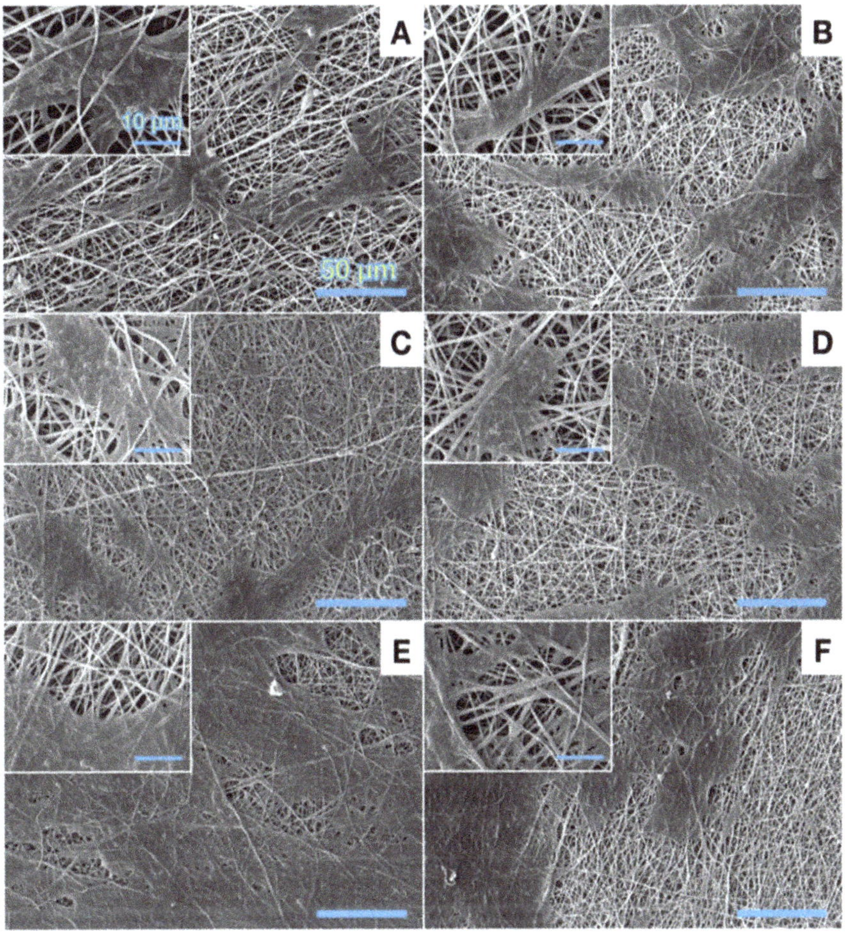

Figure 3.22. SEM micrographs of electrospun nanofibre–cell interaction after seven days of incubation: (a) PVA, (b) PVA/PEDOT(0.1 wt%), (c) PVA/PEDOT(0.3 wt%), (d) PVA/PEDOT(0.6 wt%), (e) PVA/PEDOT(1 wt%), and (f) PVA/PEDOT(3). Scale bars = 50 μm (mains) and 10 μm (inlets). Reprinted from [136], Copyright (2020), with permission from Elsevier.

The hydrophilicity or hydrophobicity of a drug affects its solubility, the solvent environment, and thus loading capacity and encapsulation efficiency. The wide variety of polymer–solvent pairs that can be used with EHD makes it possible to design systems containing active substances for a wide range of use cases, ranging from antibiotics, anticancer drugs, growth factors, and proteins to genetic material (DNA, RNA, etc.) and metal particles [11, 138].

Nano- and microfibre production is the most frequent use of EHD systems. Among the important parameters in the design of drug delivery fibre systems produced with EHD are the drug–polymer-solvent compatibility, the biological application, and the biological area. In addition, the method of application of the produced fibre also affects the release mechanism. The release mechanisms of fibres

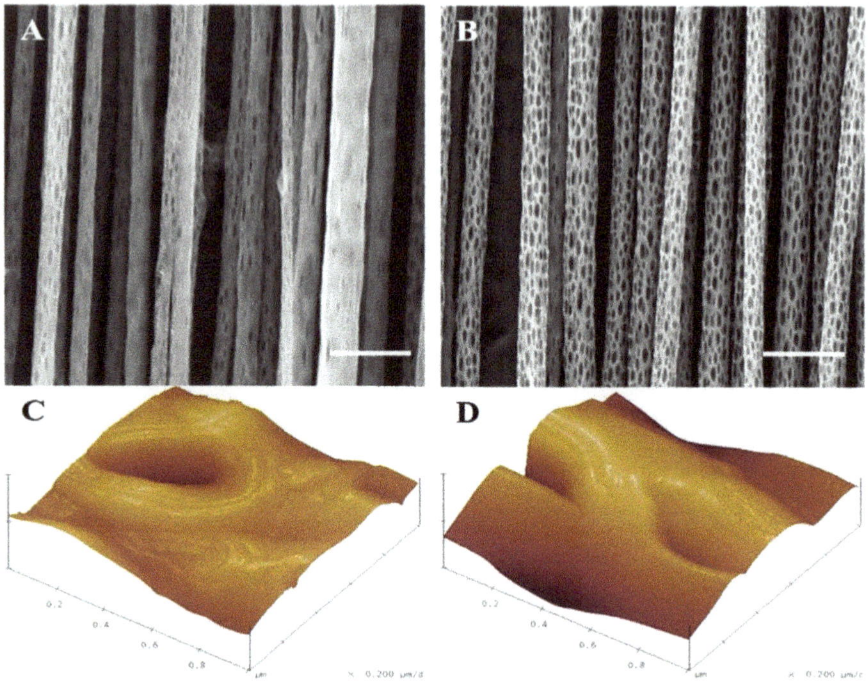

Figure 3.23. Electrospun PLA fibres: (a) SEM micrographs (scale bar = 5μm), and (b) atomic force microscopy (AFM) micrographs at 40% and 70% ambient humidity, respectively. Reproduced from [137]. CC BY 4.0.

in topical, transdermal, transmucosal, submucosal, and other application areas depend on the application site as well as the solubility and degradation characteristics of the drug and the polymer type [139, 140]. Because of this, the characteristics of the application site (temperature, presence of inflammation, type and amount of drug, etc.) also affect the release mechanism.

In drug-releasing nanofibre applications, the drug release mechanism can occur by diffusion or the degradation of the polymer. The release profiles used in controlled drug release, which are affected by diffusion and the degradation rate of the polymer, are grouped into four main categories. These nanofibre controlled drug release mechanisms are known as immediate, prolonged, biphasic, and stimulus-activated drug release (figure 3.24) [141].

In the immediate drug release profile, after the rapid burst effect is observed, the amount of drug released is then constant. In the prolonged release profile, the drug is released over a longer time frame. In biphasic drug release, fast (immediate) release is followed by slow (prolonged) release; this is a release type commonly observed in multilayered structures. On the other hand, in stimulus-activated drug release systems, no release profile is observed in the absence of a stimulus effect, whereas a rapid release profile is observed in the presence of a stimulus. When the stimulus is removed, the release mechanism is stopped. Stimulus-sensitive release can be performed in a thermoresponsive, pH-responsive, or electro-responsive manner.

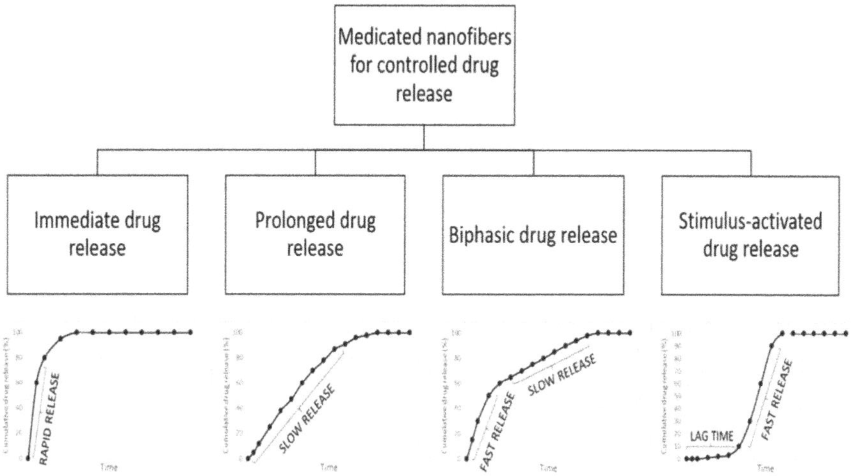

Figure 3.24. Nanofibre drug release classification according to drug release profile. Reprinted from [141], Copyright (2019), with permission from Elsevier.

In addition to the polymer and drug properties used, the method used to produce fibre structures also affects drug release mechanisms. Co-electrospinning is the simplest production strategy for drug-loaded fibres. This method relies on dissolving the drug and the polymer in the same solution and spinning it using a single-nozzle spinneret. The product includes the fibre-drug blend, and the release is performed by simple diffusion from the bulk fibre structure.

In a study, Xue *et al* produced blended metronidazole (MNA)-loaded PCL and gelatine fibres for antibacterial bone tissue engineering. PCL, gelatine, and MNA were dissolved in a common solvent (a methanol, trifluoroethanol, and acetic acid mixture). MNA-loaded hybrid fibres are an example of the simple diffusion mechanism. The fibre membrane production was performed by electrospinning using a single-needle spinning setup. The drug encapsulation efficiency reached a maximum of 93.6% and an anti-inflammatory response was observed in both *in vitro* antibacterial tests and *in vivo* histological haematoxylin and eosin (H&E) stains [142].

In another strategy, polymer nanofibres are produced and the drug is loaded into the fibres by physical absorption or chemical immobilisation. In the physical absorption of drug into the fibres, release occurs by simple diffusion (figure 3.25) [143]. On the other hand, chemically immobilised drugs need the linker between the drug and fibre to be cleaved in order for drug release to occur [144]. Immobilisation of the drug on the polymer surface may be preferable when there are common solvent incompatibility conditions between the drug and the polymer [143].

Multilayer fibre structures can be produced by core–axial and layer-by-layer electrospinning techniques. The effect of these techniques on drug release mechanisms is that they can help to produce prolonged or biphasic release profiles that prevent

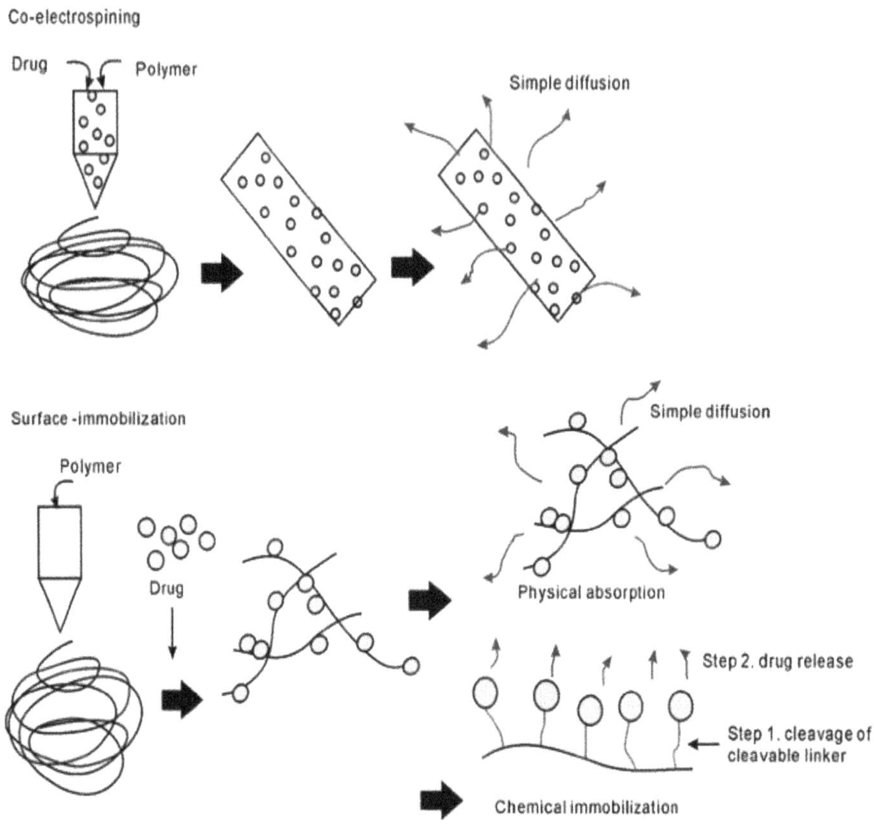

Figure 3.25. Illustrative representations of simple diffusion-based drug release from nanofibres produced using co-electrospinning and surface immobilisation techniques to load drug into the fibre structure. Reprinted by permission from Springer Nature [143], Copyright (2014).

immediate release. In addition, double-effect treatment applications can be provided by loading different drugs into each layer of the multilayer structure (figure 3.26) [143]. The prolonged and biphasic release mechanisms are also induced by blending drug-loaded nanoparticles into the polymer solution prior to electrospinning (figure 3.27). Studies have described hydrogels with tissue-like water-holding capacity that are surrounded by nanofibres with hydrogels, which can be used to control and prolong the release and penetration of the drug into the tissue. In a study by Liu *et al*, doxorubicin hydrochloride (DOX)-loaded poly(l-lactide-co-ε-caprolactone)/gelatine core–shell fibres were produced by a coaxial spinneret as shown in figure 3.28. The fibre diameters and release kinetics were evaluated by varying the loaded drug concentration (0.5, 1.5, 2.0, and 2.5%) (figure 3.29). The DOX was loaded into the core layer and the sustained release profile was prolonged for up to 480 h. It was determined that the release kinetics of DOX from nanofibres was compatible with the Fickian diffusion mechanism and the Ritger–Peppas model [145].

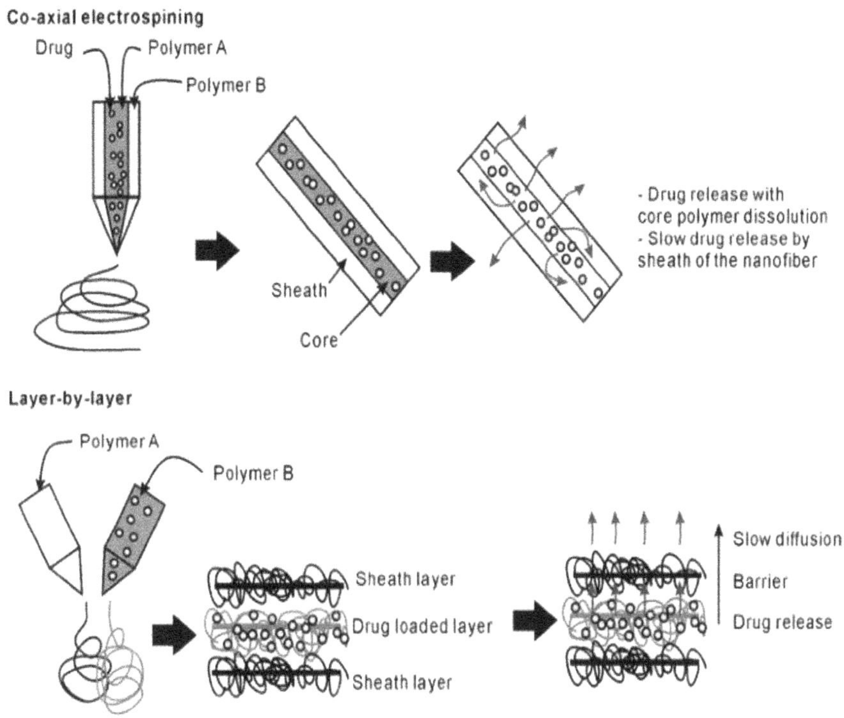

Figure 3.26. An illustrative representation of drug-loaded core–shell and layer-by-layer nanofibre production methods and drug release strategies. Reprinted by permission from Springer Nature [143], Copyright (2014).

3.5.3 Wound dressings

Since the skin is our largest organ and has a high surface area that covers the body, it is most exposed to acute or chronic injuries. Therefore, the need for wound dressings is always evolving. Although it is expected that a dressing material will meet the specific requirements of the area it is applied to, it should be able to permit the passage of oxygen and water vapour, thereby helping to maintain the optimum moisture balance of the wound area. It should also have adequate mechanical properties; for example, it should be conformable around moving joints and have a high enough tensile strength to resist deformation. Remarkable skin treatments are available, such as wound dressings, transdermal regenerations, and cosmetics due to the porosity, permeability, and mechanical strength of nonwoven nanofibre mats obtained by electrospinning.

Studies of wound healing and its development are increasing daily. Nanofibre structures can be used to produce porous mats with small fibre diameters and large surface areas. These structures, which allow for the protection of moisture balance and oxygen transfer, also act as barriers against the risk of infection that can be induced by external effects. They can also provide drainage by absorbing and removing the exudate that may occur in the wound area. In addition to their physical functions, they can prevent infection through the use of antibacterial agents

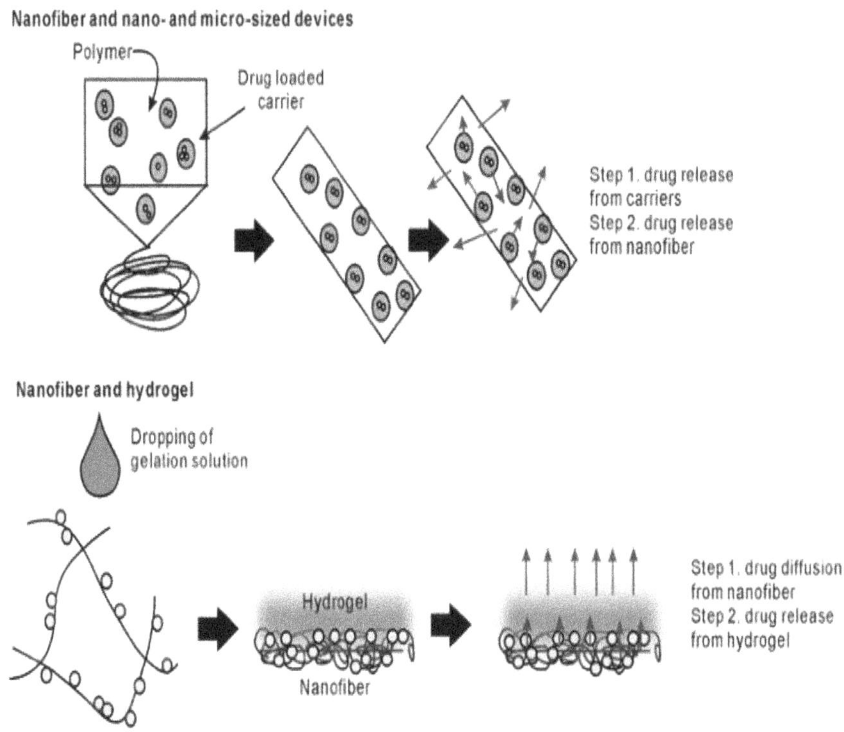

Figure 3.27. A schematic representation of the production of drug-loaded nanofibre hybrid systems via drug-loaded carrier blending and hydrogel coating strategies. Reprinted by permission from Springer Nature [143], Copyright (2014).

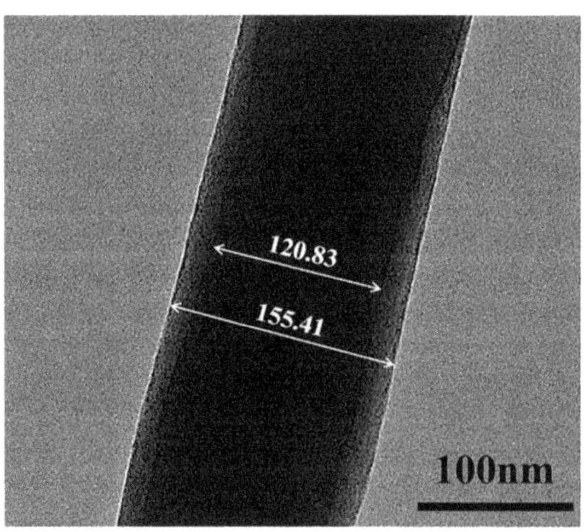

Figure 3.28. A TEM micrograph of a DOX/PLCL/GE (2.5%) nanofibre [145] John Wiley & Sons. [2023].

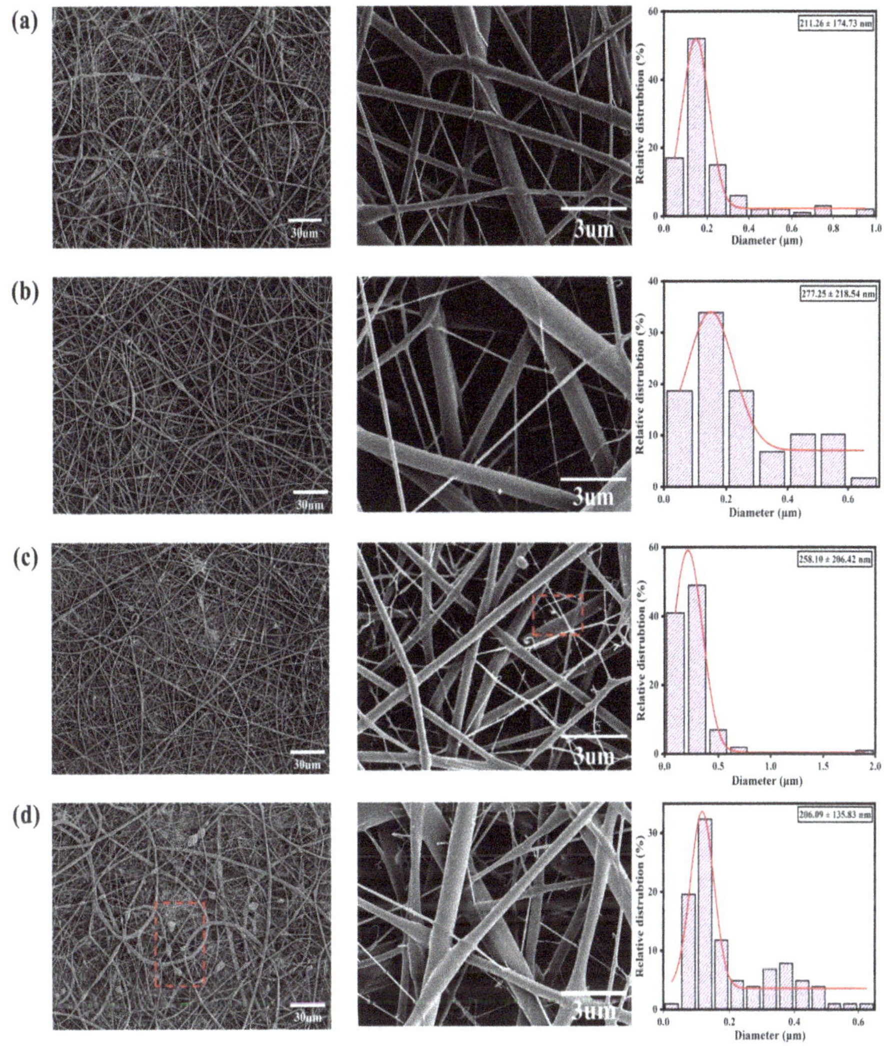

Figure 3.29. SEM micrographs and the size distribution graphs of PLCL/GE nanofibres with different DOX loading rates: (a) 0.5%, (b) 1.5% (c) 2.0%, and (d) 2.5% [145] John Wiley & Sons. [2023].

that can be loaded into the fibre structure and can induce cell regeneration through the use of growth factors.

In studies that aim to add antibacterial properties to nanofibre dressings, the most popular approach is silver ion and tetracycline loading; however, prednisolone-loaded nanofibres are preferred for anti-inflammatory purposes. On the other hand, anti-oxidant and anti-inflammatory activities are obtained by loading natural substances such as curcumin onto fibres. Various studies have loaded fibres with epidermal growth factor (EGF), vascular endothelial growth factor (VEGF), and transforming growth factor (TGF) in tissue engineering applications (figure 3.30) [146].

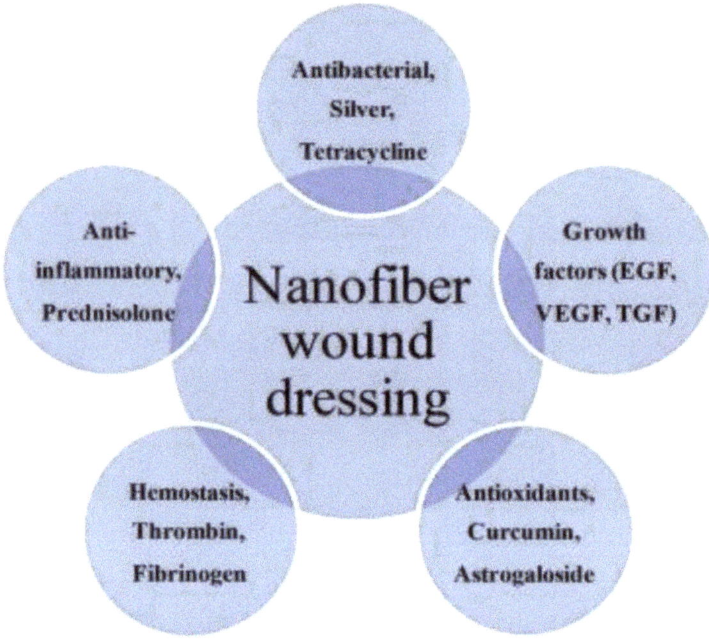

Figure 3.30. The classification of nanofibre-based wound-dressing materials in terms of biological efficiency and the loaded active ingredient. Reprinted from [146], Copyright (2017), with permission from Elsevier.

In the production of antibacterial wound dressings, many molecules are loaded into the structure through blending, immobilisation, or impregnation. In a study, Sofokleous *et al* produced amoxicillin-loaded PLGA fibres for wound-dressing applications [147]. In addition to antibiotics, one of the antibacterial agents most frequently used for antibacterial wound dressings is silver (Ag) [148–150]. When silver is used in a dose-controlled manner, it is a biocompatible molecule with antibacterial activity against both Gram-negative and Gram-positive bacterial species. In addition, Ag is preferred to antibiotics since it does not develop bacterial resistance.

In one particular study, Dubey and co-workers produced poly(ethylene oxide (PEO))–PCL blended nanofibres by electrospinning. In addition, AgNPs were loaded into the PEO–PCL solution to produce antibacterial nanofibre wound dressings (figure 3.31) [150]. The synthesis of the AgNPs was conducted using the solvent N,N-dimethylformamide, which was used as both a solvent for the polymers and a reducing agent for the Ag (average size:15–20 nm). The average size distributions of the nanofibres were calculated to be 224.4±74.2 nm for the PEO–PCL and 116.6±26.8 nm for the AgNP/PEO–PCL nanofibres. Antibacterial disc diffusion assay results showed that increasing AgNP concentrations showed higher antibacterial efficiency against antibiotic-resistant *Escherichia coli* bacteria species (figure 3.32).

In a 2019 study by Zhang *et al*, chitosan (CS):PVA nanofibre 2D membranes were produced by electrospinning and layered as 3D nanofibre sponges to induce blood

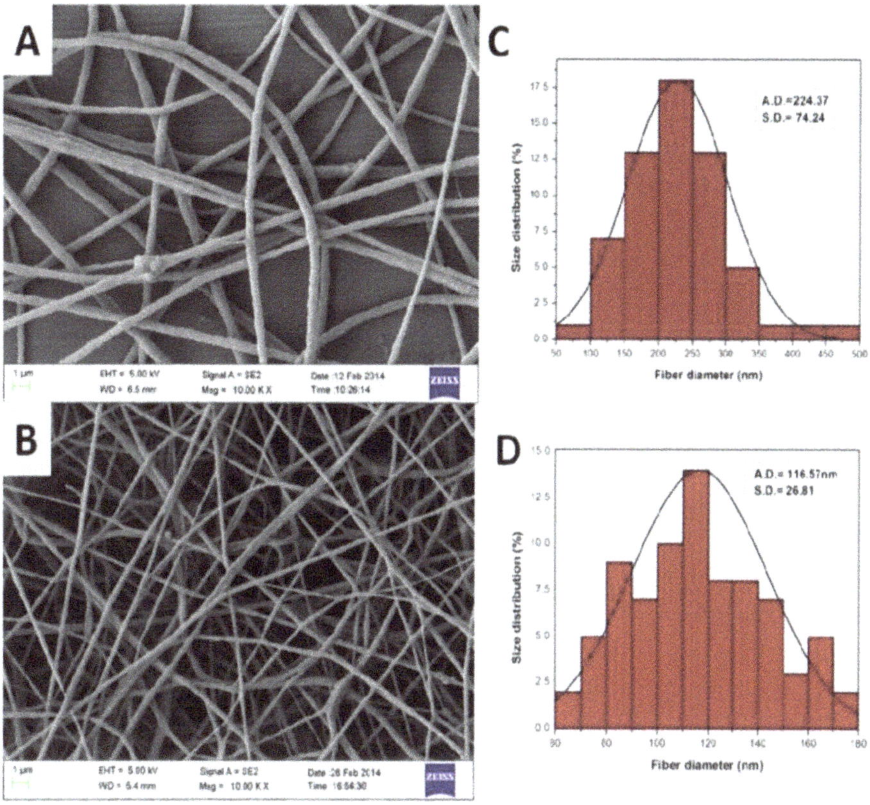

Figure 3.31. SEM micrographs of (a) PEO–PCL and (b) AgNP/PEO–PCL nanofibres. Size distribution histograms of (c) PEO–PCL and (d) AgNP/PEO–PCL nanofibres. (A.D.:average diameter; S.D.: standard deviation) [150] John Wiley & Sons. [2015].

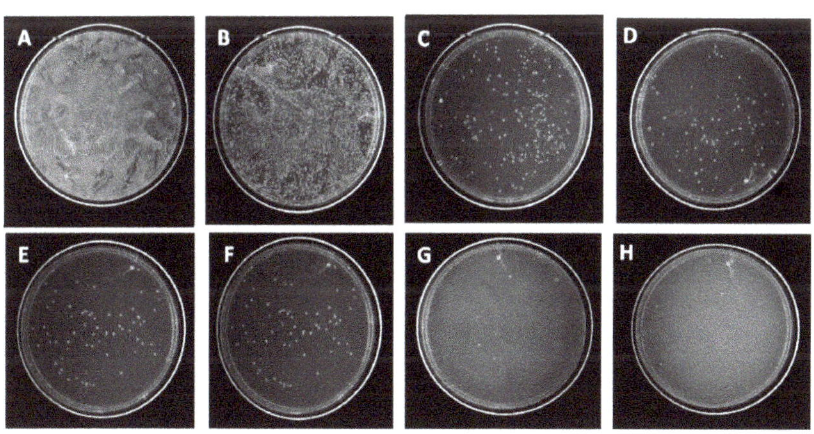

Figure 3.32. Optical images of antibacterial agar diffusion tests using antibiotic-resistant green fluorescent protein-expressing *E. coli*: (a) PEO–PCL nanofibres and (b-h) AgNP/PEO–PCL nanofibres with increasing AgNP concentrations (0 mg, 1 mg, 2 mg, 4 mg, 6 mg, 7 mg, 8 mg, and 10 mg) [150]. John Wiley & Sons. [2015].

coagulation and wound healing. The results showed that 3D CS-PVA nanofibre sponges exhibited high water retention and blood coagulation with high mechanical resistance, elasticity, and integrity upon wetting (figure 3.33). In addition, the 3D nanofibre sponges also reduced the scarring area compared to control and 2D fibres, which reduced collagen III deposition. Cell proliferation also took place in a more controlled manner in the 3D nanofibre sponges. After the seventh day, the cell proliferation rate decreased in the 3D nanofibre sponges, but scar formation was greater in the control and 2D fibres because high-speed proliferation continued

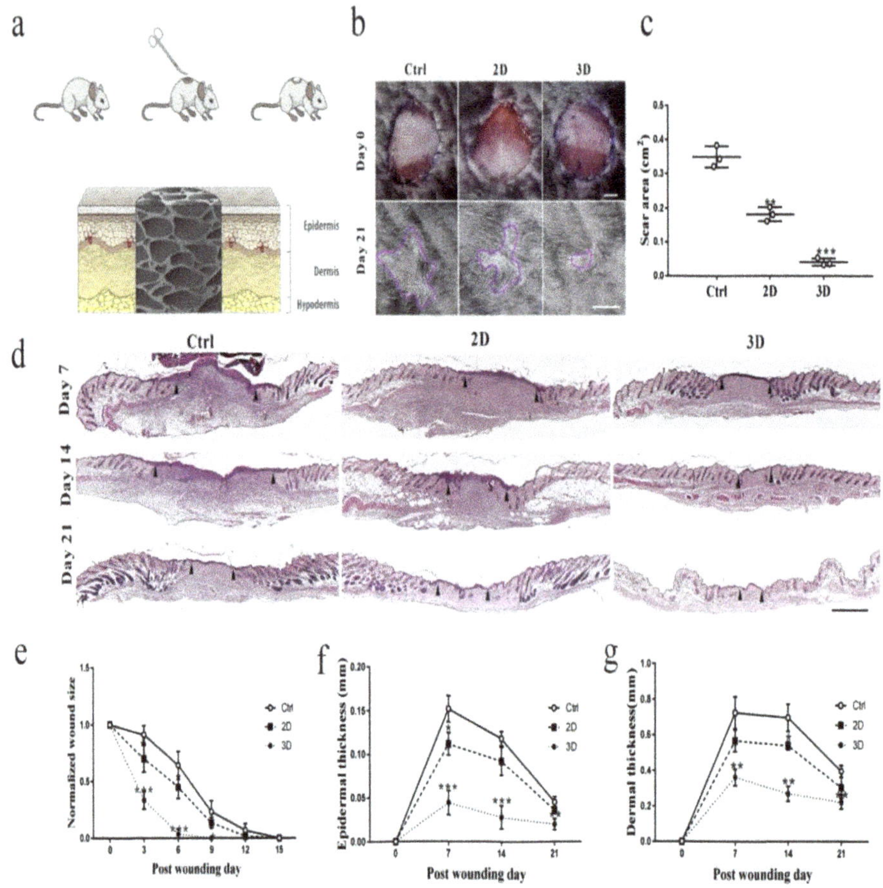

Figure 3.33. The performance of CS:PVA 3D nanofibre sponges in wound healing. (a) An illustrative image of the CS:PVA 3D nanofibre sponge in the full-thickness skin model. (b) Optical images of wound healing and scar formation on days zero and 21 for the full-thickness wound model on mice for the control group, the 2D fibre membrane, and the 3D nanofibre sponge (scale bar = 2.5 mm). (c) Scar size distributions for the control group, the 2D fibre membrane, and the 3D nanofibre sponge. (d) H&E staining of regenerated tissue for the control group, the 2D fibre membrane and the 3D nanofibre sponge at 7, 14, and 21 days (scale bar = 1 mm). (e–g) Wound size distribution graphs at different time points for normalised wound, epidermal, and dermal thicknesses, respectively (*$p < 0.05$, **$p < 0.01$, and ***$p < 0.001$ vs. control). Reprinted from [151], Copyright (2019), with permission from Elsevier.

in them. The *in vitro* cell culture results were supported by *in vivo* animal experiment results, and the 3D nanofibre sponges were found to be promising for clinical study [151].

3.5.4 Implant modification

In addition to their use as the abovementioned biodegradable materials in tissue scaffolds or dressings, the deposition of nanofibre structures on biomaterials' surfaces by electrospinning for biomimetic modification is a relatively new approach. The first studies of this new approach, which is carried out for both nanoscale modification and biochemical activation of the surface, date back to the early 2010s. Using this approach, it is possible to imitate nanofibrillar proteins, which are found in the structure of native tissues, mainly collagen structures [152]. Electrospinning also allows for the incorporation of bioactive molecules, such as growth factors or drugs, into the scaffold structure. These molecules can be encapsulated within the fibres or surface functionalised, enabling controlled release and localised delivery to support cellular functions and enhance tissue regeneration [153].

Electrospun nanofibre structures were formed to modify the titanium (Ti) surfaces of implants that are frequently used in hard-tissue applications, and the relevant cell phenotypes and stem cell differentiations were tested on these surfaces. In these studies, which aimed to increase the biomimetic property of the surface (i.e. its ability to imitate natural tissues), biopolymers were used as ECM analogues. PLGA, PCL, PLA, and SF have been used for surface functionalisation achieved via electrospinning [154, 155].

The periodic arrangement of hydroxyapatite nanocrystals and collagen fibres plays an important role in the hierarchical structure of bone. SF is frequently employed as a collagen analogue in tissue engineering because of its long-term stability, biodegradability, and good mechanical properties, along with its spatial similarity to collagen. Bayram *et al* reported the surface modification of Ti surfaces with electrospun silk nanofibres to increase the biomimetic property of an implant. As a result of this study, it was observed that the presence of the electrospun SF nanofibres increased alkaline phosphatase (ALP) activity and calcium accumulation, which are the leading indicators of early osteointegration, and resulted in more cell adhesion and proliferation compared to those of the control group (figure 3.34) [155].

An important developmental stage in bone healing is the formation of apatitic calcium phosphates. The acceleration of this stage, and therefore early healing, can be enabled by a bioactive implant surface. After examining the deposition of mineralisation-inducing nanofibre structures on titanium substrates, Abdal-hay *et al* reported that apatitic calcium phosphates were seen in the samples coated with PCL/PLA after they were kept in simulated body fluid but no mineralisation was observed for the control groups [156]. Another case study in which mineralisation increased was reported by Ravichadran *et al*; it similarly confirmed that a nanofibre surface morphology increased intracellular mineralisation. In this study, which used human stem cells, PLGA and PLGA/collagen hybrid nanofibre structures were found on the surface [154].

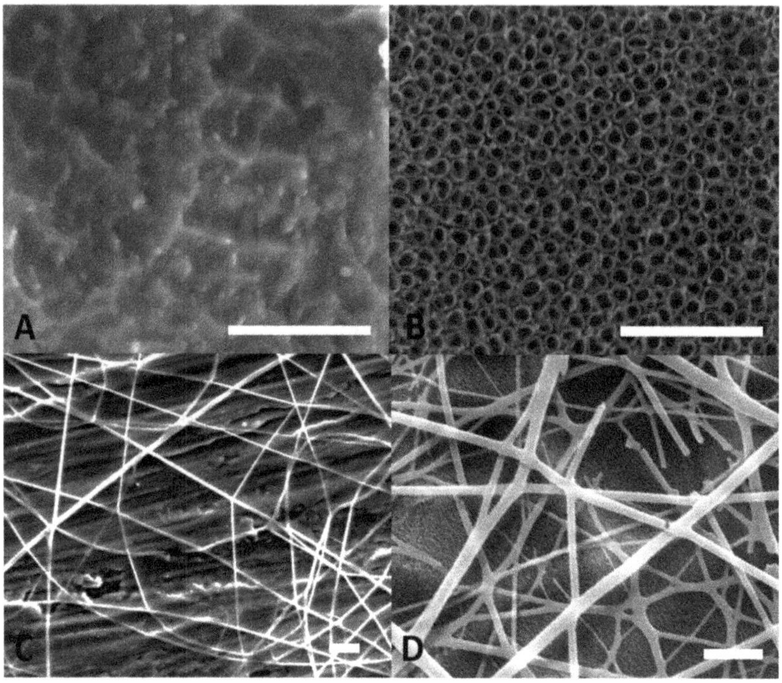

Figure 3.34. SEM micrographs of (a) an unanodized Ti surface, (b) an anodised titanium surface with individual 45 nm nanotubes, (c and d) unanodized and anodised Ti surfaces, respectively, with 350–400 nm nanofibre SF (scale bar = 1 μm). Reprinted from [155], Copyright (2014), with permission from Elsevier.

In addition to studies in which the tissue healing time was accelerated and ossification was induced, many studies have also investigated the preparation of antibacterial surfaces using electrospun fibres. Although these studies [157, 158] previously focused on the use of small molecules and drugs with antimicrobial effects as an inhibitor of infection in the local area by confirming delayed release properties, studies of coatings that physiochemically prevent bacterial attachment and biofilm formation have been more dominant due to the discovery of bacterial mutations that are resistant to antibacterial agents over time. The basis of these coatings is in their hydrophilic nature, which are used to reduce the protein adsorption that plays a role in bacterial binding pathways. Since it is known that extremely hydrophilic surfaces inhibit cell adhesion along with bacterial adhesion, Şimşek *et al* proposed a surface coating that consisted of crosslinked polyethylene oxide electrospun nanofibres in a study published in 2019. Although it was observed that the presence of *S. aureus* decreased significantly on nanofibre-coated rough surfaces compared to the control group, the study concluded that highly hydrophilic surfaces also reduced osteoblast adhesion (figure 3.35) [159].

In addition to their biological uses, such as biologically mimicking the ECM, increasing the surface area in a biomimetic way, or mediating the release of a bioactive organic compound, nanofibre coatings can also be applied to protect medical devices from chemical reactions.

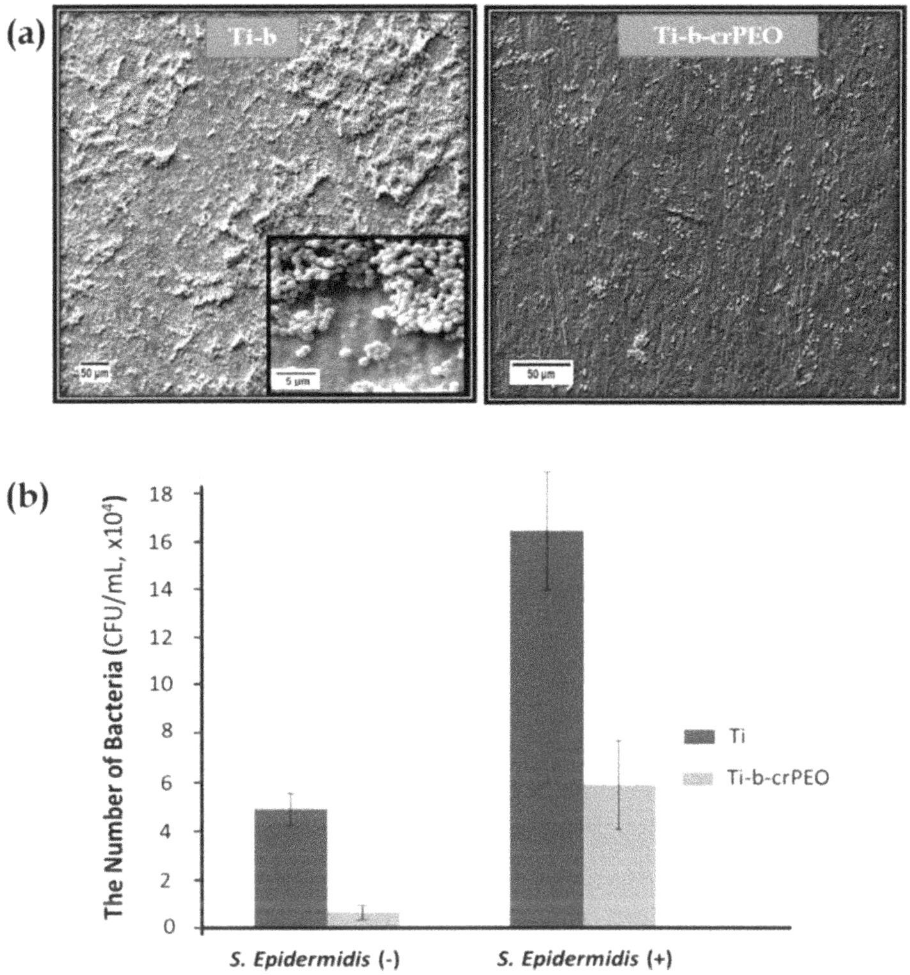

Figure 3.35. The antibacterial activity of polyethylene oxide nanofibres: (a) SEM micrographs of bacterial species on fibre surfaces (scale bar = 50μm), (b) the number of adhered bacteria. Reprinted by permission from Springer Nature [159], Copyright (2019).

Implant success may decrease as a result of undesirable reactions such as corrosion, oxidation, and the release of metal ions that may occur between an implant and the tissues in the area where it is used (figure 3.36) [160, 161]. As a result of the corrosion of a biomaterial that has both mechanical and biological functions, implant failure may occur before the tissue heals. Here, anticorrosion coatings can also be applied via electrospinning in the form of nanofibres to prevent these scenarios that are likely to occur with titanium alloy implants [162].

These anticorrosion coatings can be made from biocompatible and biodegradable polymeric nanofibres which can retain their form for the first few weeks (this is especially critical in implant applications). After a few weeks, these fibres disappear,

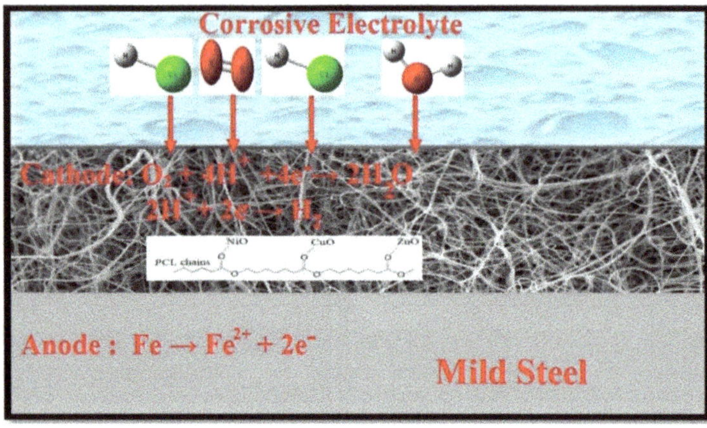

Figure 3.36. Illustrative representation of a nanofibre-based anticorrosion strategy implemented using PCL/ZnO-NiO-CuO coatings. Reprinted from [160], Copyright (2020), with permission from Elsevier.

which accompanies the appearance of healthy tissue. To evaluate the corrosion performance, PCL and ZnO, NiO, and CuO nanofibres were electrospun onto steel surfaces, and corrosion inhibition of up to 95% was obtained due to the presence of ohmic resistance coatings [160].

3.5.5 Surface patterning

Although lithography and its derivatives are accepted as the gold standard in surface patterning, alternative approaches are needed due to lithography's strict working conditions, device infrastructure, and materials with limited applicability that can be used in the relevant techniques. Electrohydrodynamic direct writing is a technique that can be used to write structures in nanofibre form directly onto a substrate in a continuous and controllable manner, offering a high-efficiency and cost-effective solution. It combines techniques such as dip-pen, inkjet, and electrospinning for fabrication at the micrometre and submicrometre scales, overcoming the disadvantages of expensive lithographic techniques that involve relatively slow, complex methodology.

Electrohydrodynamic direct writing allows the printing resolution and pattern positioning flexibility to be easily adjusted via the motion of a digitally controlled sub-table, the distance from the nozzle to the sub-table, and the applied voltage. Therefore, it is a highly versatile and low-cost method for the development of large-scale flexible/stretchable bio-electronics and the direct writing of materials to form soft sensors [99, 163]. In recent years, remarkable progress has been made in sensor systems for the collection of real-time data through the use of miniaturised, low-cost, high-performance, flexible wearable devices produced using flexible and soft bio-electronics technologies. Compared to lithography, which requires a clean room and a complex production process, printing methods have many advantages such as low cost, good reproducibility, and easy procedures. Non-stencil printing methods include inkjet and 3D printing techniques. The fabrication technology used in the stencil-based methods is highly dependent on the printing inks that can be deposited in the substrate layers to form the target pattern. Template-free printing methods include a range of advanced technologies such as piezoelectric, pneumatic, and electrohydrodynamic printing. Electrohydrodynamic printing, a subfield of electrospinning and electrospraying, has recently been used in the high-resolution micro/nanofabrication of minimally invasive electronics and particularly for biomedical device fabrication such as bio-electrodes (figures 3.37 and 3.38) [164, 165]. It also has enormous potential for applications in supercapacitors [166], field-effect transistors [167], etc. These micro/nanofibres composed of electrically conductive, semiconducting, photoelectric, piezoelectric, or dielectric materials or their composite structures have been extensively investigated for use as light emitters, energy harvesters, supercapacitors, and sensors [168–170].

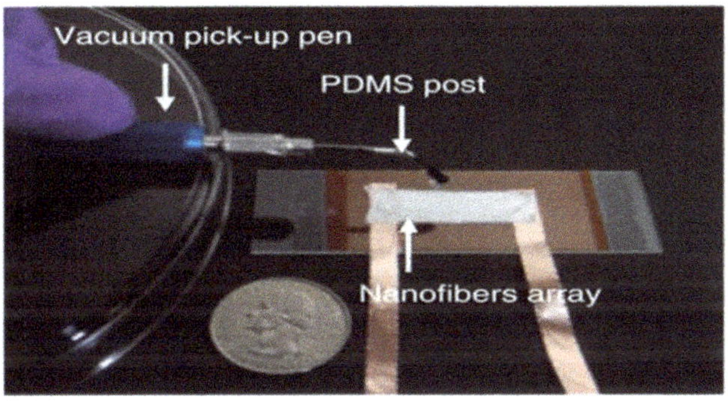

Figure 3.37. A photograph of a nanofibre-decorated pressure sensor setup. Reprinted by permission from Springer Nature [164], Copyright (2013).

By directly writing electrically active micro/nanofibres onto flexible substrates at ambient conditions, it is possible to fabricate low-cost, flexible/stretchable electronics without the use of conventional photolithographic processes. The direct writing of smooth microstructures using viscous inks has received considerable attention for use in flexible/stretchable electronics [83, 98, 167]. By adjusting the processing parameters (e.g. the electrospinning voltage, electrospinning distance, and substrate speed), the helical motion of the jet formed in the spinning head can be controlled and complex circuit patterns with different geometries can be written on the substrate. As a result of the rapid development of electronic skin studies, organic/inorganic materials [171, 172], polymer composite materials [173], hybrid composite materials [174], and nanomaterial components [175] have been tested extensively. Nanomaterial-based applications were investigated by Cai and co-workers [175]: here, silver nanowires (AgNWs) were directly printed on different substrates (Si wafer, glass slide, polyimide film, and very high bond tape) to obtain highly stretchable and conductive sensors (figure 3.39).

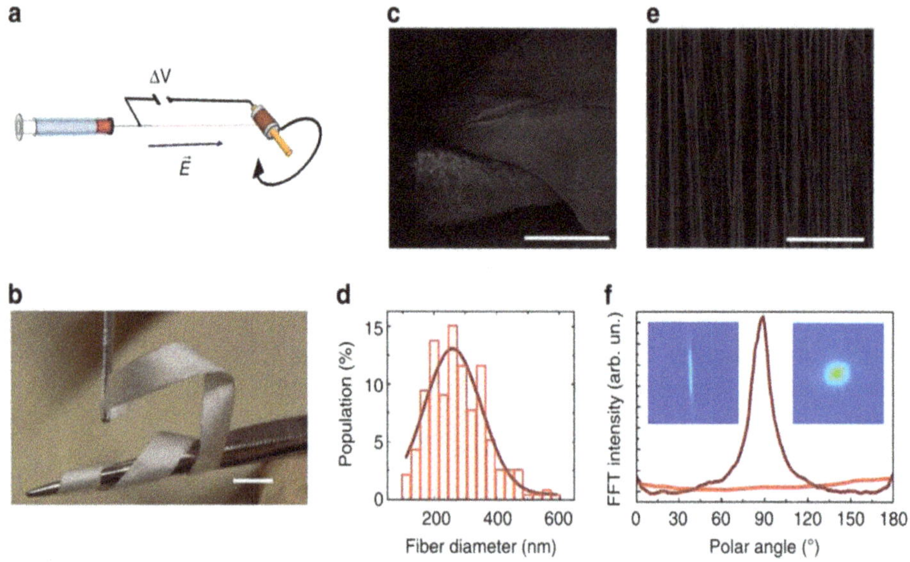

Figure 3.38. Piezoelectric poly[(vinylidenefluoride)-co-trifluoroethylene] nanofibres: (a) setup, (b) a photograph of a film structure composed of aligned nanofibres (scale bar = 1 cm), (c) an SEM micrograph of a folded nanofibre, (d) a size distribution graph for nanofibres, (scale bar = 400μm), (e) an SEM micrograph of highly aligned nanofibres (scale bar = 10μm), and (f) intensity/polar angle distributions for aligned and non-aligned fibres. Reprinted by permission from Springer Nature [164], Copyright (2013).

3.6 Perspectives on the future development of electrohydrodynamic technology

EHD is an important fabrication technique that is based on the manipulation of an electrical field and solution flow components. It has a wide product range that extends to particles, microbubbles, fibres, and patterned combinations. The diverse nature of the physicochemical properties of the materials used also provides the ability to manipulate the optimisation step of production. Precise control of the parameters used gives the produced structures unique features such as repeatability and a narrow size distribution. Materials produced using the EHDA technique support a wide variety of applications including drug delivery systems, tissue engineering products, filtration membranes, wound dressings, implant surface modifications, patterning studies, and even wearable electronics. On the other hand, it is known that particle-, bubble-, and fibre-based biofabrication products produced using EHD still have a low production rate, making them difficult to scale industrially. The production of polymers via EHD has achieved successful results on the research and development scale. However, in order to achieve commercial success in the systems used, it is necessary to design these systems in such a way that they can produce on an industrial scale. Parameters such as the voltage and the distance to the collector used when producing in low quantities require different optimisation conditions for industrial production. At the same time, as the layer thickness of the fibres accumulated in the collector system increases, it becomes

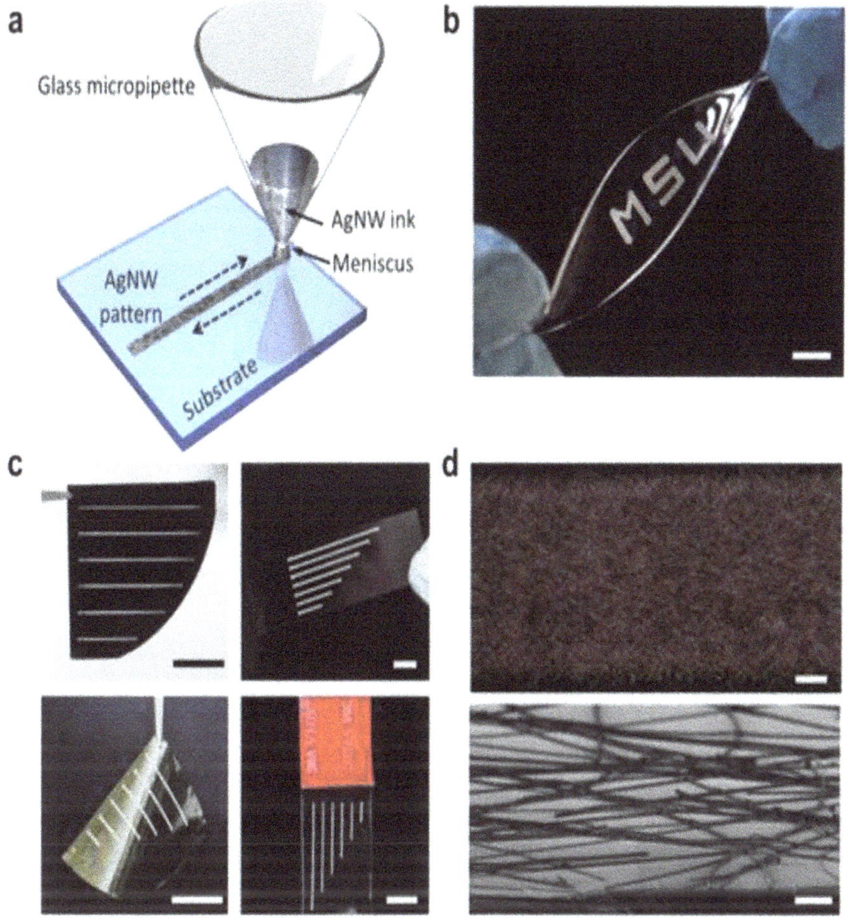

Figure 3.39. Direct printing/patterning for stretchable sensor applications based on AgNWs. (a) Illustration of the direct printing setup, (b) AgNW:PDMS (scale bar = 1 cm), (c) AgNW:Si wafer/glass slide/polyimide film/ VHB tape, respectively (scale bar = 2 cm), (d) optic image (top, scale bar = 50 μm) and SEM (bottom, scale bar = 1μm) micrographs of AgNW:Si wafer [175] John Wiley & Sons. [2018].

harder to maintain the potential difference. For these reasons, customised production condition improvements for the industrial-scale use of EHD systems, which offer commercialisation potential and unique advantages in applications in the biomedical field, will become a necessity in the future.

Another potential development that will be offered by EHD systems in the future is miniaturised, portable EHD guns; these have been an increasing research topic in recent years (figure 3.40) [176]. With the anticipated arrival of portable EHD guns that can operate using alkaline batteries without the need for a high-voltage source, wound-dressing applications will offer great potential in the form of personalised medical products that can be directly applied to wound areas. With these new types of devices, it will be possible in the near future to overcome the difficulties experienced in the extensive commercialisation of wound dressings.

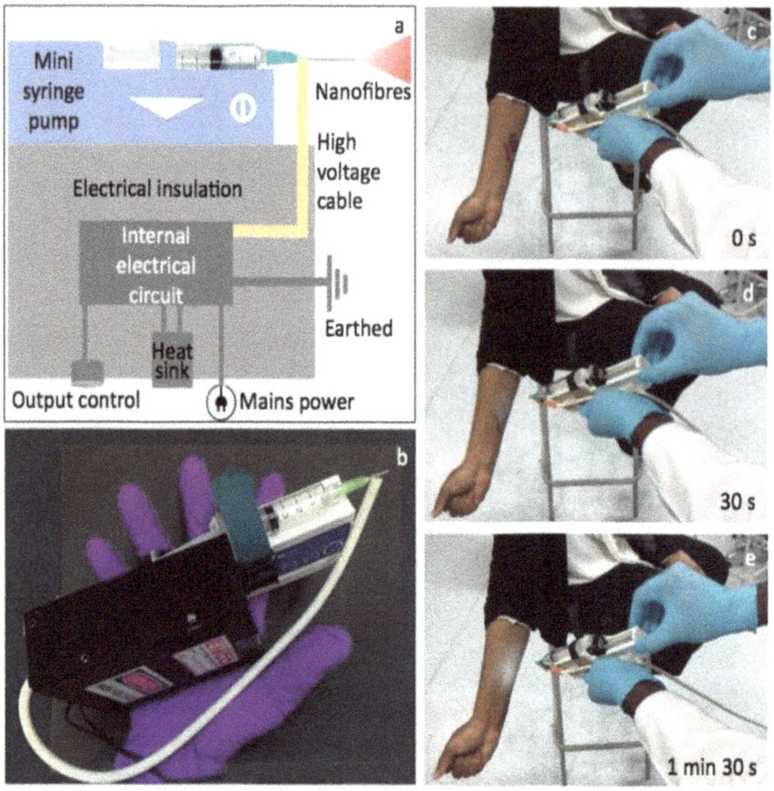

Figure 3.40. (a) An illustrative image of a portable EHD device, (b) an optical image of a handheld portable EHD device, and (c–e) photographs of the *in situ* application of a portable EHD device over a period of time. Reproduced from [176]. CC BY 4.0.

References

[1] Park J-U, Hardy M, Kang S J, Barton K, Adair K, Mukhopadhyay D K, Lee C Y, Strano M S, Alleyne A G and Georgiadis J G 2007 High-resolution electrohydrodynamic jet printing *Nat. Mater.* **6** 782–9

[2] Cloupeau M and Prunet-Foch B 1994 Electrohydrodynamic spraying functioning modes: a critical review *J. Aerosol Sci.* **25** 1021–36

[3] Lim L-T, Mendes A C and Chronakis I S 2019 Electrospinning and electrospraying technologies for food applications *Adv. Food Nutr. Res.* **88** 167–234

[4] Rayleigh L 1917 VIII. On the pressure developed in a liquid during the collapse of a spherical cavity *Lond., Edinb., Dublin Philos. Mag. J. Sci.* **34** 94–8

[5] Rayleigh L 1879 On the capillary phenomena of jets *Proc. R. Soc. London* **29** 71–97

[6] Taylor G I 1953 Dispersion of soluble matter in solvent flowing slowly through a tube *Proc. Roy. Soc. Lond.* A **219** 186–203

[7] Davies R and Taylor G I 1950 The mechanics of large bubbles rising through extended liquids and through liquids in tubes *Proc. R. Soc. Lond.* A **200** 375–90

[8] Taylor G I 1964 Disintegration of water drops in an electric field *Proc. R. Soc. Lond.* A **280** 383–97

[9] Fernández de La Mora J 2007 The fluid dynamics of Taylor cones *Annu. Rev. Fluid Mech.* **39** 217–43

[10] Kang Y, Wang C, Qiao Y, Gu J, Zhang H, Peijs T, Kong J, Zhang G and Shi X 2019 Tissue-engineered trachea consisting of electrospun patterned scPLA/GO-g-IL fibrous membranes with antibacterial property and 3D-printed skeletons with elasticity *Biomacromolecules* **20** 1765–76

[11] Zamani M, Prabhakaran M P and Ramakrishna S 2013 Advances in drug delivery via electrospun and electrosprayed nanomaterials *Int. J. Nanomed.* **8** 2997–3017

[12] Shin J, Lee W H, Nothnagle C and Wijesundara M B 2014 EHD as sensor fabrication technology for robotic skins *Proc. SPIE* **9116** 91160F

[13] Vu T-H, Nguyen H T, Fastier-Wooller J W, Tran C-D, Nguyen T-H, Nguyen H-Q, Nguyen T, Nguyen T-K, Dinh T and Bui T T 2022 Enhanced electrohydrodynamics for electrospinning a highly sensitive flexible fiber-based piezoelectric sensor *ACS Appl. Electron. Mater.* **4** 1301–10

[14] Han Y and Dong J 2018 Electrohydrodynamic (EHD) printing of molten metal ink for flexible and stretchable conductor with self-healing capability *Adv. Mater. Technol.* **3** 1700268

[15] Gungordu S, Kelly E A, Jayasuriya S B W and Edirisinghe M 2022 Nanofiber based on electrically conductive materials for biosensor applications *Biomed. Mater. Devices* 1–16

[16] Laohalertdecha S, Naphon P and Wongwises S 2007 A review of electrohydrodynamic enhancement of heat transfer *Renew. Sustain. Energy Rev.* **11** 858–76

[17] Mestel A 1994 The electrohydrodynamic cone-jet at high Reynolds number *J. Aerosol Sci.* **25** 1037–47

[18] Paschkewitz J and Pratt D 2000 The influence of fluid properties on electrohydrodynamic heat transfer enhancement in liquids under viscous and electrically dominated flow conditions *Exp. Therm Fluid Sci.* **21** 187–97

[19] Shanko E-S, van de Burgt Y, Anderson P D and den Toonder J M 2019 Microfluidic magnetic mixing at low reynolds numbers and in stagnant fluids *Micromachines* **10** 731

[20] Kirby B J 2010 *Micro-and Nanoscale Fluid Mechanics: Transport In Microfluidic Devices* (Cambridge: Cambridge University Press)

[21] Mark D, Haeberle S, Roth G, Von Stetten F and Zengerle R 2010 Microfluidic lab-on-a-chip platforms: requirements, characteristics and applications *Microfluidics Based Microsystems* (Dordrecht: Springer) pp 305–76

[22] Nikoleli G-P, Siontorou C G, Nikolelis D P, Bratakou S, Karapetis S and Tzamtzis N 2018 Biosensors based on microfluidic devices lab-on-a-chip and microfluidic technology *Nanotechnology and biosensors* (Amsterdam: Elsevier) pp 375–94

[23] Atten P, McCluskey F M and Lahjomri A C 1987 The electrohydrodynamic origin of turbulence in electrostatic precipitators *IEEE Trans. Ind. Appl.* **4** 705–11

[24] Ramos A 2007 Electrohydrodynamic and magnetohydrodynamic micropumps *Microfluidic Technologies for Miniaturized Analysis Systems* (Boston, MA: Springer) pp 59–116

[25] Stuetzer O M 1962 Magnetohydrodynamics and electrohydrodynamics *Phys. Fluids* **5** 534–44

[26] Webb G 2018 *Magnetohydrodynamics and Fluid Dynamics: Action Principles and Conservation Laws* (Berlin: Springer)

[27] Ahn C H and Choi J-W 2010 Microfluidic devices and their applications to lab-on-a-chip *Springer Handbook of Nanotechnology* (Berlin, Heidelberg: Springer) pp 503–30
[28] Constantin P and Foias C 2020 *Navier–Stokes Equations* (Chicago, IL: University of Chicago Press) https://press.uchicago.edu/ucp/books/book/chicago/N/bo5973146.html
[29] Saville D 1997 Electrohydrodynamics: the Taylor-Melcher leaky dielectric model *Annu. Rev. Fluid Mech.* **29** 27–64
[30] Castellanos A 1998 *Electrohydrodynamics* (Berlin: Springer Science & Business Media)
[31] Nezarati R M, Eifert M B and Cosgriff-Hernandez E 2013 Effects of humidity and solution viscosity on electrospun fiber morphology *Tissue Eng.* C **19** 810–9
[32] Augustine R, Kalarikkal N and Thomas S 2016 Clogging-free electrospinning of polycaprolactone using acetic acid/acetone mixture *Polym.-Plast. Technol. Eng.* **55** 518–29
[33] Jayasinghe S and Townsend-Nicholson A 2006 Stable electric-field driven cone-jetting of concentrated biosuspensions *Lab Chip* **6** 1086–90
[34] Smeets A, Clasen C and Van den Mooter G 2017 Electrospraying of polymer solutions: study of formulation and process parameters *Eur. J. Pharm. Biopharm.* **119** 114–24
[35] Ku B K and Kim S S 2002 Electrospray characteristics of highly viscous liquids *J. Aerosol Sci.* **33** 1361–78
[36] Al-Oqla F M, Sapuan S, Anwer T, Jawaid M and Hoque M 2015 Natural fiber reinforced conductive polymer composites as functional materials: a review *Synth. Met.* **206** 42–54
[37] Dang Z M, Yuan J K, Yao S H and Liao R J 2013 Flexible nanodielectric materials with high permittivity for power energy storage *Adv. Mater.* **25** 6334–65
[38] Luo C, Stride E and Edirisinghe M 2012 Mapping the influence of solubility and dielectric constant on electrospinning polycaprolactone solutions *Macromolecules* **45** 4669–80
[39] Sun Z, Deitzel J M, Knopf J, Chen X and Gillespie J W 2012 The effect of solvent dielectric properties on the collection of oriented electrospun fibers *J. Appl. Polym. Sci.* **125** 2585–94
[40] Collins G, Federici J, Imura Y and Catalani L H 2012 Charge generation, charge transport, and residual charge in the electrospinning of polymers: a review of issues and complications *J. Appl. Phys.* **111** 044701
[41] Subbiah T, Bhat G S, Tock R W, Parameswaran S and Ramkumar S S 2005 Electrospinning of nanofibers *J. Appl. Polym. Sci.* **96** 557–69
[42] Chien A-T, Cho S, Joshi Y and Kumar S 2014 Electrical conductivity and Joule heating of polyacrylonitrile/carbon nanotube composite fibers *Polymer* **55** 6896–905
[43] Theodossiou G, Nelson J, Lee M and Odell G 1988 The influence of electrohydrodynamic motion on the breakdown of dielectric liquids *J. Phys.* D **21** 45
[44] Valizadeh A and Mussa Farkhani S 2014 Electrospinning and electrospun nanofibres *IET Nanobiotechnol.* **8** 83–92
[45] Pham Q P, Sharma U and Mikos A G 2006 Electrospinning of polymeric nanofibers for tissue engineering applications: a review *Tissue Eng.* **12** 1197–211
[46] Kim M K, Lee J Y, Oh H, Song D W, Kwak H W, Yun H, Um I C, Park Y H and Lee K H 2015 Effect of shear viscosity on the preparation of sphere-like silk fibroin microparticles by electrospraying *Int. J. Biol. Macromol.* **79** 988–95
[47] Douglas J F, Gasiorek J M, Swaffield J A and Jack L B 2005 *Fluid Mechanics* (London: Pearson Education)
[48] Yang S M, Lee Y S, Jang Y, Byun D and Choa S-H 2016 Electromechanical reliability of a flexible metal-grid transparent electrode prepared by electrohydrodynamic (EHD) jet printing *Microelectron. Reliab.* **65** 151–9

[49] Ibrahim H M and Klingner A 2020 A review on electrospun polymeric nanofibers: production parameters and potential applications *Polym. Test.* **90** 106647

[50] Atik D S, Bölük E, Bildik F, Altay F, Torlak E, Kaplan A A, Kopuk B and Palabıyık İ 2022 Particle morphology and antimicrobial properties of electrosprayed propolis *Food Packag. Shelf Life* **33** 100881

[51] Nguyen D N, Clasen C and Van den Mooter G 2016 Pharmaceutical applications of electrospraying *J. Pharm. Sci.* **105** 2601–20

[52] Bair S and Winer W 1992 The high pressure high shear stress rheology of liquid lubricants *J. Tribol.* **114** 1–9

[53] Yamamoto T and Velkoff H 1981 Electrohydrodynamics in an electrostatic precipitator *J. Fluid Mech.* **108** 1–18

[54] Wagner H D and Vaia R A 2004 Nanocomposites: issues at the interface *Mater. Today* **7** 38–42

[55] Keirouz A, Chung M, Kwon J, Fortunato G and Radacsi N 2020 2D and 3D electrospinning technologies for the fabrication of nanofibrous scaffolds for skin tissue engineering: a review, *Wiley Interdiscip. Rev. Nanomed. Nanobiotechnol.* **12** e1626

[56] Coelho S C, Estevinho B N and Rocha F 2021 Encapsulation in food industry with emerging electrohydrodynamic techniques: electrospinning and electrospraying—a review *Food Chem.* **339** 127850

[57] Chakraborty S, Liao I-C, Adler A and Leong K W 2009 Electrohydrodynamics: a facile technique to fabricate drug delivery systems *Adv. Drug Delivery Rev.* **61** 1043–54

[58] Esa Z, Abid M, Zaini J H, Aissa B and Nauman M M 2022 Advancements and applications of electrohydrodynamic printing in modern microelectronic devices: a comprehensive review *Appl. Phys.* A **128** 780

[59] Zhang W, Liu H, Zhang X, Li X, Zhang G and Cao P 2021 3D printed microelectrochemical energy storage devices: from design to integration *Adv. Funct. Mater.* **31** 2104909

[60] Castrovilli M C, Bolognesi P, Chiarinelli J, Avaldi L, Cartoni A, Calandra P, Tempesta E, Giardi M T, Antonacci A and Arduini F 2020 Electrospray deposition as a smart technique for laccase immobilisation on carbon black-nanomodified screen-printed electrodes *Biosens. Bioelectron.* **163** 112299

[61] Grant J J, Pillai S C, Hehir S, McAfee M and Breen A 2021 Biomedical applications of electrospun graphene oxide *ACS Biomater. Sci. Eng.* **7** 1278–301

[62] Mehta P, Haj-Ahmad R, Rasekh M, Arshad M S, Smith A, van der Merwe S M, Li X, Chang M-W and Ahmad Z 2017 Pharmaceutical and biomaterial engineering via electrohydrodynamic atomization technologies *Drug Discov. Today* **22** 157–65

[63] Wu Y and Clark R L 2008 Electrohydrodynamic atomization: a versatile process for preparing materials for biomedical applications *J. Biomater. Sci. Polym. Ed.* **19** 573–601

[64] Xie J, Lim L K, Phua Y, Hua J and Wang C-H 2006 Electrohydrodynamic atomization for biodegradable polymeric particle production *J. Colloid Interface Sci.* **302** 103–12

[65] Jaworek A 2007 Electrospray droplet sources for thin film deposition *J. Mater. Sci.* **42** 266–97

[66] Jaworek A and Sobczyk A T 2008 Electrospraying route to nanotechnology: an overview *J. Electrostat.* **66** 197–219

[67] Hogan C J, Yun K M, Chen D-R, Lenggoro I W, Biswas P and Okuyama K 2007 Controlled size polymer particle production via electrohydrodynamic atomization *Colloids Surf.* A **311** 67–76

[68] Wang J, Dong T, Cheng Y and Yan W-C 2022 Machine learning assisted spraying pattern recognition for electrohydrodynamic atomization system *Ind. Eng. Chem. Res.* **61** 8495–503
[69] Gungordu S, Tabish E T, Edirisinghe M and Matharu R K 2022 Antiviral properties of porous graphene, graphene oxide and graphene foam ultrafine fibers against Phi6 bacteriophage *Front. Med.* **9** 3466
[70] Faraji S, Nowroozi N, Nouralishahi A and Shayeh J S 2020 Electrospun poly-caprolactone/graphene oxide/quercetin nanofibrous scaffold for wound dressing: evaluation of biological and structural properties *Life Sci.* **257** 11
[71] Khan M K I, Nazir A and Maan A A 2017 Electrospraying: a novel technique for efficient coating of foods *Food Eng. Rev.* **9** 112–9
[72] De La Mora J F and Loscertales I G 1994 The current emitted by highly conducting Taylor cones *J. Fluid Mech.* **260** 155–84
[73] Rosell-Llompart J, Grifoll J and Loscertales I G 2018 Electrosprays in the cone-jet mode: from Taylor cone formation to spray development *J. Aerosol Sci.* **125** 2–31
[74] De Juan L and De La Mora J F 1997 Charge and size distributions of electrospray drops *J. Colloid Interface Sci.* **186** 280–93
[75] Tanhaei A, Mohammadi M, Hamishehkar H and Hamblin M R 2021 Electrospraying as a novel method of particle engineering for drug delivery vehicles *J. Control. Release* **330** 851–65
[76] Yang L, Wang X, Yu Y, Shang L, Xu W and Zhao Y 2022 Bio-inspired dual-adhesive particles from microfluidic electrospray for bone regeneration *Nano Res.* **16** 5292–9
[77] Wang H, Zhao Z, Liu Y, Shao C, Bian F and Zhao Y 2018 Biomimetic enzyme cascade reaction system in microfluidic electrospray microcapsules *Sci. Adv.* **4** eaat2816
[78] Tang H, Yang C, Lin Z, Yang Q, Kang F and Wong C P 2015 Electrospray-deposition of graphene electrodes: a simple technique to build high-performance supercapacitors *Nanoscale* **7** 9133–9
[79] Teo W E and Ramakrishna S 2006 A review on electrospinning design and nanofibre assemblies *Nanotechnology* **17** R89
[80] Bhardwaj N and Kundu S C 2010 Electrospinning: a fascinating fiber fabrication technique *Biotechnol. Adv.* **28** 325–47
[81] Wang B, Wang Y, Yin T and Yu Q 2010 Applications of electrospinning technique in drug delivery *Chem. Eng. Commun.* **197** 1315–38
[82] Li Y, Zhu J, Cheng H, Li G, Cho H, Jiang M, Gao Q and Zhang X 2021 Developments of advanced electrospinning techniques: a critical review *Adv. Mater. Technol.* **6** 2100410
[83] Agarwal S, Wendorff J H and Greiner A 2008 Use of electrospinning technique for biomedical applications *Polymer* **49** 5603–21
[84] Diez-Pascual A M and Diez-Vicente A L 2017 Multifunctional poly(glycolic acid-co-propylene fumarate) electrospun fibers reinforced with graphene oxide and hydroxyapatite nanorods *J. Mater. Chem.* B **5** 4084–96
[85] Horzum N, Arik N and Truong Y B 2017 Nanofibers for fiber-reinforced composites *Fiber Technology for Fiber-Reinforced Composites* (Amsterdam: Elsevier) 251–75
[86] Jiang S, Chen Y, Duan G, Mei C, Greiner A and Agarwal S 2018 Electrospun nanofiber reinforced composites: a review *Polym. Chem.* **9** 2685–720
[87] Shakil U A, Hassan S B, Yahya M Y and Nauman S 2020 Mechanical properties of electrospun nanofiber reinforced/interleaved epoxy matrix composites—a review *Polym. Compos.* **41** 2288–315

[88] El-Sayed H, Vineis C, Varesano A, Mowafi S, Andrea Carletto R, Tonetti C and Abou Taleb M 2019 A critique on multi-jet electrospinning: state of the art and future outlook *Nanotechnol. Rev.* **8** 236–45
[89] Varesano A, Carletto R A and Mazzuchetti G 2009 Experimental investigations on the multi-jet electrospinning process *J. Mater. Process. Technol.* **209** 5178–85
[90] Hosseini Ravandi S A, Sadrjahani M, Valipouri A, Dabirian F and Ko F K 2022 Recently developed electrospinning methods: a review *Textile Res. J.* **92** 5130–45
[91] Yousefzadeh M and Ghasemkhah F 2019 Design of porous, core–shell, and hollow nanofibers *Handbook of Nanofibers* (Berlin: Springer) pp 157–214
[92] Song W, Tang Y, Qian C, Kim B J, Liao Y and Yu D-G 2023 Electrospinning spinneret: a bridge between the visible world and the invisible nanostructures *Innovation* **4** 100381
[93] SalehHudin H S, Mohamad E N, Mahadi W N L and Muhammad Afifi A 2018 Multiple-jet electrospinning methods for nanofiber processing: a review *Mater. Manuf. Processes* **33** 479–98
[94] Cam M E, Crabbe-Mann M, Alenezi H, Hazar-Yavuz A N, Ertas B, Ekentok C, Ozcan G S, Topal F, Guler E and Yazir Y 2020 The comparision of glybenclamide and metformin-loaded bacterial cellulose/gelatin nanofibres produced by a portable electrohydrodynamic gun for diabetic wound healing *Eur. Polym. J.* **134** 109844
[95] Liu M, Wang Y and Lu D 2019 Sensitive and selective non-enzymatic glucose detection using electrospun porous CuO–CdO composite nanofibers *J. Mater. Sci.* **54** 3354–67
[96] Hon K, Li L and Hutchings I 2008 Direct writing technology—advances and developments *CIRP Ann.* **57** 601–20
[97] Huot B 1990 The literature of direct writing assessment: major concerns and prevailing trends *Rev. Educ. Res.* **60** 237–63
[98] Huang Y, Bu N, Duan Y, Pan Y, Liu H, Yin Z and Xiong Y 2013 Electrohydrodynamic direct-writing *Nanoscale* **5** 12007–17
[99] Rasekh M, Ahmad Z, Day R, Wickam A and Edirisinghe M 2011 Direct writing of polycaprolactone polymer for potential biomedical engineering applications *Adv. Eng. Mater.* **13** B296–305
[100] Gibson I, Rosen D, Stucker B, Khorasani M, Gibson I, Rosen D, Stucker B and Khorasani M 2021 Direct write technologies *Additive Manufacturing Technologies* (Boston, MA: Springer) pp 319–45
[101] Samarasinghe S, Pastoriza-Santos I, Edirisinghe M, Reece M and Liz-Marzán L M 2006 Printing gold nanoparticles with an electrohydrodynamic direct-write device *Gold Bull.* **39** 48–53
[102] Coppola S, Nasti G, Todino M, Olivieri F, Vespini V and Ferraro P 2017 Direct writing of microfluidic footpaths by pyro-EHD printing *ACS Appl. Mater. Interfaces* **9** 16488–94
[103] Han Y and Dong J 2018 Electrohydrodynamic printing for advanced micro/nanomanufacturing: current progresses, opportunities, and challenges *J. Micro Nano-Manuf.* **6** 040802
[104] Qu X, Li J, Yin Z and Zou H 2019 New lithography technique based on electrohydrodynamic printing platform *Org. Electron.* **71** 279–83
[105] Piqué A and Chrisey D B 2002 *Direct-Write Technologies for Rapid Prototyping Applications: Sensors, Electronics, and Integrated Power Sources* (New York: Academic) https://shop.elsevier.com/books/direct-write-technologies-for-rapid-prototyping-applications/pique/978-0-12-174231-7

[106] Zhang Y, Shi G, Qin J, Lowe S E, Zhang S, Zhao H and Zhong Y L 2019 Recent progress of direct ink writing of electronic components for advanced wearable devices *ACS Appl. Electron. Mater.* **1** 1718–34

[107] Ghosh S, Parker S T, Wang X, Kaplan D L and Lewis J A 2008 Direct-write assembly of microperiodic silk fibroin scaffolds for tissue engineering applications *Adv. Funct. Mater.* **18** 1883–9

[108] Barry R A, Shepherd R F, Hanson J N, Nuzzo R G, Wiltzius P and Lewis J A 2009 Direct-write assembly of 3D hydrogel scaffolds for guided cell growth *Adv. Mater.* **21** 2407–10

[109] O'Neill P F, Ben Azouz A, Vazquez M, Liu J, Marczak S, Slouka Z, Chang H C, Diamond D and Brabazon D 2014 Advances in three-dimensional rapid prototyping of microfluidic devices for biological applications *Biomicrofluidics* **8** 052112

[110] Shen X, Yu Z, Huang F, Gu J and Zhang H 2022 Fabrication of 3D microstructures for flexible pressure sensors based on direct-writing printing *AIP Adv.* **12** 105205

[111] Husain O, Lau W, Edirisinghe M and Parhizkar M 2016 Investigating the particle to fibre transition threshold during electrohydrodynamic atomization of a polymer solution *Mater. Sci. Eng.* C **65** 240–50

[112] Nie H, Dong Z, Arifin D Y, Hu Y and Wang C H 2010 Core/shell microspheres via coaxial electrohydrodynamic atomization for sequential and parallel release of drugs *J. Biomed. Mater. Res.* A **95** 709–16

[113] Ahmad Z, Rasekh M and Edirisinghe M 2010 Electrohydrodynamic direct writing of biomedical polymers and composites *Macromol. Mater. Eng.* **295** 315–9

[114] Keshvardoostchokami M, Majidi S S, Huo P, Ramachandran R, Chen M and Liu B 2020 Electrospun nanofibers of natural and synthetic polymers as artificial extracellular matrix for tissue engineering *Nanomaterials* **11** 21

[115] Mikos A G, Sarakinos G, Lyman M D, Ingber D E, Vacanti J P and Langer R 1993 Prevascularization of porous biodegradable polymers *Biotechnol. Bioeng.* **42** 716–23

[116] Biswal T 2021 Biopolymers for tissue engineering applications: a review *Mater. Today Proc.* **41** 397–402

[117] Bose S, Koski C and Vu A A 2020 Additive manufacturing of natural biopolymers and composites for bone tissue engineering *Mater. Horizons* **7** 2011–27

[118] Abbasian M, Massoumi B, Mohammad-Rezaei R, Samadian H and Jaymand M 2019 Scaffolding polymeric biomaterials: are naturally occurring biological macromolecules more appropriate for tissue engineering? *Int. J. Biol. Macromol.* **134** 673–94

[119] Rahmati M, Mills D K, Urbanska A M, Saeb M R, Venugopal J R, Ramakrishna S and Mozafari M 2021 Electrospinning for tissue engineering applications *Prog. Mater Sci.* **117** 100721

[120] Peranidze K, Safronova T V and Kildeeva N R 2021 Fibrous polymer-based composites obtained by electrospinning for bone tissue engineering *Polymers* **14** 96

[121] Yang C, Shao Q, Han Y, Liu Q, He L, Sun Q and Ruan S 2021 Fibers by electrospinning and their emerging applications in bone tissue engineering *Appl. Sci.* **11** 9082

[122] Lin W, Chen M, Qu T, Li J and Man Y 2020 Three-dimensional electrospun nanofibrous scaffolds for bone tissue engineering *J. Biomed. Mater. Res.* B **108** 1311–21

[123] Dong C, Qiao F, Chen G and Lv Y 2021 Demineralized and decellularized bone extracellular matrix-incorporated electrospun nanofibrous scaffold for bone regeneration *J. Mater. Chem.* B **9** 6881–94

[124] Ranganathan S, Balagangadharan K and Selvamurugan N 2019 Chitosan and gelatin-based electrospun fibers for bone tissue engineering *Int. J. Biol. Macromol.* **133** 354–64
[125] Chahal S, Kumar A and Hussian F S J 2019 Development of biomimetic electrospun polymeric biomaterials for bone tissue engineering: a review *J. Biomater. Sci. Polym. Ed.* **30** 1308–55
[126] Nukavarapu S P and Dorcemus D L 2013 Osteochondral tissue engineering: current strategies and challenges *Biotechnol. Adv.* **31** 706–21
[127] Pan Y, Shen Q, Pan C and Wang J 2013 Compressive mechanical characteristics of multi-layered gradient hydroxyapatite reinforced poly (vinyl alcohol) gel biomaterial *J. Mater. Sci. Technol.* **29** 551–6
[128] Harley B A, Lynn A K, Wissner-Gross Z, Bonfield W, Yannas I V and Gibson L J 2010 Design of a multiphase osteochondral scaffold III: fabrication of layered scaffolds with continuous interfaces *J. Biomed. Mater. Res.* A **92** 1078–93
[129] Armiento A, Stoddart M, Alini M and Eglin D 2018 Biomaterials for articular cartilage tissue engineering: learning from biology *Acta Biomater.* **65** 1–20
[130] Reboredo J W, Weigel T, Steinert A, Rackwitz L, Rudert M and Walles H 2016 Investigation of migration and differentiation of human mesenchymal stem cells on five-layered collagenous electrospun scaffold mimicking native cartilage structure *Adv. Healthcare Mater.* **5** 2191–8
[131] Wise J K, Yarin A L, Megaridis C M and Cho M 2009 Chondrogenic differentiation of human mesenchymal stem cells on oriented nanofibrous scaffolds: engineering the superficial zone of articular cartilage *Tissue Eng.* A **15** 913–21
[132] Stankus J J, Soletti L, Fujimoto K, Hong Y, Vorp D A and Wagner W R 2007 Fabrication of cell microintegrated blood vessel constructs through electrohydrodynamic atomization *Biomaterials* **28** 2738–46
[133] Gil-Castell O, Ontoria-Oviedo I, Badia J, Amaro-Prellezo E, Sepúlveda P and Ribes-Greus A 2022 Conductive polycaprolactone/gelatin/polyaniline nanofibres as functional scaffolds for cardiac tissue regeneration *React. Funct. Polym.* **170** 105064
[134] Ahmadi P, Nazeri N, Derakhshan M A and Ghanbari H 2021 Preparation and characterization of polyurethane/chitosan/CNT nanofibrous scaffold for cardiac tissue engineering *Int. J. Biol. Macromol.* **180** 590–8
[135] Flaig F, Ragot H, Simon A, Revet G, Kitsara M, Kitasato L, Hebraud A, Agbulut O and Schlatter G 2020 Design of functional electrospun scaffolds based on poly (glycerol sebacate) elastomer and poly (lactic acid) for cardiac tissue engineering *ACS Biomater. Sci. Eng.* **6** 2388–400
[136] Babaie A, Bakhshandeh B, Abedi A, Mohammadnejad J, Shabani I, Ardeshirylajimi A, Moosavi S R, Amini J and Tayebi L 2020 Synergistic effects of conductive PVA/PEDOT electrospun scaffolds and electrical stimulation for more effective neural tissue engineering *Eur. Polym. J.* **140** 110051
[137] Xuan H, Li B, Xiong F, Wu S, Zhang Z, Yang Y and Yuan H 2021 Tailoring nano-porous surface of aligned electrospun poly (L-lactic acid) fibers for nerve tissue engineering *Int. J. Mol. Sci.* **22** 3536
[138] Khodadadi M, Alijani S, Montazeri M, Esmaeilizadeh N, Sadeghi-Soureh S and Pilehvar-Soltanahmadi Y 2020 Recent advances in electrospun nanofiber-mediated drug delivery strategies for localized cancer chemotherapy *J. Biomed. Mater. Res.* A **108** 1444–58

[139] Deepak A, Goyal A K and Rath G 2018 Nanofiber in transmucosal drug delivery *J. Drug Deliv. Sci. Technol.* **43** 379–87

[140] Goyal R, Macri L K, Kaplan H M and Kohn J 2016 Nanoparticles and nanofibers for topical drug delivery *J. Control. Release* **240** 77–92

[141] Kajdič S, Planinšek O, Gašperlin M and Kocbek P 2019 Electrospun nanofibers for customized drug-delivery systems *J. Drug Deliv. Sci. Technol.* **51** 672–81

[142] Xue J, He M, Liu H, Niu Y, Crawford A, Coates P D, Chen D, Shi R and Zhang L 2014 Drug loaded homogeneous electrospun PCL/gelatin hybrid nanofiber structures for anti-infective tissue regeneration membranes *Biomaterials* **35** 9395–405

[143] Son Y J, Kim W J and Yoo H S 2014 Therapeutic applications of electrospun nanofibers for drug delivery systems *Arch. Pharm. Res.* **37** 69–78

[144] Yoo H S, Kim T G and Park T G 2009 Surface-functionalized electrospun nanofibers for tissue engineering and drug delivery *Adv. Drug Deliv. Rev.* **61** 1033–42

[145] Liu Y, Wang L, Huang Y, Hou C, Xin B, Li T and Jiang Q 2023 Electrospun poly(l-lactide-co-ε-caprolactone)/gelatin core–shell nanofibers encapsulated with doxorubicin hydrochloride as a drug delivery system *Polym. Int.* **72** 166–75

[146] Kamble P, Sadarani B, Majumdar A and Bhullar S 2017 Nanofiber based drug delivery systems for skin: a promising therapeutic approach *J. Drug Deliv. Sci. Technol.* **41** 124–33

[147] Sofokleous P, Stride E and Edirisinghe M 2013 Preparation, characterization, and release of amoxicillin from electrospun fibrous wound dressing patches *Pharm. Res.* **30** 1926–38

[148] Bozkaya O, Arat E, Gök Z G, Yiğitoğlu M and Vargel I 2022 Production and characterization of hybrid nanofiber wound dressing containing *Centella asiatica* coated silver nanoparticles by mutual electrospinning method *Eur. Polym. J.* **166** 111023

[149] Alven S, Buyana B, Feketshane Z and Aderibigbe B A 2021 Electrospun nanofibers/nanofibrous scaffolds loaded with silver nanoparticles as effective antibacterial wound dressing materials *Pharmaceutics* **13** 964

[150] Dubey P, Bhushan B, Sachdev A, Matai I, Uday Kumar S and Gopinath P 2015 Silver-nanoparticle-incorporated composite nanofibers for potential wound-dressing applications *J. Appl. Polym. Sci.* **132** 42473

[151] Zhang K, Bai X, Yuan Z, Cao X, Jiao X, Li Y, Qin Y, Wen Y and Zhang X 2019 Layered nanofiber sponge with an improved capacity for promoting blood coagulation and wound healing *Biomaterials* **204** 70–9

[152] Nandakumar A, Birgani Z T, Santos D, Mentink A, Auffermann N, van der Werf K, Bennink M, Moroni L, van Blitterswijk C and Habibovic P 2012 Surface modification of electrospun fibre meshes by oxygen plasma for bone regeneration *Biofabrication* **5** 015006

[153] Nhlapo N, Dzogbewu T C and de Smidt O 2022 Nanofiber polymers for coating titanium-based biomedical implants *Fibers* **10** 36

[154] Ravichandran R, Ng C C, Liao S, Pliszka D, Raghunath M, Ramakrishna S and Chan C K 2011 Biomimetic surface modification of titanium surfaces for early cell capture by advanced electrospinning *Biomed. Mater.* **7** 015001

[155] Bayram C, Demirbilek M, Yalçın E, Bozkurt M, Doğan M and Denkbaş E B 2014 Osteoblast response on co-modified titanium surfaces via anodization and electrospinning *Appl. Surf. Sci.* **288** 143–8

[156] Abdal-hay A, Lim J, Hassan M S and Lim J K 2013 Ultrathin conformal coating of apatite nanostructures onto electrospun nylon 6 nanofibers: mimicking the extracellular matrix *Chem. Eng. J.* **228** 708–16

[157] Weng L and Xie J 2015 Smart electrospun nanofibers for controlled drug release: recent advances and new perspectives *Curr. Pharm. Design* **21** 1944–59
[158] Zhang L, Yan J, Yin Z, Tang C, Guo Y and Li D *et al* 2014 Electrospun vancomycin-loaded coating on titanium implants for the prevention of implant-associated infections *Int. J. Nanomed.* **9** 3027–36
[159] M, Şimşek, S D, Aldemir, M and Gümüşderelioğlu 2019 Anticellular PEO coatings on titanium surfaces by sequential electrospinning and crosslinking processes *Emerg. Mater.* **2** 169–79
[160] AlFalah M G K, Kamberli E, Abbar A H, Kandemirli F and Saracoglu M 2020 Corrosion performance of electrospinning nanofiber ZnO–NiO–CuO/polycaprolactone coated on mild steel in acid solution *Surf. Interfaces* **21** 100760
[161] Sasikumar Y, Indira K and Rajendran N 2019 Surface modification methods for titanium and its alloys and their corrosion behavior in biological environment: a review *J. Bio-Tribo-Corr.* **5** 1–25
[162] Mohammed M T, Khan Z A and Siddiquee A N 2014 Surface modifications of titanium materials for developing corrosion behavior in human body environment: a review *Proc. Mater. Sci.* **6** 1610–8
[163] Rasekh M, Ahmad Z, Frangos C C, Bozec L, Edirisinghe M and Day R M 2013 Spatial and temporal evaluation of cell attachment to printed polycaprolactone microfibres *Acta Biomater.* **9** 5052–62
[164] Persano L, Dagdeviren C, Su Y, Zhang Y, Girardo S, Pisignano D, Huang Y and Rogers J A 2013 High performance piezoelectric devices based on aligned arrays of nanofibers of poly (vinylidenefluoride-co-trifluoroethylene) *Nat. Commun.* **4** 1633
[165] Duan Y, Huang Y, Yin Z, Bu N and Dong W 2014 Non-wrinkled, highly stretchable piezoelectric devices by electrohydrodynamic direct-writing *Nanoscale* **6** 3289–95
[166] Li X, Wang G, Wang X, Li X and Ji J 2013 Flexible supercapacitor based on MnO_2 nanoparticles via electrospinning *J. Mater. Chem.* A **1** 10103–6
[167] Min S-Y, Kim T-S, Kim B J, Cho H, Noh Y-Y, Yang H, Cho J H and Lee T-W 2013 Large-scale organic nanowire lithography and electronics *Nat. Commun.* **4** 1773
[168] Li Y, Fu Z Y and Su B L 2012 Hierarchically structured porous materials for energy conversion and storage *Adv. Funct. Mater.* **22** 4634–67
[169] Yang H, Lightner C R and Dong L 2012 Light-emitting coaxial nanofibers *ACS Nano* **6** 622–8
[170] Gumennik A, Stolyarov A M, Schell B R, Hou C, Lestoquoy G, Sorin F, McDaniel W, Rose A, Joannopoulos J D and Fink Y 2012 All-in-fiber chemical sensing *Adv. Mater.* **24** 6005–9
[171] He H, Fu Y, Zang W, Wang Q, Xing L, Zhang Y and Xue X 2017 A flexible self-powered T-ZnO/PVDF/fabric electronic-skin with multi-functions of tactile-perception, atmosphere-detection and self-clean *Nano Energy* **31** 37–48
[172] Hatakeyama-Sato K, Wakamatsu H, Yamagishi K, Fujie T, Takeoka S, Oyaizu K and Nishide H 2019 Ultrathin and stretchable rechargeable devices with organic polymer nanosheets conformable to skin surface *Small* **15** 1805296
[173] Wang M, Baek P, Akbarinejad A, Barker D and Travas-Sejdic J 2019 Conjugated polymers and composites for stretchable organic electronics *J. Mater. Chem.* C **7** 5534–52

[174] Li X-P, Li Y, Li X, Song D, Min P, Hu C, Zhang H-B, Koratkar N and Yu Z-Z 2019 Highly sensitive, reliable and flexible piezoresistive pressure sensors featuring polyurethane sponge coated with MXene sheets *J. Colloid Interface Sci.* **542** 54–62

[175] Cai L, Zhang S, Zhang Y, Li J, Miao J, Wang Q, Yu Z and Wang C 2018 Direct printing for additive patterning of silver nanowires for stretchable sensor and display applications *Adv. Mater. Technol.* **3** 1700232

[176] Brako F, Luo C, Craig D Q M and Edirisinghe M 2018 An inexpensive, portable device for point-of-need generation of silver-nanoparticle doped cellulose acetate nanofibers for advanced wound dressing *Macromol. Mater. Eng.* **303** 1700586

IOP Publishing

Biomaterials
Innovation for world healthcare
Mohan Edirisinghe, Merve Gultekinoglu and Jubair Ahmed

Chapter 4

Gyratory processes for manufacturing

Centrifugal spinning is a way of rapidly generating small-diameter fibres for use in healthcare applications using a range of biomaterials. Over the decades, centrifugal spinning has shown that that it can produce fine polymeric structures that have the ability to be scaled up industrially. This technique has also given rise to newer fibre manufacturing approaches which utilise centrifugal spinning and an applied gas pressure, such as pressurised gyration (PG), which has been used to produce polymeric structures for a wide range of biomedical applications, such as drug delivery, tissue engineering, and antimicrobial air and water filtration.

4.1 Centrifugal spinning

The utilisation of a centrifugal force to drive the production of fibres is not a new process and has been available for over a century; during this time, it has been used to produce glass wool for applications including thermal insulation and filtration [1, 2]. More recently however, the technology has been featured extensively in the realm of biomedical engineering for the production of various biomaterials which see applications ranging from tissue engineering to drug delivery. As the focal point of this book is biomaterials for healthcare, this chapter explores the recent developments in this field, cases in which this technology has inspired others based on it, and the impact that these processes have had on the production of functional biomaterials.

The basic principle behind centrifugal spinning involves the use of a driving motor, which allows a vessel or polymer reservoir to rotate at high speed. This high-speed rotation generates a centrifugal force which in turn drives the polymer solution within the rotating vessel into instability, causing it to exit the nozzles at high velocity [3]. A polymer jet is formed when the centrifugal force exceeds the surface tension of the solution. The polymer jet allows the solution to be focused in a singular path, which is akin to extrusion. As the solvent evaporates, the exiting polymer jet solidifies and fibres are created.

A basic centrifugal spinning setup therefore consists of a rotating vessel with nozzles or orifices which guide the fibre production. An electrical motor is typically

doi:10.1088/978-0-7503-5187-4ch4

used to rotate the vessel with enough centrifugal force to form a polymer jet and thus fibres [4]. Figure 4.1 shows a diagram of a basic centrifugal spinning setup (variations of this basic design may exist).

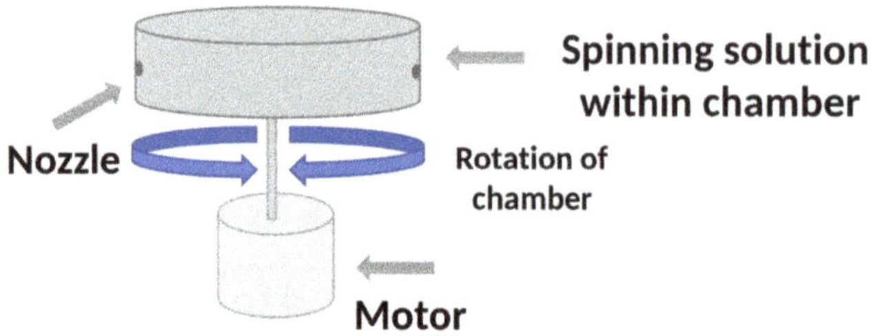

Figure 4.1. A diagram showing an overview of the basic centrifugal spinning setup.

The main benefit of utilising a technique such as centrifugal spinning is its high production rate, which is typically several orders of magnitude higher than those of other comparable methods, such as electrospinning. This increase in production rate is heavily influenced by the use of a high-speed motor, the ability to spin larger volumes, and the absence of limiting syringe pumps and other polymer feed approaches. Due to its simple design, centrifugal spinning can also be scaled up to obtain a higher production rates of polymeric fibres, in contrast to the scale-up of electrospinning, which typically faces the issue of nozzle-to-nozzle interference that can cause a loss of production yield.

One of the most notable iterations of centrifugal spinning is a method called Forcespinning™, which was introduced in 2010 as a new process for the manufacture of nanofibres from a wide range of materials [5]. Forcespinning was developed as process to rival electrospinning in terms of fibre quality and morphology, but to overcome its main limitations in scaling up to match high industrial demands. This technology can produce ultrafine fibres from solutions or from solid materials which are heated into a melt. Forcespinning offers great control over the morphology of the produced fibres because its key parameters can easily be changed; these include control over the rotational speed, the collection temperature, and even the geometry of the spinnerets, allowing a high degree of customisation over the final product. Forcespinning has been incredibly successful in producing biomaterials for a wide range of healthcare-related applications and numerous articles have been published to describe its use. For example, Forcespinning has been used to produce polyacrylonitrile fibres for lithium-ion battery components, polyamide fibres for applications such as filtration and wound healing, and silver-nanoparticle-reinforced polylactic acid fibres for potential applications such as tissue engineering [6–8].

Centrifugal spinning has also inspired the formation of other fibre manufacturing technologies which aim to improve upon the fibre production rate and provide additional control over the final fibre morphology, a key determinant in the suitability of biomaterials for their intended healthcare applications. One technology, which the authors have unique experience with, is called PG. The rest of the chapter details how this technology has changed the landscape of fibre production for healthcare applications. It is important to note, however, that PG can also be operated in centrifugal-spinning-only mode; therefore, any advancements made in centrifugal spinning alone can also be applied to PG.

4.2 Pressurised gyration

PG was first invented in 2013 due to a desire to mass-produce fibrous products without the limitations of prior techniques [9]. The name 'pressurised gyration' combines centrifugal spinning (the 'gyration' portion of the name) with an infused gas pressure (the 'pressurised' portion of the name). In its essence, centrifugal spinning involves the high-speed rotation of a perforated spinneret into which a polymer solution is placed. The centrifugal force built up during the high-speed rotation acts on the solution and extrudes it out of the small-diameter orifices [10]. Solution blow spinning is an alternative nanofibre production route which integrates a high-velocity gas flow into the polymer solution. The pressurised gas is therefore responsible for extruding the polymer solution through the small opening of the nozzle; as the solvent evaporates, dried nanofibres are formed in a simple one-step process [11]. PG combines both centrifugal force and pressurised gas to further drive down the size of the generated fibres, allowing structures with greater surface areas to be created. Because PG does not rely on electric fields for the production of fibres, it can be scaled up without the fear of needle interference; this makes it an excellent fibre production choice for biomedical materials.

4.2.1 The principles of pressurised gyration

The PG setup is integral to the fibre production mechanism. The gyrating vessel can be regarded as the principal component [12]. The setup is composed and centred around an aluminium vessel 35 mm in height and with a diameter of 60 mm. This vessel is used as a reservoir where the polymer solution is stored before spinning. The vessel is special because it contains 24 very small (0.5 mm) holes in its walls, which act as exit apertures for the fibres. The vessel is also connected to a high-speed DC motor which is capable of providing a rotational speed of up to 36 000 rpm. In addition, the vessel has a lid which is connected to an external pressurised gas supply, which provides a nitrogen gas infusion from 0.1 to 0.3 MPa. The speed of the motor can be adjusted using a variable-speed controller which is placed in between the power supply and the motor. Figure 4.2 diagrammatically shows the principal components of the basic PG setup required for fibre production.

In order to form fibres using PG, a polymer solution, which is one part polymer and another part solvent, is required. The key mechanism which leads to fibre production in PG is the centrifugal force that acts on the vessel, manipulating the polymer solution within it. At the fundamental level, this force manipulates the Rayleigh–Taylor instability of the polymer solution: when the centrifugal force exceeds the surface tension of the polymer, the solution escapes from the exit apertures [13]. If the critical minimum energy of the polymer solution is not exceeded by the rotation of the motor, the solution may exit the orifices but only with enough velocity to create droplets. Droplets contain excess solvent and do not form into fibres. However, if the critical minimum energy of the polymer solution is exceeded,

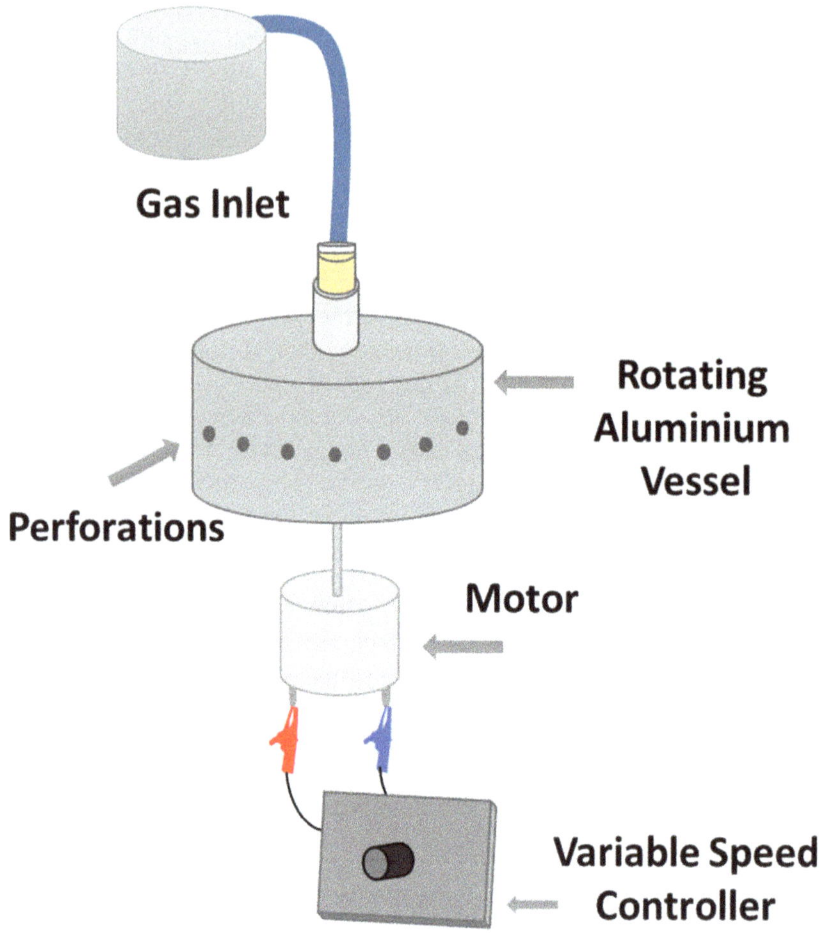

Figure 4.2. A diagrammatic representation of the basic PG setup, depicting the key components which are responsible for the fibre production mechanism.

the centrifugal force becomes the external driving force and the polymer solution initially exits the apertures in the form of small droplets [14]. As the droplets traverse the orifice, a surface tension gradient is created along the liquid–air interface, prompting the separation of the polymer solution from the surrounding air and creating a polymer jet. This gradient triggers a Gibbs–Marangoni stress which is tangential to the liquid–gas interface, instigating a flow to the tip of the polymer droplet [15]. The polymer jet, which is essential for fibre production, is a highly focused stream of solution that has sufficient velocity to atomise the solvent portion of the polymer solution [16]. As the solvent rapidly evaporates from the polymer jet, the polymer dries in the form in which it is extruded through the apertures, and polymeric fibres are deposited. Figure 4.3 visually demonstrates the role of the polymer jet in fibre production.

This principle can be understood in more detail by looking at the following equation. Equation (4.1) shows the relationship between the different variables of

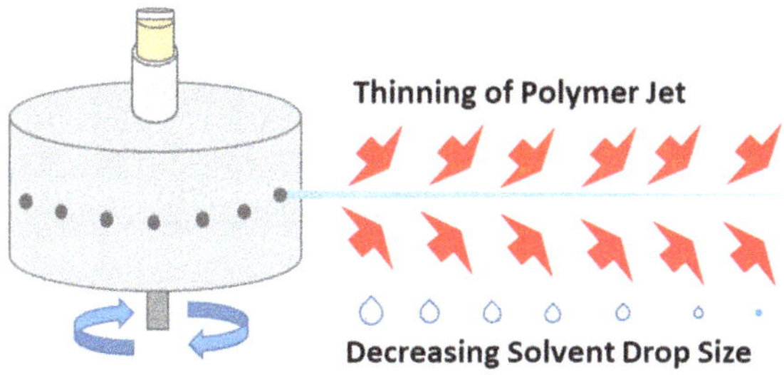

Figure 4.3. A diagram showing the role of the polymer jet in fibre production. A bead exits an orifice with sufficient energy to create a polymer jet. As the jet dries, the solvent evaporates, producing polymeric fibres.

the spinning process and the Rayleigh–Taylor instability. Here, λ corresponds to the wavelength of the Rayleigh–Taylor instability, h is the height of the liquid film, γ is the surface tension of the liquid–gas surface, $\rho\omega^2 R$ is the destabilising centrifugal force, and Δp is the pressure differential at the aperture of the gyration vessel [13].

$$\lambda = \left(\frac{h\gamma}{(\rho\omega^2 R) + \Delta p}\right)^{\frac{1}{3}} \tag{4.1}$$

Although the centrifugal force generated by the high-speed motor plays the major role in fibre production, PG also has the ability to infuse external gas pressure into the gyration vessel, creating up to 0.3 MPa of pressurisation. This external gas pressure exerts a secondary force on the polymer solution, increasing the escape energy of the initial bead and causing a thinning effect on fibre production as the polymer jet elongates and solvent evaporation becomes easier. Even without the application of centrifugal force, the external gas pressure is able to provide enough energy to the gyration vessel to cause the solution to escape through the orifices, as can be seen in figure 4.4. In the absence of the centrifugal force, however, the critical

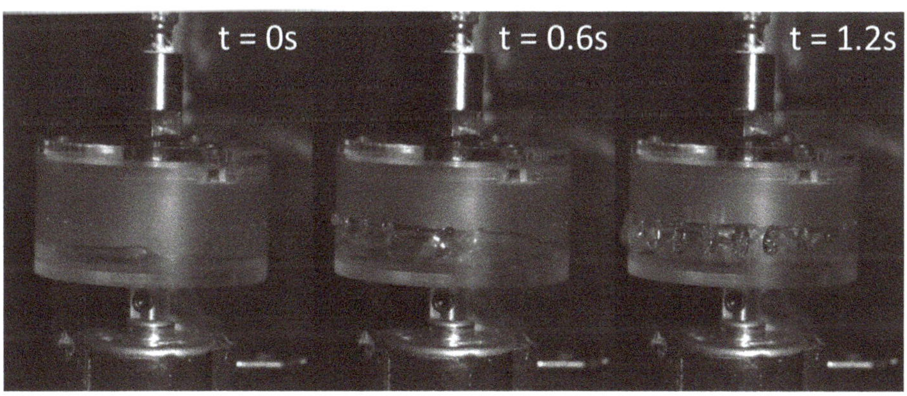

Figure 4.4. Close-up images taken with a high-speed camera depicting a transparent version of the aluminium PG vessel at three different time intervals. In response to the application of 0.1 MPa of external pressure to the vessel and in the absence of centrifugal rotation, the polymer solution can be seen to have sufficient energy to escape the gyration orifices in the form of large droplets (at t = 0.6 onwards).

minimum energy required to create a polymer jet is not reached and fibres cannot be produced as a result.

PG is beneficial in a few key ways. First, it allows for a high production rate of fibres to meet the demands of many biomedical applications. It is a single-step process with very small initial setup and low long-term maintenance costs. PG is able to operate perfectly under ambient conditions and does not rely on a high-voltage electric field. As a result, it can spin a wide range of natural and synthetic polymers without requiring a direct electrical current [17]. Through the utilisation of multiple operating parameters, such as the rotational speed and the applied gas pressure, PG can produce highly customisable polymeric fibres, as their morphology can be easily tuned.

4.3 The operating parameters of pressurised gyration

The morphology of the produced polymeric fibres is of highest importance when the application of the fibres is considered in a biomedical scenario. The PG setup and its various operating parameters allow for the tailoring of the fibre morphology. Although solution properties have a major influence in producing polymeric products, this is common to all techniques including microfluidics and electrospinning [18, 19]. Therefore, it is important to understand the various operating parameters and their effect on the fibre morphology.

4.3.1 Rotational speed

At higher rotational speeds of the motor, the centrifugal force acting upon the polymer solution in the vessel intensifies. The centrifugal force exerts a stretching effect on the emerging droplets leaving the orifices; greater stretching of the polymer jet leads to more rapid evaporation of the solvent and the deposition of thinner fibres.

As mentioned previously, there is a critical minimum rotational speed that must be met in order for fibre production to ensue. When this minimum rotational speed is not met, the surface tension of the polymer solution typically prohibits the escape of the polymer solution from the orifices. At lower speeds and especially as the motor is in its accelerating phase, the solvent can occasionally separate from the polymer due to its low surface tension [20]. In these scenarios, a polymer jet is not established, and the solution is lost to the surrounding collectors as undried droplets. Therefore, it is vital to ensure that a homogeneous and completely dissolved polymer solution is used and that the ideal rotational speed is utilised. The PG system incorporates a DC motor speed controller which can adjust the speed of the gyration vessel and even provide a higher starting torque that can minimise solution loss.

As mentioned previously, the physical properties of the polymer solution (predominately the surface tension) influence the critical minimum rotational speed. Once this speed has been reached, subsequent increases in the rotational speed will cause thinner fibres to be deposited as the polymer jet stretches further. However, the effect of even greater speeds is yet to be determined, as there are difficulties caused by motor designs that can generate a greater rotational force.

4.3.2 Gas pressure

Nitrogen gas is used as the gas supply that provides a pressurised gas input into the gyration vessel. Nitrogen gas is used due to its high abundance but principally because it is an inert gas. As a wide range of biological materials and solvents are used with PG, it is necessary to eliminate the possibility of causing a chemical reaction within the vessel. This high-pressure supply of gas separates this fibre manufacturing technology from others and works in two main ways. First, the supply of gas into the vessel causes the polymer solution to expand further inside the vessel, adding to the pressure differential. This extra force increases the energy with which the polymer jet escapes, causing further stretching and therefore leading to the deposition of thinner fibres. Second, the gas input acts to replenish the volume of gas within the vessel that is lost to the surrounding environment.

It is important to understand the relationship between the rotational speed and the applied gas pressure. In order to obtain total control over the fibre yield and the resulting fibre morphology, the gas pressure should be applied after reaching the critical rotational speed that is required to form the polymer jet. If the gas pressure is applied before the critical rotational speed is reached, the solution will be forced through the orifices without forming a polymer jet and droplets will be collected instead. The gas pressure therefore acts as the secondary driving force. The morphology of the product can be controlled by controlling the magnitude of the applied gas pressure.

By utilising the gas pressure in addition to the rotational forces, certain fibre morphologies can be selected. For example, the applied gas pressure can influence the surface topography of the produced fibrous products. When spinning polymer solutions are made with highly volatile solvents, surface nanopores appear due to the formation of condensation droplets. The applied gas pressure can cause a more rapid evaporation of these droplets, creating different surface designs [21].

4.3.3 Collection setup

Just as in the other fibre manufacturing technologies such as electrospinning, the method through which the products are deposited and collected plays a crucial role in the final fibre morphology. The working distance, i.e. the measured gap between the orifices to the collector, can influence the morphology of the produced fibres. There needs to be a sufficient distance to allow the emerging polymer jet to dry. Volatile solvents require smaller distances to dry. If the collection distance is too short, the polymer is deposited as droplets which do not form uniform structures. If the collection distance is too great, other structures can be formed, such as a bead-on-a-string morphology.

By adjusting the collection distance, the average fibre diameter can be controlled. Within specific ranges, an increase in collection distance can lead to further drying and thinning of the polymer jet, leading to the deposition of thinner fibres. The standard gyration setup includes a custom-made enclosure which provides a collection distance of about 75 mm to the walls of the collection unit. However, these collectors can easily be customised, and there are limitless possibilities.

Many different modifications to the standard collection setup can be made in order to exercise control over the types of fibres that can be created. The airflow of the gyration system plays a pivotal role in how the polymer is manipulated within the gyration vessel. The centrifugal force and the applied gas pressure act directly on the liquid–air interface between the polymer solution and the environment. Without sufficient replenishment of air within the vessel, the polymer jet does not fully form, and the fibre morphology can be adversely affected. A higher airflow around the gyration vessel also works to increase the drying of the polymer jet, leading to thinner deposited fibres. For this reason, PG can be performed with little to no collection walls, which could otherwise interfere with the amount of air that reaches the inside of the vessel.

The ability of PG to achieve a range of morphologies even when spinning the same polymer is an advantage and can be easily achieved based on the collection method. For example, highly aligned nonwoven fibres, which are desired in many different biomedical applications (such as nerve tissue engineering), can be achieved by utilising a collector similar to that depicted in figure 4.5 [22]. Highly unidirectionally aligned fibres can be created through the incorporation of protruding fins centred around the gyration pot, as the fins serve to catch the emerging polymer jets and guide them to the neighbouring fins, whilst preserving the unidirectionality of the fibre collection.

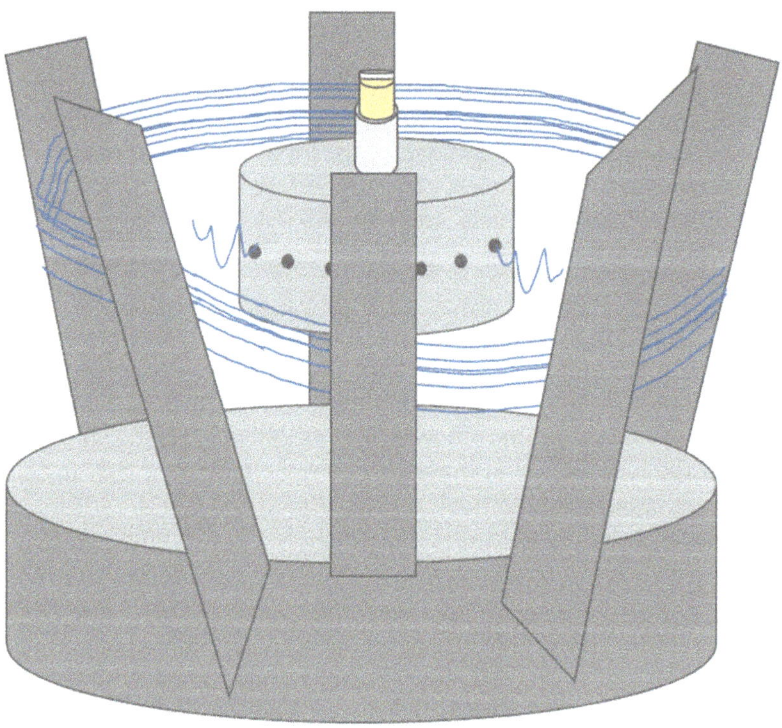

Figure 4.5. A diagrammatic representation of a modified PG collector with several protruding fins centred around the gyration vessel. As the vessel spins, polymer solution is forced out as a polymer jet which is caught by one fin. The placement of the subsequent fins ensures that there is unidirectionality in the final fibre morphology.

4.4 The physics behind pressurised gyration

Since the discovery of PG in 2013, much work has been done to optimise this technology for the mass production of polymeric fibres in their various morphologies. In order to further understand the mechanisms of the fibre production process, advanced approaches have been used, such as high-speed cameras, computational modelling, and transparent replicas of the PG vessel. In this section, the physics of PG is explained in order to better gauge the effects of the factors which play a role in the fibre manufacturing process. The behaviour of a viscous polymer solution within the PG vessel has been previously investigated experimentally and via computational fluid dynamics [23].

In this study, poly(ethylene oxide) (PEO) that had a molecular weight of 200 000 g mol^{-1} was used and dissolved in distilled water at a concentration of 21 wt%. PEO was specifically chosen since it is water soluble and would not react with the transparent gyration pot. The transparent gyration pot was designed to be an exact dimensional replica of the PG vessel and had an outer diameter of 60 mm and an inner diameter of 58 mm. Just like the original gyration pot, the transparent pot had 24 0.5 mm apertures drilled into its walls, which acted as the orifices. A high-speed camera recording at 5400 frames per second was used to capture motion images for later analysis. Numerical analysis based on computational fluid dynamics (CFD) was utilised to simulate the flow inside the gyration vessel and the outlets of the orifices to determine the influences of the rotational speed and applied gas pressure.

4.4.1 The effects of rotational speed without gas pressure

The pressured gyration vessel is capable of achieving very high rotational speeds. In the absence of the infusion of additional gas pressure, it behaves similarly to centrifugal spinning. At a lower rotational speed of 7000 revolutions per minute (rpm), the physics of the PEO polymer solution with the vessel was analysed via high-speed camera imagery. The corresponding images can be seen in figure 4.6. With zero rotation of the motor, the polymer solution forms a thin layer at the bottom of the gyration vessel because PEO is a Newtonian fluid and assumes the shape of the vessel. About 215 ms after rotation starts, the polymer solution within the vessel is observed to begin moving, following the acceleration of the motor. Interestingly, the polymer assumes a distinctive parabolic profile, indicating that the other side of the vessel also has the same shape. Although the polymer solution can be seen to have reached the level of the orifices, it does not escape from them, as

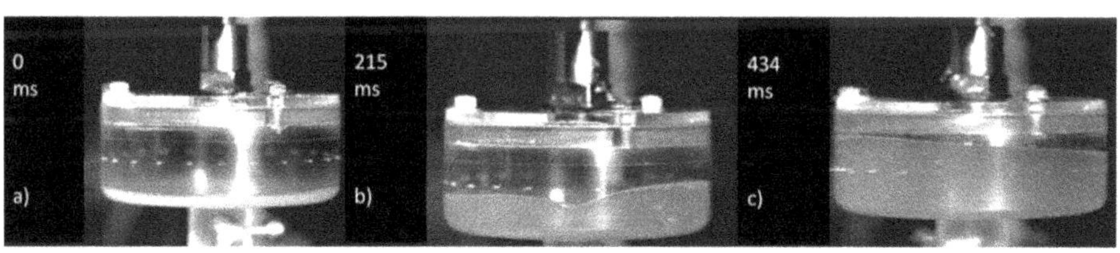

Figure 4.6. Still pictures obtained from high-speed camera footage showing the PEO solution spun at 7000 rpm: (a) at rest, $t = 0$ ms, (b) $t = 215$ ms, (c) $t = 434$ ms. Reproduced from [23]. CC BY 4.0.

surface tension prevents such behaviour at the low angular velocities encountered as the motor begins to accelerate.

Numerical analysis of the effects of low rotational speed without applied gas pressure shows that the movement of the polymer solution due to centrifugal force, which acts against surface tension and gravitational forces, leads to the deformation of the solution at the orifices. Images taken from the computer simulation of the vessel at 7000 rpm at different times after the start of rotation are shown in figure 4.7. The greater the rotational speed of the vessel, the higher the centrifugal force, which promotes solution deformation. The measured value for the surface tension of the analysed PEO solution was 57 ± 5 mN m^{-1}, and the solution had a measured viscosity of 3000 ± 30 N m^{-1}, making it a relatively viscous liquid. The polymer solution within the vessel therefore responded to two opposing forces, namely the normal stresses and shear stresses. In response to these forces, the solution elongated towards the orifices as the motor accelerated. The computer simulations show the volume fraction of the PEO polymer solution at different times following the start of rotation. These simulations show that the profile of the surface is not flat, reflecting experimental observations, and that the fluid shifts towards the sides of the vessel to form the expected parabolic shape due to centrifugal force. At lower rotational speeds, it takes about 6 ms to form the parabola; however, these simulations assume that the rotation of the motor is instantaneous, whereas in the laboratory, the motor has an acceleration phase.

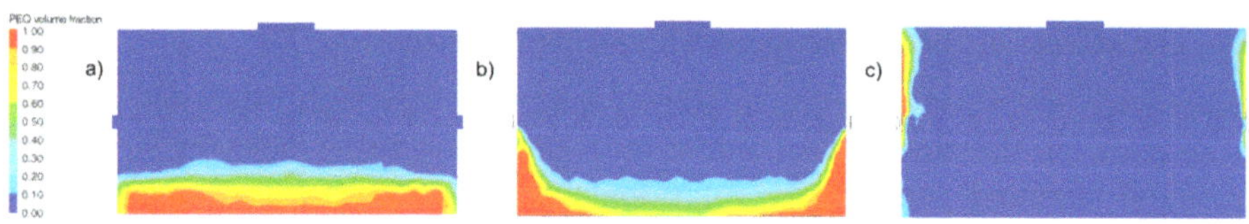

Figure 4.7. Computational modelling images from an ANSYS-Fluent simulation of the PEO polymer solution spun at 7000 rpm: (a) rest, t = 0, (b) t = 6 ms after the start of rotation and (c) t = 20 ms after the start of rotation. Reproduced from [23]. CC BY 4.0.

4.4.2 The effects of gas pressure on fluid physics

What sets PG apart from centrifugal spinning and other fibre generation methods is that it incorporates an infused gas pressure capable of providing up to 0.3 MPa of additional pressure within the vessel. At the maximum tested rotational speed of 10 000 rpm, high-speed camera images have been used to understand the physics of additional gas pressure within the vessel. Figure 4.8 shows still images of the transparent pot at different applied gas pressures. At rest, the profile of the polymer solution appears to be flat. At about 370 ms after the start of rotation of the pot, the solution reaches the orifices and the jet can be seen to be formed. Compared to centrifugal spinning, the additional gas pressure creates a supplementary driving force for the polymer solution, and the time taken to form the polymer jet reduces. Figure 4.8(e) clearly shows the effect of the additional gas

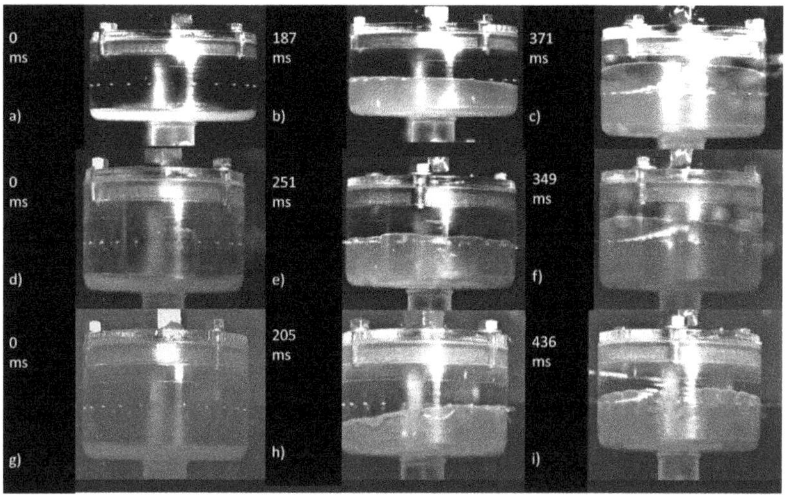

Figure 4.8. Still images taken from high-speed camera videos showing: a PEO solution spun at 10 000 rpm and 0.1 MPa additional gas pressure at (a) rest, t = 0 ms, (b) t = 187 ms, (c) t = 371 ms; (d) a PEO solution spun at 10 000 rpm and 0.2 MPa additional gas pressure when t = 0 ms, (e) t = 251 ms, (f) t = 349 ms; and a PEO solution spun at 10 000 rpm and 0.3 MPa additional gas pressure when (g) t = 0 ms, (h) t = 205 ms and (i) t = 436 ms after the start of rotation of the vessel. Reproduced from [23]. CC BY 4.0.

pressure in controlling the profile of the viscous polymer solution. The parabolic nature of the polymer solution seen with centrifugal spinning is not observed here. The gas pressure ensures that the polymer solution reaches the orifices at the same time, which leads to a more balanced output speed and altitude. At the very high applied gas pressure of 0.3 MPa (figure 4.8(g,h,i)), the time taken for the polymer solution to reach the orifice and produce a polymer jet is reduced. The gas pressure therefore contributes to earlier jetting and increases jet elongation, which can result in the production of thinner fibres.

4.5 The applications of pressurised gyration fibres

Polymeric small-diameter fibres produced by any fibre manufacturing technique offer a wide range of physical characteristics which make them beneficial for biomedical applications. Thin fibres benefit from a high surface-area-to-volume ratio as well as other useful topological features such as the presence of nanopores or grooves [24, 25]. PG is especially useful in producing a range of polymeric fibrous constructs and has the ability to closely tailor the final product dimensions and morphology. Since its first appearance in 2013, many publications have highlighted the benefits of this technology and the various applications of its fibres in biomedical and healthcare applications. In this section, the key applications of the fibres produced by electrospinning will be described along with their developments over the years.

4.5.1 Drug delivery

The administration of drugs plays a colossal role in healthcare. The pharmaceutical industry faces a common problem when delivering drugs to the intended user. The method of drug delivery must be minimally invasive, and patient compliance is always at the forefront of their concerns. Unfortunately, the easiest method of drug delivery, which is buccal delivery, is also one of the least compatible with many drug formulations. Drug delivery engineering via the use of polymeric matrices allows for the enhancement of oral drug solubility by leveraging amorphic solid dispersions. A solid dispersion is essentially created when a drug, in its amorphic and easy-to-dissolve state, is embedded into a degradable polymer. Such polymers are typically hydrophilic; when they contact an aqueous environment, this increases the solubility of the active pharmaceutical ingredient [26, 27].

4.5.1.1 The development and characterisation of amorphous nanofibre drug dispersions prepared using pressurised gyration

Drugs which belong to class II of the Biopharmaceutics Classification System have the ability to be highly permeable but have the problem of low oral solubility [28]. Thinner fibres exhibit a greater available surface area, making them more suitable for drug delivery applications in which dissolution plays a key role. PG offers the ability to mass-produce fine fibres which can be used to deliver pharmaceuticals.

PG allows hydrophilic polymers such as poly(vinylpyrrolidone) (PVP) and PEO to be spun into small-diameter fibres for the purpose of increasing the oral solubility of certain active pharmaceutical ingredients. In one early study of PG, dispersions of ibuprofen (a BSC class II drug) were prepared at up to 50% weight loadings of PVP as a drug dispersion and characterised using a range of imaging and spectroscopic techniques and drug release profiles [17]. The effect of increasing drug content was observed, which was that higher loadings of drugs led to differences in the final fibre morphology (figure 4.9). Having the ability to customise the drug percentage of fibres allows for more control over the release profile of the drug inside the body; for example, it is possible to obtain a quick burst release or a prolonged sustained release by modifying the drug content and morphology of the fibres. Without any drug loading, PG was able to produce 10% w/v PVP fibres in ethanol with an average diameter of about 795 nm. This shows that PG has the ability to produce fibres in the nanometre range, especially with more environmentally friendly solvents such as water and ethanol. With drug loading, the fibre diameter of the produced ibuprofen-PVP fibres increased, reaching average fibre diameters of 1.2 μm, 4.2 μm, and 5.4 μm for drug loadings of 10%, 30%, and 50%, respectively. From figure 4.9, we can see from the high-magnification images that the surfaces of the drug-loaded fibres appear to be smooth and devoid of surface features. Although surface features such as grooves, pits, and roughness are not necessarily an undesirable characteristic, the use of smooth surfaces in drug delivery can ensure that doses are administered more reliably. The fibre diameter increase seen here is consistent with increases seen in other fibre manufacturing techniques as the drug content of the system is increased [29].

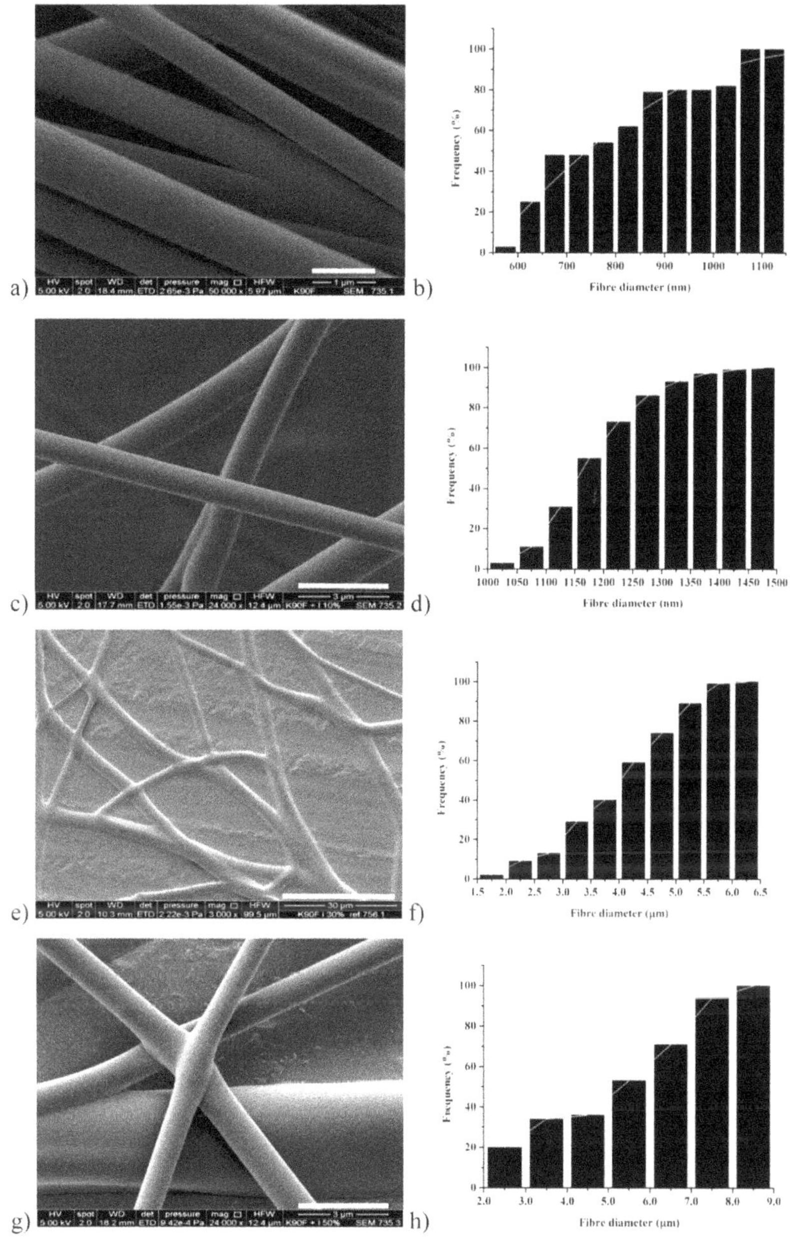

Figure 4.9. Scanning electron microscopy (SEM) images of: (a) virgin PVP fibres, (b) the corresponding fibre diameter frequency (cumulative %) distribution graph, (c) 10% PVP–ibuprofen fibres, (d) the corresponding fibre diameter frequency (cumulative %) distribution graph, (e) 30% PVP–ibuprofen fibres, (f) the corresponding fibre diameter frequency (cumulative %) distribution graph, (g) 50% PVP–ibuprofen fibres, (h) the corresponding fibre diameter frequency (cumulative %) distribution graph. Reproduced from [17]. CC BY 4.0.

The active pharmaceutical ingredient, ibuprofen, was present within the fibre in its amorphous, easy-to-dissolve form, as confirmed by x-ray diffraction and Fourier transform infra-red (FTIR) spectroscopy patterns. Dissolution tests are *in vitro* tests that measure the rate of dissolution or drug release in an aqueous medium under specified conditions. They can be used to compare the drug release patterns of the original formulation with those of new methods of delivery [30]. The PVP–ibuprofen fibres displayed an increase in dissolution rate compared to ibuprofen alone (figure 4.10). The drug contents of all the fibres produced using PG were between 98.4% and 100.2% of the theoretical values.

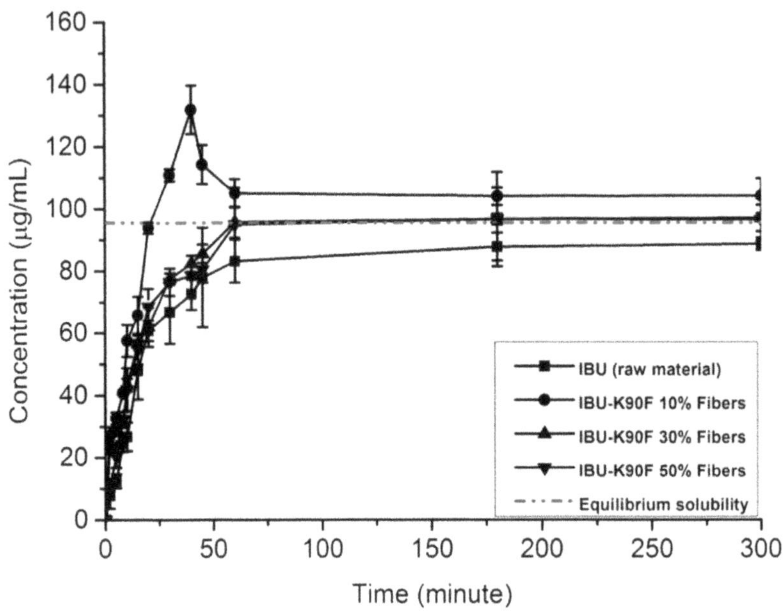

Figure 4.10. *In vitro* dissolution profiles of PVP–ibuprofen fibres. Ibuprofen 10%, 30%, and 50% fibres produced using PG were evaluated under non-sink conditions at pH 1 (0.1 M HCl). Reproduced from [17]. CC BY 4.0.

The most rapid dissolution occurred in 10% PVP–ibuprofen fibres, in which the peak concentration was higher and more rapid than that achieved using ibuprofen alone. PVP is able to successfully inhibit the crystallisation of ibuprofen and other amorphous drugs. The 30% and 50% PVP–ibuprofen fibres had slower dissolution rates than the 10% fibres, as an increase in polymer content is known to slow down crystallisation. By changing the concentration of polymer within the solid dispersion, the dissolution rate can be controlled further.

PVP has also been used to deliver antifungal pharmaceuticals belonging to the BSC class II classification in a study in which fibres produced using PG were compared to those produced using the industry-standard method of electrospinning [31]. Electrospinning is an excellent technology for producing ultrafine fibres which are especially suited for drug delivery applications. PG-spun fibres also have specific benefits in such applications. A comparison between PVP fibres produced by electrospinning and those produced by PG is shown in figure 4.11; 10% (w/v) PVP dissolved in ethanol was spun using both techniques.

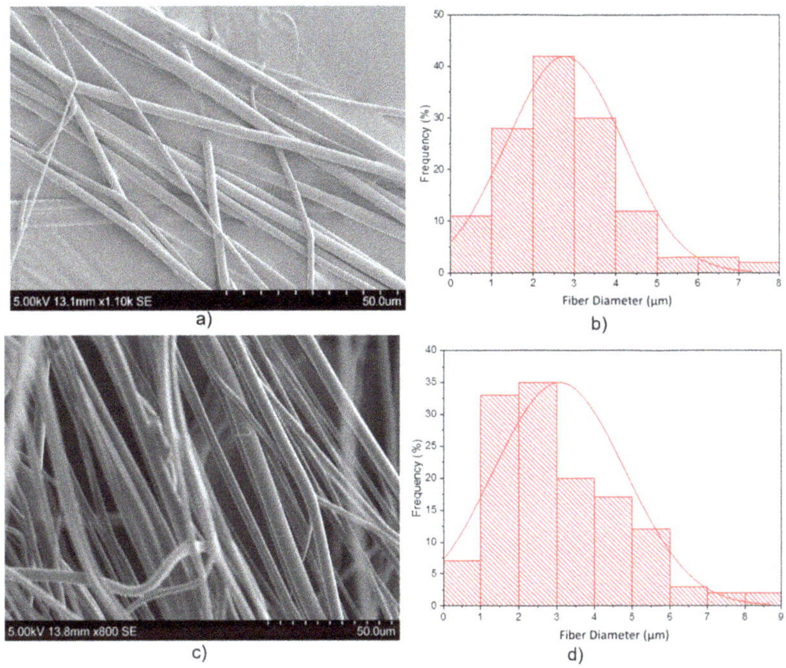

Figure 4.11. SEM images and fibre diameter distribution of PVP fibres prepared by (a and b) electrospinning and (c and d) PG [31] John Wiley & Sons. [2018].

This comparison of the two formation methods shows that they both produced fibres with a smooth, pore-free surface; the electrospun fibres had a more cross-woven structure and the fibres produced using gyration demonstrated a more uniaxial alignment. Because of the way the gyration pot rotates, it can easily produce aligned fibres, depending on the method of collection, although advanced collection setups for electrospinning exist as well. The average diameter of the PVP fibres produced by electrospinning was 3.13 ± 1.34 μm and for the fibres produced using PG, the average was 3.53 ± 1.70 μm, indicating that both technologies can produced fine fibres. When it is necessary to achieve a higher fibre production output through electrospinning, a higher flowrate is required; this in turn increases the average fibre diameter. However, in the case of PG, the production rate is considerably higher.

Antifungal drugs, namely itraconazole and amphotericin B, were loaded into PVP fibres in order to compare the difference between the drug release profiles of electrospinning and PG. High-magnification images of these drug-loaded fibres are presented in figure 4.12. Finer polymeric structures are more desirable for drug delivery because they offer a greater surface area for the release of amorphous drug molecules. Electrospinning produced thinner drug-loaded fibres when compared with PG; the addition of the drug to the fibre resulted in the production of fewer fibres,

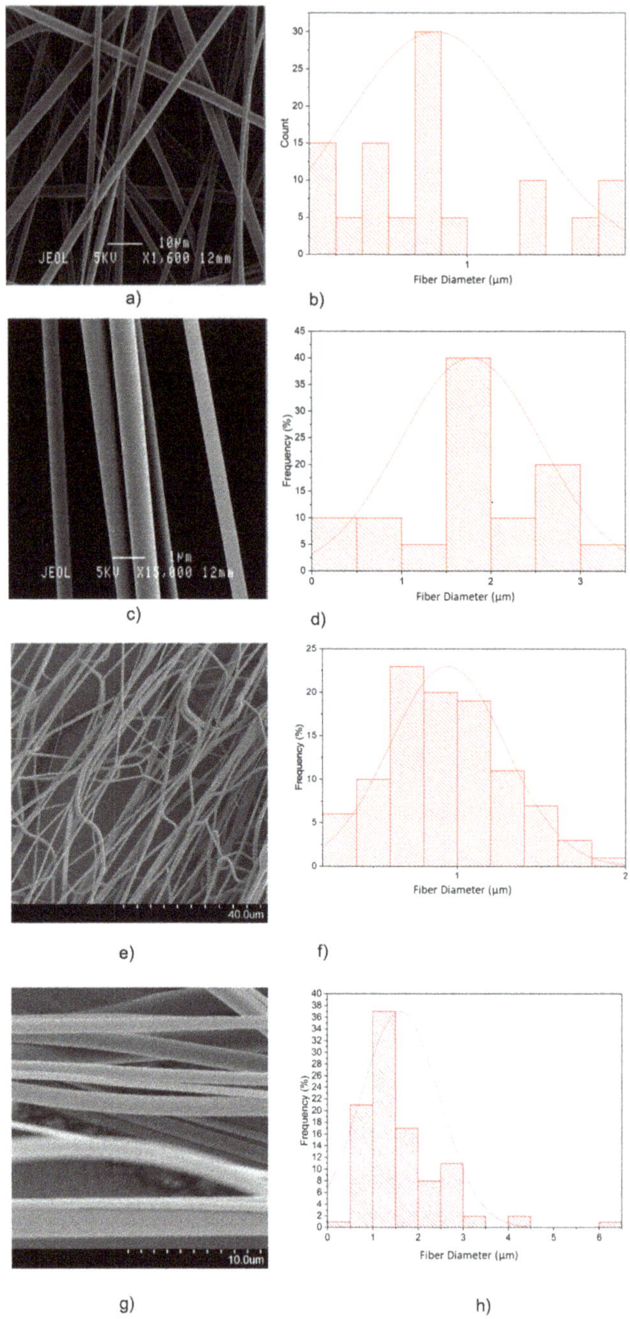

Figure 4.12. SEM images and fibre diameter distributions of: amphotericin B-loaded PVP fibres prepared by electrospinning (a) and pressurised gyration (c), itraconazole-loaded PVP fibres produced by (e) electrospinning and (g) pressurised gyration. (b, d, f, and h) The fibre diameter distributions for the corresponding fibre types [31] John Wiley & Sons. [2018].

as the drug interacts with the polymer chains. In a comparison of itraconazole-loaded PVP fibres, electrospun fibres had an average diameter of 0.94 ± 0.34 μm compared to 1.60 ± 0.87 μm for the PG fibres. While these values are close, the added surface area afforded by the thinner electrospun fibres could be advantageous in drug release scenarios, should all other factors be equal. In a comparison of amphotericin B-loaded PVP fibres, electrospun fibres had an average diameter of 0.88 ± 0.35 μm, while PG fibres had an average diameter of 1.78 ± 0.81 μm.

The morphological differences between these fibres play a role in dissolution. Figure 4.13 shows the drug release profiles of the itraconazole–PVP and amphotericin B–PVP fibres produced by electrospinning and PG.

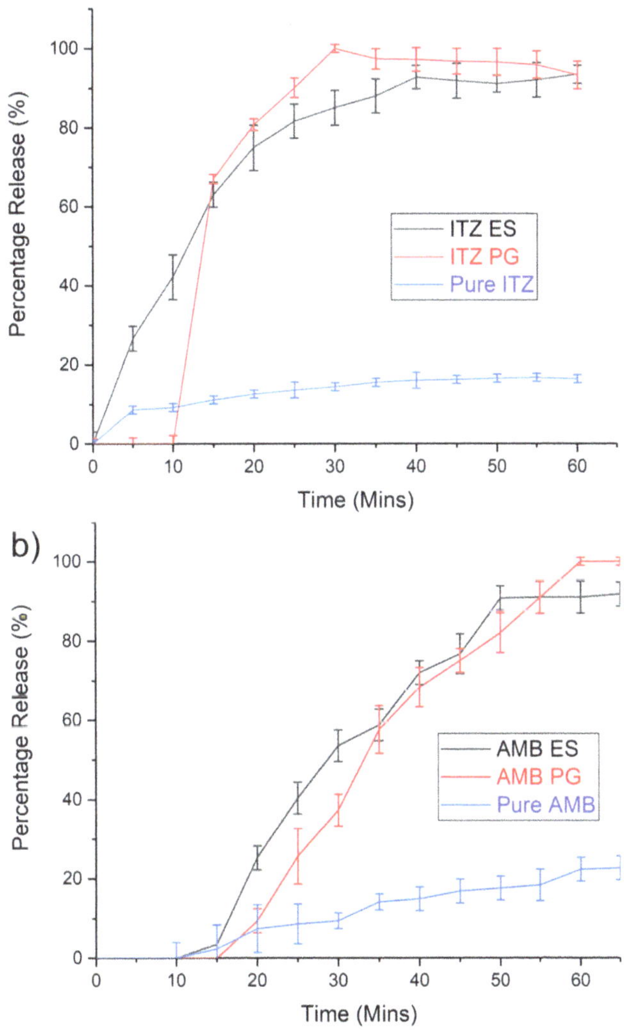

Figure 4.13. Drug dissolution profiles: (a) itraconazole-loaded PVP fibres and (b) amphotericin B-loaded PVP fibres [31] John Wiley & Sons. [2018].

Upon comparing the drug release profiles of itraconazole- and amphotericin B-loaded PVP fibres, it can be seen that both fibre types show a significant increase in drug dissolution rate compared to the raw drug alone in the same aqueous environment of phosphate buffered saline at a pH of 7.4. Interestingly, fibres spun using PG showed a higher maximum release, and compared to the electrospun itraconazole fibres, they showed a more rapid burst release profile. Therefore, the structure and morphology of the fibres play contributory roles in the drug release kinetics, whereas the average fibre diameter alone cannot be used to predict the mode of dissolution. Electrospun fibres have the benefit of being finer and more uniform but pressure-spun fibres are more uniaxially aligned and produce fibres as a much faster rate; for example, for 10% PVP fibres, the production rate was 30 g min^{-1} of dry fibre. The production rate is dependent on the polymer used, the concentration and the solvent used to dissolve it.

4.5.1.2 Intra-vaginal progesterone-loaded fibrous patches

The supply of essential pharmaceuticals and hormones to the targeted site is a field of drug delivery that is contributing to the advancement of healthcare for the masses. Preterm birth, as defined by the World Health Organisation as birth before 37 weeks of pregnancy, is the leading cause of death for children under the age of five years [32]. The majority of global preterm births occur in low-income countries due to a lack of proper medical care, something that could be more preventable with a better supply of medicine. Progesterone is a steroidal hormone naturally produced by the body and is crucial for reproduction in humans. Low levels of progesterone have been linked with an increased occurrence of neonatal morbidity and mortality in women [33]. Progesterone can be administered via many routes, including oral, parenteral, and topical routes, via the use of pessaries, creams, and vaginal gels. The vaginal mucosal cavity offers a feasible and safe site for drug delivery and is desirable in terms of its drug interactions, which include high absorption, metabolism, and elimination [34]. However, existing methods of progesterone vaginal delivery have been hindered by poor retention, leakages, and poor bioavailability [35].

A nanofibrous system capable of carrying and delivering progesterone could overcome many of the current limitations with the administration of progesterone to pregnant women. The system should be able to be transported easily and administered simply and it should be able to release progesterone over a prolonged period of time. As early as 2015, work was carried out using PG to identify and analyse the optimal conditions required to produce mucoadhesive nanofibres using blends of polymers with differing adhesive properties. Mucoadhesive systems are able to provide intimate contact between the vaginal mucosa and the drug to be administered; this can lead to a high drug concentration in the local area and thus high drug flux throughout the vaginal mucosa [34]. In 2015, Brako *et al* examined several polymers with mucoadhesive properties for their ability to be spun using PG into nanofibres capable of vaginal delivery [36]. In this work, four polymers were used and blended: sodium carboxymethylcellulose (CMC), PEO, polyacrylic acid (PAA) and sodium alginate in addition to purified water as the solvent of choice. Simulated vaginal fluid was created for these studies which contained a range of substances including mucin from porcine stomachs and bovine serum albumin. Nanofibres were produced as part of this work. Nanofibres are especially coveted due to their more numerous beneficial physical properties that become apparent at that scale; however, nanofibres are thus also more difficult to produce. Using water as a solvent, nanofibres can be produced through the use of PG. Blends containing 25 wt% CMC produced the finest fibres, which had an average diameter of only 266 ± 49 nm. It was found that for this blend, increasing the applied pressure from 0.1 to 0.2 MPa led to a reduction in the average fibre diameter.

The fibres produced in this study are displayed in figure 4.14. The fibres appear to have well-defined structures and smooth topographies. The uniformity of these fibres was also good; for example, PAA blends had a polydispersity index of only 15%. FTIR analysis of the fibres confirmed the presence of both individual polymers in the blended solution.

The fibre blends were then subjected to mucoadhesive studies in which they were placed in a simulated vaginal environment. Their breaking properties were assessed by measuring the force required to detach the polymer from the simulated mucosal environment. The results of this study can be found in figure 4.15.

It was found that compared to using the powder-only form of the polymers, the nanofibre form could significantly increase the force required to detach the polymer from the simulated vaginal environment. Alginate and CMC, when used as polymer blends, are more likely to offer strong contact by adhesion on mucosal surfaces. Utilising this materials-based approach offers great potential when mucoadhesion is desired; in addition, the thin diameter of the fibres also offers great benefits in drug release. The dried residue of the fibre/mucin complexes was later analysed via atomic force microscopy (AFM) to analyse the surface roughness; smoother surfaces indicated greater mucoadhesion. The results of the surface topography analysis were in line with the results of the previous mucoadhesion tests, in which the PEO–alginate mixture produced the roughest surface and the PEO–CMC mixture produced the smoothest surface.

A follow-up study was carried out based on the promising results of the initial mucoadhesion study with PEO polymer blends. In the follow-up study, progesterone-loaded nanofibres were produced using PG [37]. Progesterone was added to these PEO–CMC polymer blends in ascending concentrations from 0.5 to 7.7 (w w^{-1} %). Ethanol was used to dissolve the progesterone, while water was used as the main solvent of the blend. These polymer solutions were then spun via PG at an applied working pressure of 0.15 MPa and a rotational speed of 24 000 rpm. The fibres thus produced can be seen in figure 4.16.

The progesterone-loaded PEO–CMC blends produced ultrafine fibres with what appears to be a mostly smooth surface with some visible ridges on the surface. The progesterone–PEO fibres had an average diameter of 349 nm and a polydispersity index of 22% in the absence of CMC. The progesterone-loaded PEO–CMC blend had an average fibre diameter of 404 nm and a polydispersity index of only 15%. Adding CMC into the complex results in an increase in the average fibre diameter due to the increase in overall solution viscosity; however, the CMC provides the additional mucoadhesive properties and it must therefore be applied. FTIR

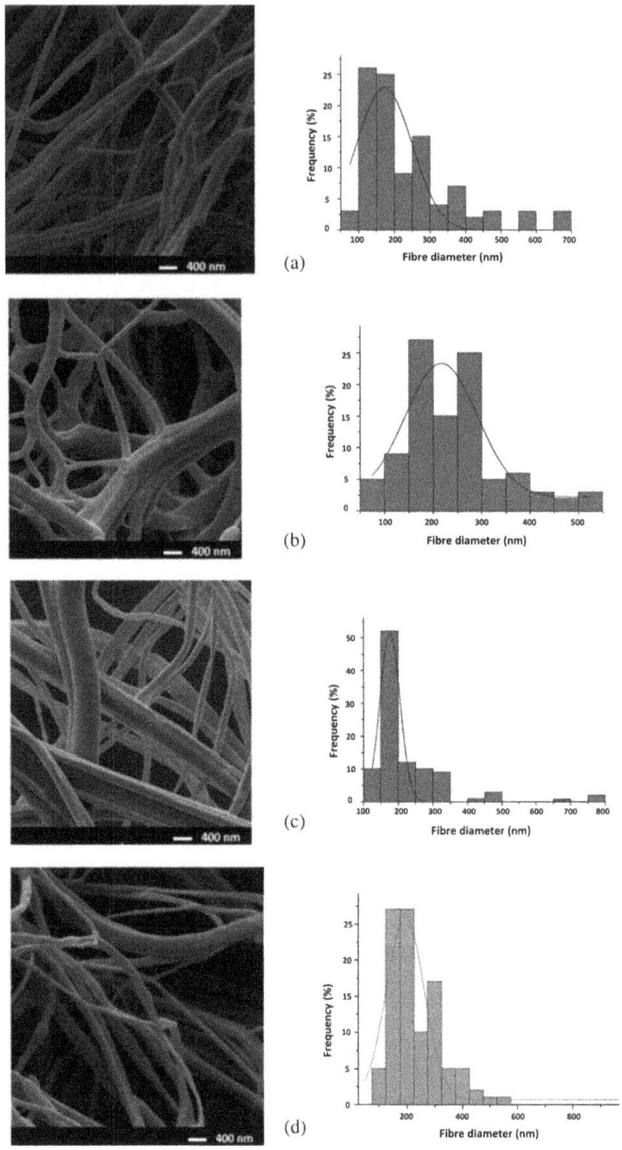

Figure 4.14. SEM micrographs and size distributions of fibre patches produced from 15% w w^{-1} PEO and blends incorporating: (a) 15 wt% w w^{-1} of polyethylene oxide, (b) 5% w w^{-1} alginate, (c) 5% w w^{-1} polyacrylic acid, and (d) 4% w w^{-1} carboxymethylcellulose. A gyration speed of 24 000 rpm and a working pressure of 0.15 MPa were used. Reprinted from [36], Copyright (2015), with permission from Elsevier.

analysis confirmed that the characteristic peaks of progesterone were present in the progesterone-loaded PEO–CMC blend. Hot stage microscopy (figure 4.17) visually showed the presence of progesterone encapsulated within the fibre strands. At a temperature of 95 °C, the PEO melted and the drug molecules were left exposed.

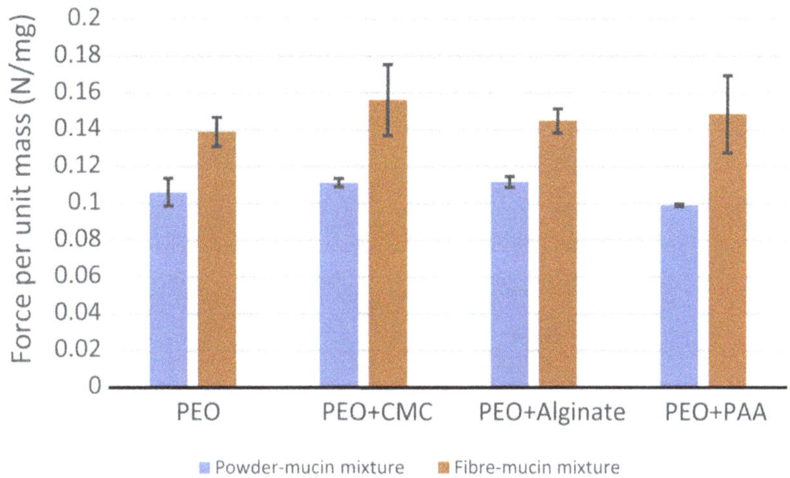

Figure 4.15. The forces required to separate the samples from the simulated environment. The bars compare the powder form and the fibre form for each polymer blend. Reprinted from [36], Copyright (2015), with permission from Elsevier.

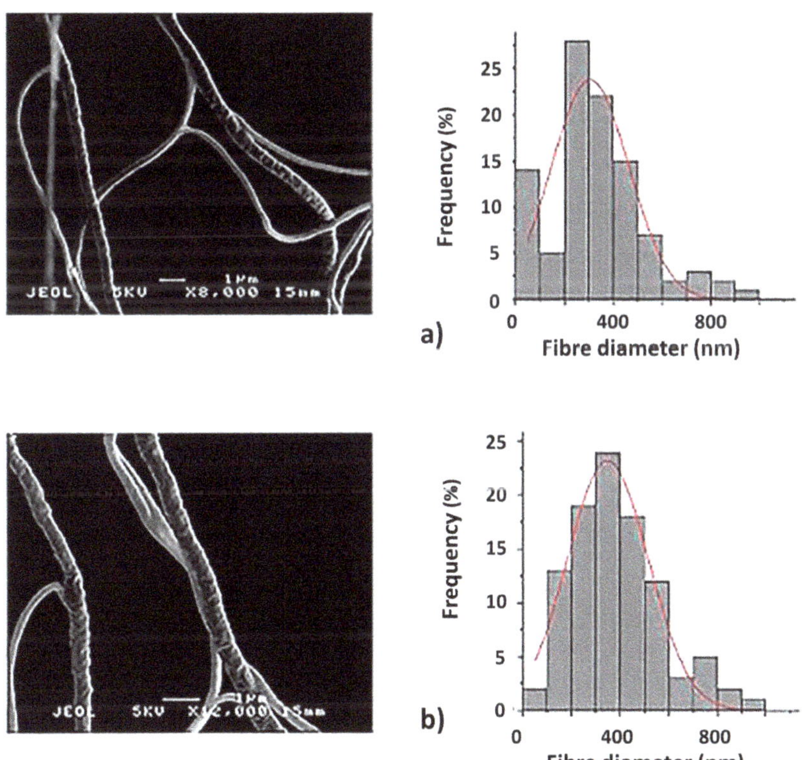

Figure 4.16. SEM images and size distribution for (a) PEO progesterone-loaded fibres (produced using a solution containing 5 wt% progesterone and 15 wt% PEO and (b) progesterone-loaded PEO/CMC (produced using a solution containing 5 wt% progesterone, 13.75 wt% PEO, and 1.25 wt% CMC). Reprinted from [37], Copyright (2018), with permission from Elsevier.

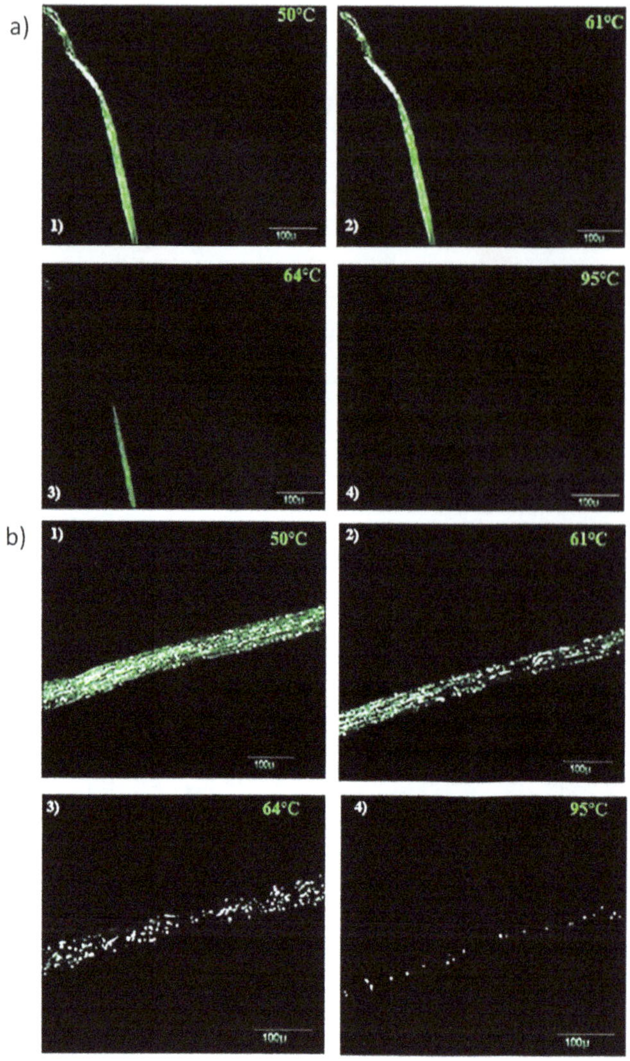

Figure 4.17. Hot-stage microscopy images showing: (a) melting of PEO fibres without progesterone and the corresponding temperatures, (b) melting of PEO fibres with 5 wt% progesterone and the corresponding temperatures. The numbers represent the different stages. Reprinted from [37], Copyright (2018), with permission from Elsevier.

Cyclogest is trademark name of a clinically approved and currently available 400 mg pessary which provides progesterone to the patient intravaginally [38]. The progesterone-loaded PEO and progesterone-loaded PEO–CMC nanofibres were compared with Cyclogest; the results are shown in figure 4.18. The drug release profiles of the progesterone-loaded nanofibres and the commercially available pessary are comparable; however, the nanofibres release the drug content more rapidly than the Cyclogest. Given the high surface area of the fibres, this is not surprising. By controlling the crystalline form of the progesterone within the fibre

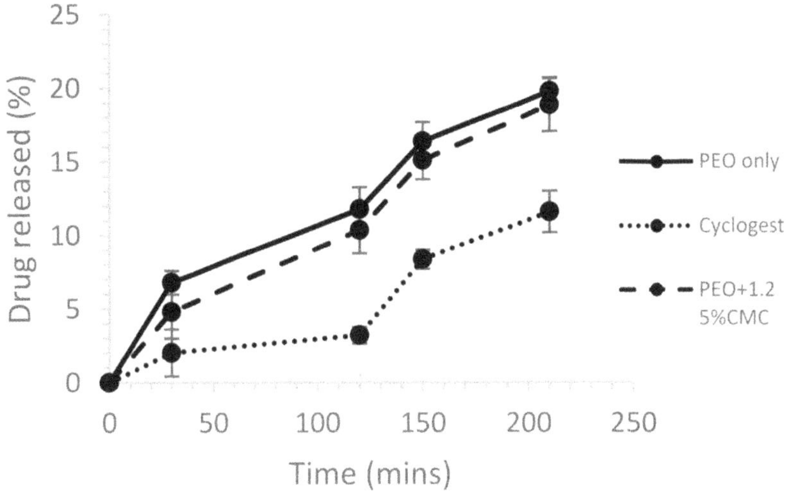

Figure 4.18. A graph showing the drug release profiles of progesterone–PEO fibres, progesterone-loaded PEO–CMC fibres and Cyclogest in simulated vaginal fluid. Reprinted from [37], Copyright (2018), with permission from Elsevier.

matrix, the release can be altered, allowing a more sustained release of the hormone throughout the day. The addition of CMC to the drug complex had little effect on the drug release profile when compared to the use of PEO alone; this is beneficial because the CMC adds to the mucoadhesive properties of the complex.

The potential to produce mucoadhesive nanofibres with PG was further explored in a study which analysed the mucoadhesive interactions between progesterone-loaded fibres made with PEO and CMC polymer blends [39]. Mucoadhesion can be defined as an interactive state between two material surfaces, one of which is biological in nature (typically a mucosa), in which these surfaces are held for an extended time period by interfacial forces [40]. Mucoadhesion can be said to occur in two stages: (1) first there is spreading and swelling of the mucoadhesive material to allow contact with the mucosa, (2) second, the mucoadhesive materials interact with the membrane; in the second stage, moisture plasticises the systems, causing molecules to break free and form van der Waals and hydrogen bonds with the mucins [41].

This study produced nanofibres using progesterone-loaded mixtures of PEO and CMC. Figure 4.19 shows micrographs and the diametric distributions of the produced fibres. The fibres present a mostly smooth surface that includes some surface roughness in the form of grooves. Progesterone-loaded PEO (13.75 wt%)/CMC (1.25 wt%) fibres had an average fibre diameter of 404 nm and a polydispersity index of 22%, whilst PEO (13.75 wt%)/CMC (1.25 wt%) fibres without any drug had an average fibre diameter of 194 nm and a polydispersity index of 12%. The addition of progesterone leads to an increase in the average fibre diameter.

The mucoadhesive properties of the PEO–CMC fibre blends were assessed using both artificial and biological membranes. Both the adhesion and permeation

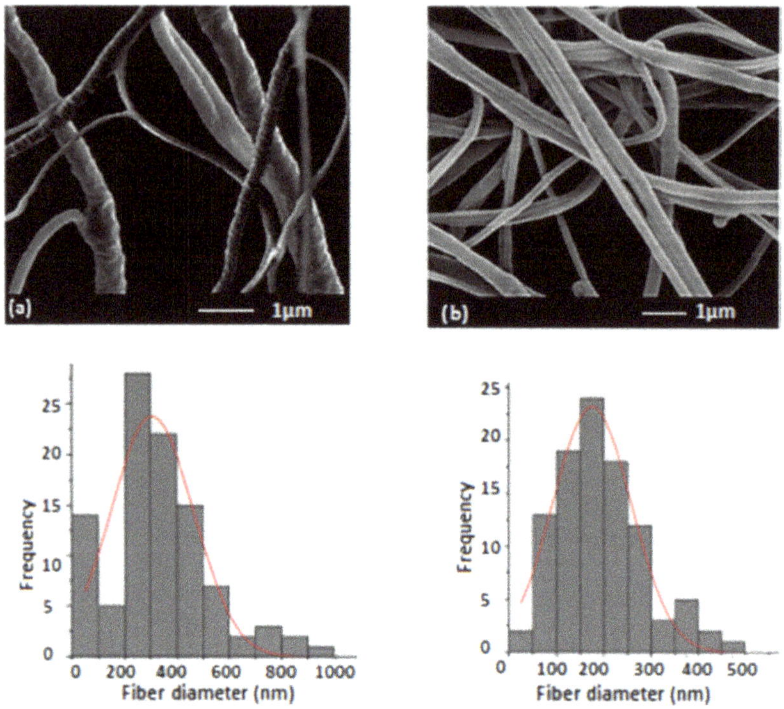

Figure 4.19. SEM images and size distributions ($n = 100$) of: (a) progesterone-loaded PEO (13.75 wt%)/CMC (1.25 wt%) fibres, (b) PEO (13.75 wt%)/CMC (1.25 wt%) fibres without drug content. Reproduced from [39]. CC BY 4.0.

properties of mucoadhesive delivery systems should be assessed to determine their performance; for this reason, artificial cellulose acetate membranes were selected, as they are not prone to inconsistencies during the tissue preparation process and they also correlate well with animal mucosa tissues [42]. The effect on the mucoadhesive properties of increasing the CMC content in the progesterone-loaded fibres was assessed using both cellulose acetate membranes and lamb oesophagus mucosa. Figure 4.20 shows a summary of the findings. With higher CMC content, there is a clear link to increasing mucoadhesion for both artificial and natural mucosa membranes. The carboxylic groups found in the CMC are able to form strong hydrogen bonds with the mucin chains, creating a stronger interfacial bond between the fibres and the mucosa [43]. The mucoadhesive properties are significantly more apparent in the cellulose acetate material; this is thought to be due to the adhesive behaviour of cellulose-based materials, which facilitates the easy formation of strong hydrogen bonding by their hydroxyl groups.

AFM was also utilised to observe the effect of increasing CMC content on the mucoadhesion of freshly slaughtered lamb esophagus mucosa. Figure 4.21 shows AFM images of progesterone-loaded PEO fibres with increasing CMC content. Interfacial roughness was used as an indication of interpenetration between two surfaces, which suggests mucoadhesion. Stronger binding of the surfaces can

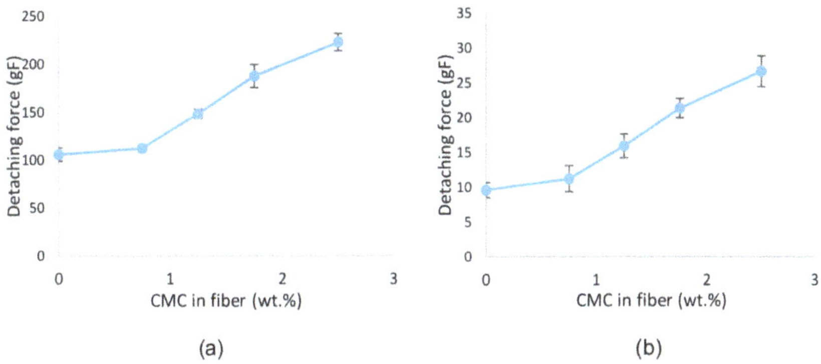

Figure 4.20. The effect of CMC content on the mucoadhesive properties of nanofibres as assessed by measuring the forces required to detach them from: (a) a cellulose acetate membrane and (b) lamb oesophageal mucosa. Reproduced from [39]. CC BY 4.0.

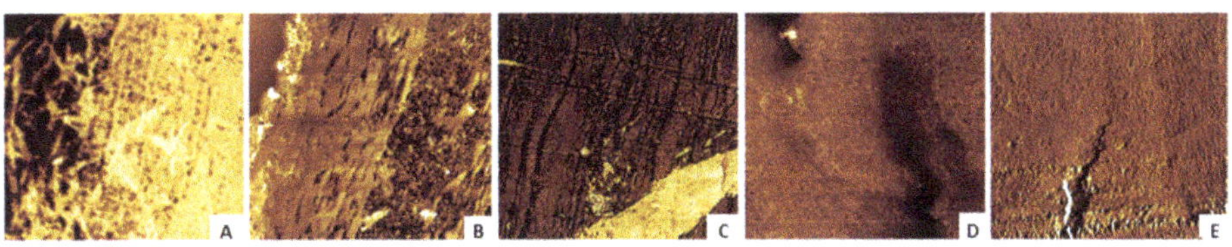

Figure 4.21. AFM phase images from the fibre–mucosa interface following a period of mucoadhesion. Homogeneity (material uniformity) is seen to increase with the CMC content of the fibres: (A) 0%, (B) 0.75%, (C) 1.25%, (D) 1.75%, (E) 2.5%. Images represent an area of 900 μm^2 with angular units between −30° and 15°. Reproduced from [39]. CC BY 4.0.

therefore be indicated by extensive penetration; therefore, a smoother cross section corresponds to more mucoadhesive samples. Fibre samples with higher CMC contents were seen to have smoother interfacial images. The images showed increasing uniformity in response to higher CMC contents in the progesterone-loaded fibres from 0% (A) to 2.5% (E). These results suggest that progesterone-loaded nanofibres produced by PG could be used to develop vaginal inserts whose performance is improved by mucoadhesion.

More recently, PG and electrospinning were used to produce intravaginal progesterone-loaded fibrous patches using poly(lactic acid) (PLA) [44]. Four concentrations of PLA solutions were prepared using chloroform as the solvent at concentrations of 8%, 10%, 12%, and 15% (w/v). These solutions were then spun, and the resulting micrographs can be seen in figure 4.22. The pure PLA fibres produced highly unidirectionally aligned fibres with PG. Increasing polymer concentrations naturally led to increases in the final fibre diameter. The addition of progesterone to the polymer solution also led to three notable observations. First, the addition of progesterone led to a small increase in average fibre diameter, as expected; second, it also resulted in a loss of unidirectional alignment; and third, it led to the formation of beads within the fibre strands.

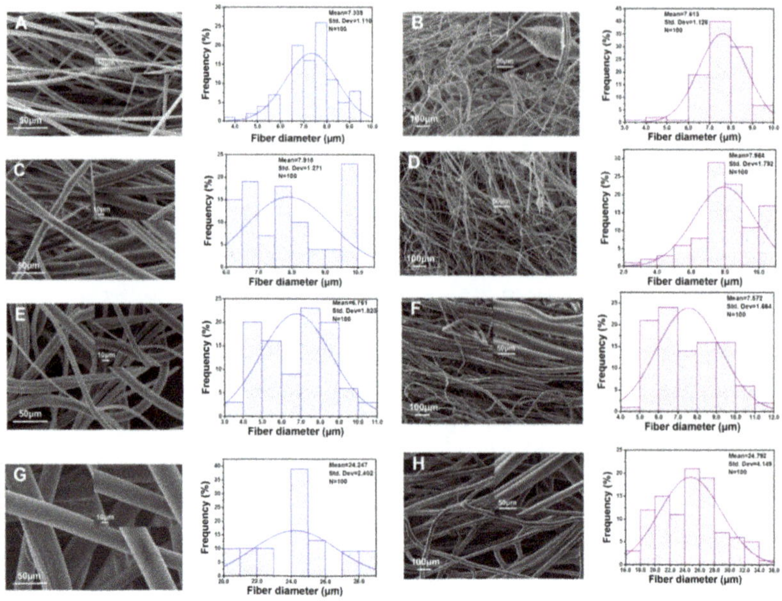

Figure 4.22. SEM images and fibre diameter distributions of pure and progesterone-loaded fibrous patches produced using PG: (A) 8% (w/v) PLA, (B) progesterone-loaded 8% PLA, (C) 10% PLA, (D) progesterone-loaded 10% PLA, (E) 12% PLA, (F) progesterone-loaded 12% PLA, (G) 15% PLA, and (H) progesterone-loaded 15% PLA. Reprinted from [44], Copyright (2018), with permission from Elsevier.

The 12% PLA fibres produced using PG had an average diameter of 6.76 ± 1.82 μm and the addition of progesterone lead to an increase in the average fibre diameter to 7.57 ± 1.79 μm. Of all the fibres spun, the 12% PLA fibres displayed the highest yield of 102.4 mg ml^{-1} when spun using PG and produced a yield of 114.7 mg ml^{-1} in the progesterone-loaded format. A sweet spot often exists between the polymer concentration and the yield; if the polymer concentration is too low, the yield can be low, but overlarge concentrations also affect the yield. Polymer concentration and the ability to spin viable fibres via PG can be attributed to polymer chain entanglement; higher concentrations and higher molecular weights contribute to higher polymer chain entanglement, therefore there is an optimal concentration at which the yield is high and the fibre diameter is low [45]. Compared to electrospun PLA fibres, PG was able to produce fibres of similar average diameters that ranged from 7.02–7.89 μm. However, due to the low solution feed rate required to obtain fine fibres using electrospinning, the production rate was significantly slower than that of PG.

When progesterone is normally administered intravaginally, its release is typically rapid, and the majority of the drug is distributed within about 3 h. The aim of the fibres produced using gyration and electrospinning is to create a delivery method that can facilitate the longer-term release of progesterone. Figure 4.23 shows the drug release profile for progesterone, gyration-spun progesterone-loaded fibrous

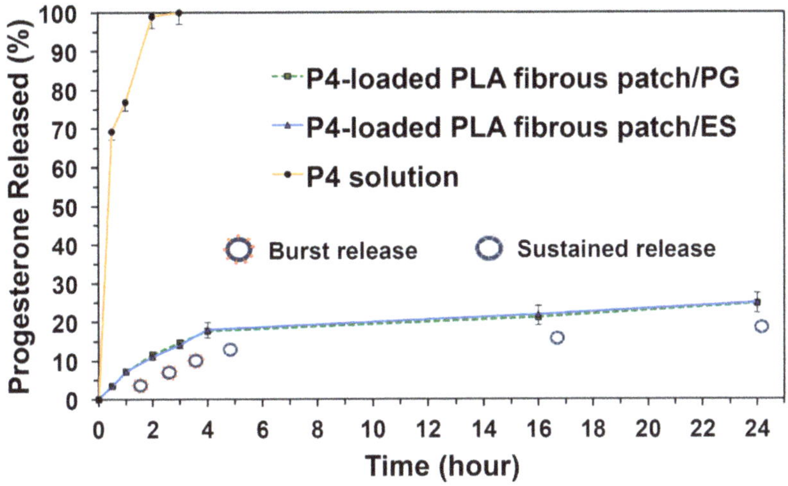

Figure 4.23. Progesterone (P4) release profiles of: progesterone-loaded fibrous patches produced by pressurised gyration and electrospinning and pure progesterone solution according to a first-order model. ES: electrospinning, PG: pressurised gyration, P4: progesterone. Reprinted from [44], Copyright (2018), with permission from Elsevier.

patches, and electrospun progesterone-loaded fibrous patches. Both of the fibrous patches demonstrated a more sustained release profile compared to the progesterone alone. The release profiles for both of the fibrous patches were very closely matched and showed a burst release profile for the first 4 h. The sustained release of progesterone is a desired feature for the treatment of preterm birth; this would also improve patient compliance, as fewer administrations would be needed in order to obtain the correct therapeutic effect.

In vitro cytotoxicity testing of the fibrous patches was investigated with the commercial Vero epithelial cell line; the results are shown in figure 4.24(a). The Vero cells were found to successfully attach to the surfaces of all the progesterone-loaded fibrous patches; within just 60 min of the initial cell seeding, almost 50% of the cells were attached to the fibres. Compared to tissue culture polystyrene (TCPS), all the fibres, with or without progesterone loading, showed a significant increase in cell attachment, indicating that the fibres were viable for maintaining cellular growth.

In order to assess the cell viability of the fibres, 3-(4,5-dimethylthiazol-2-yl)-2,5-diphenyltetrazolium bromide (MTT) colorimetric assays were conducted for a duration of seven days; the results are presented in figure 4.24(b). The MTT assay measures cell viability and proliferation via the reduction of coloured dyes; the reduction occurs in the mitochondria of cells and thus the intensity of this reduction depends on the metabolic activity of the participating cells [46]. During the seven-day test period, the fibres initially showed similar absorbance to that of the TCPS control; however, after day three, the fibre samples overtook the control samples and demonstrated significantly greater dye absorbance, indicating greater cell viability

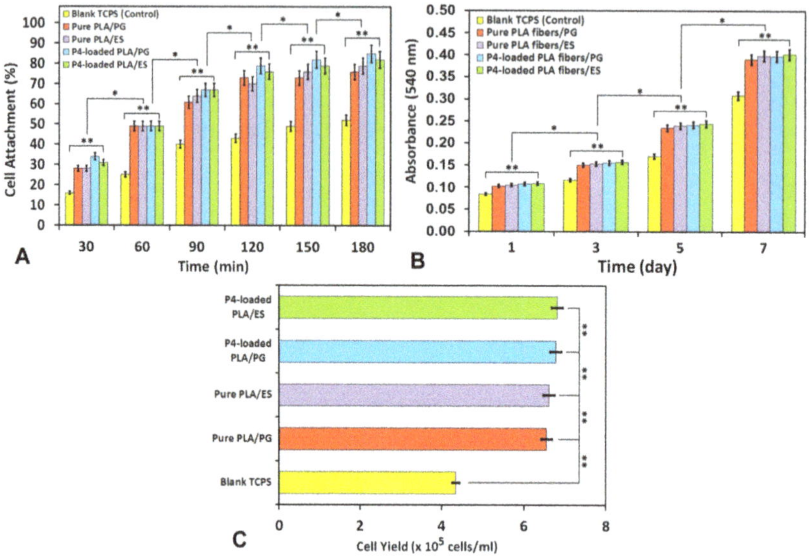

Figure 4.24. Cell culture results for fibrous patches: (A) 3 h attachment, (B) seven-day viability, and (C) cell yield (at the seventh day) performances of the pure and progesterone-loaded fibrous patches produced by PG and electrospinning, including blank TCPS control Petri dishes. The symbols '*' and '**' indicate the significant differences (* for $p < 0.05$ and ** for $p < 0.01$). ES: electrospinning, PG: pressurised gyration, P4: progesterone. Reprinted from [44], Copyright (2018), with permission from Elsevier.

and proliferation. The fibrous structure was able to facilitate greater viability and proliferation due to its superior surface-area-to-volume ratio and was able to provide additional anchorage points for the attachment and subsequent proliferation of the cells. In addition, the number of cells counted on these fibrous patches exceeded the limit of possible cell population on a flat 1 cm^2 surface.

The cell yield was also calculated following the MTT assay and is presented in figure 4.24(c). Compared to the control, all the fibre samples permitted an increase in cellular metabolic activity, which can be interpreted as increased cell number and viability. It was concluded that the fibrous patches were able to provide a more suitable environment that allowed cells to stay healthy and viable throughout the seven-day course. The results shown in this section show that PG and electrospinning are excellent ways of producing fibrous patches which could be used to administer progesterone intravaginally in an attempt to prevent preterm birth in mothers.

4.5.1.3 Remote-controlled drug delivery

Minimally invasive approaches to drug delivery have become increasingly attractive due to the development of superparamagnetic nanoparticles [47]. These nanoparticles can be fashioned into drug delivery vehicles in the form of membranes, liposomes, and even small-diameter fibres to treat certain cancers and cardiovascular diseases. The magnetic component is activated by predetermined triggers such as chemical signals or homoeostatic variations. Activation via external magnetic fields, however, is a new approach and one that could lead to great advances in pharmaceutical engineering, especially for targeted, controlled, and precise drug delivery. An efficient method utilising infusion gyration was reported for the production of biocompatible magnetically actuated fibres for targeted drug release [48]. A composite mixture of polyvinyl alcohol (PVA) at three different molecular weights (13 000, 31 000, and 146 000) was combined with iron magnetic nanoparticles (MNPs) and the drug paracetamol (acetaminophen) and fibres were generated.

Images of the produced PVA–MNP fibres can be seen in figure 4.25. At lower magnifications of the fibre surface, it was apparent that the PVA–MNP fibres contained small amounts of beads throughout their matrix, which might have arisen from the spinning conditions and the rheological properties of the polymer solution. Higher-magnification scanning electron microscopy (SEM) images (figure 4.25(c) and (d)) showed that the surface of the fibres was smooth and mostly devoid of surface features and roughness. The PVA–MNP fibres with iron-loaded nanoparticles also exhibited a bead-on-string morphology, and SEM dot mapping was used to confirm the presence of iron in the fibres. There was a good distribution of iron nanoparticles within the fibre matrix, making it suitable for use in superparamagnetic applications. The PVA–MNP-Fe fibres had average diameters of 100–300 nm; water-soluble polymers spun using gyration techniques are typically able to form fibrous structures in the nanometre range (<900 nm).

The PVA–MNP fibres successfully exhibited the ability to release controlled quantities of drugs via the application of an external magnetic field (stimulus). Drug

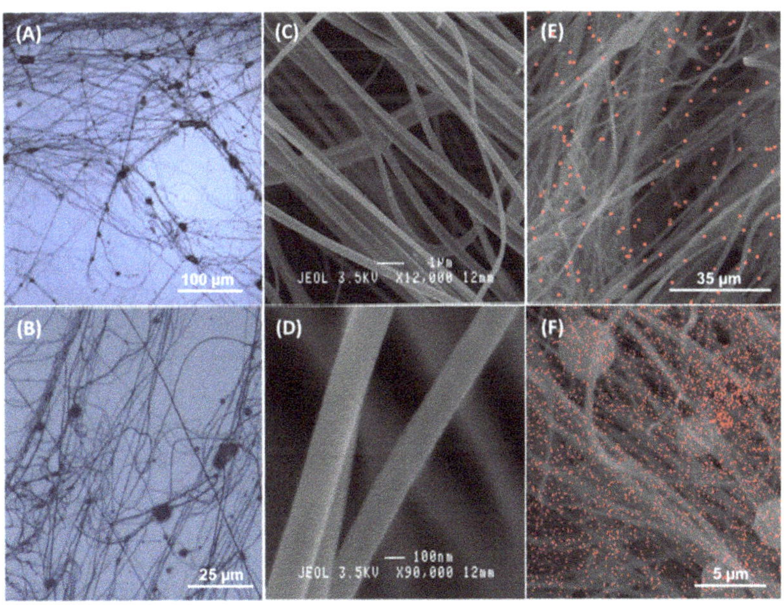

Figure 4.25. PVA–MNP fibres (5% (w w^{-1})). (A, B) Optical microscopy images, (C, D) SEM images, and (E, F) SEM dot mapping: the red dots indicate the presence of Fe in the fibres. Reproduced from [48]. CC BY 4.0.

dissolution studies were conducted to assess the release profile of these fibres without and with actuation. Non-actuated and actuated samples differed in their drug release profile, as illustrated in figure 4.26. Acetaminophen has a characteristic peak at a UV absorption of around 243 nm, as can be seen in figure 4.26(a), which confirms the uptake of acetaminophen by the fibres. Figure 4.26(b) shows an overview of the drug release profiles of the control (non-magnetically actuated) fibres and the actuated fibres. The magnetically activated fibres released significantly more acetaminophen over time compared to the non-actuated fibres. The actuated samples displayed rapid drug release during the initial 5 min, exhibiting a 'burst release' behaviour. About 50% of the acetaminophen was released within this period and over 90% was released by the end of the fifteenth minute after actuation. From the 15-minute point onwards, there was no significant difference in release between the two samples.

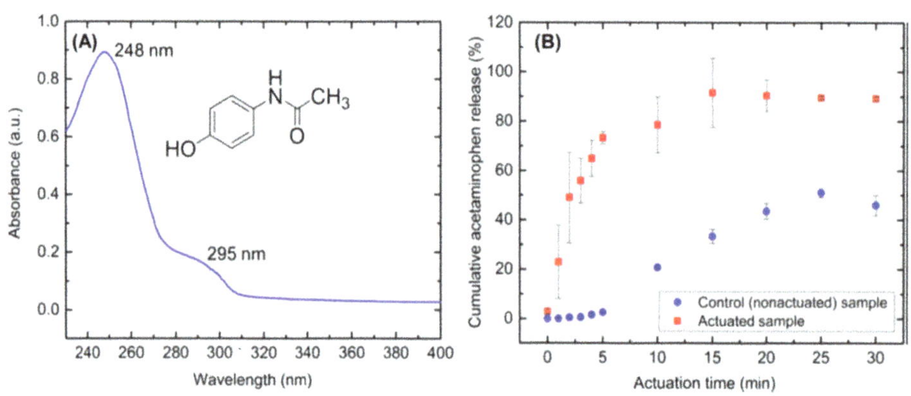

Figure 4.26. The use of magnetic fibres for the controlled release of acetaminophen with and without magnetic actuation. (A) The chemical structure and UV–vis absorption spectrum of acetaminophen, (B) cumulative weight percentages of acetaminophen released over time. Reproduced from [48]. CC BY 4.0.

This work shows that PVA nanofibres integrating magnetic Fe_3O_4 nanoparticles were successfully produced. The fibres demonstrated high levels of stability and an absence of iron leaching. These fibres maintained a good degree of nanoparticle distribution within their fibre matrix and were able to sustain sufficient magnetisation to support actuation via an external magnetic field. Compared to the non-actuated control sample, the magnetic PVA nanofibres demonstrated over 70% more release of the drug within the first 5 min. Gyration-based technologies offer a promising technique for the manufacture of efficient remote-controlled drug delivery products.

4.5.1.4 Diabetic wound healing

Diabetes is a very common disease which affects millions of adults and is a result of hyperglycaemia. Wounds associated with this disease are characterised by a lack of proper healing, and in more serious cases, severe infection may arise, leading to potential amputation [49]. Peroxisome proliferator-activated receptors (PPARs) are a superfamily of nuclear receptor proteins that includes PPAR-α, PPAR-γ, and PPAR-β/δ, which function as transcription factors in the regulation of gene expression [50]. PPARs have been found to have many roles in the wound healing process, such as during the inflammation phase, as a regulator of keratinocyte activity, and in fibroblast proliferation [51]. In particular, PPAR-γ has been a focus in many studies of diabetic wound healing due to its role in the regulation of glucose metabolism, lipid metabolism, and adipocyte differentiation. In mice, the use of PPAR-γ has been demonstrated to delay wound healing by disturbing the debris clearance of apoptotic cells [52]. Pioglitazone hydrochloride (PHR) is an orally-administered medication used to treat type 2 diabetes. It can be used in conjunction with other common diabetes medications, such as metformin [53]. PHR also acts as a synthetic agonist for PPAR-γ which can activate it and modulate its activity. PG has been used to produce PHR-loaded drug delivery patches to tackle diabetic wound healing [54].

The control of drugs can be achieved in a polymeric system that contains two or more polymers that have different degradation rates. For example, the co-polymer polylactic-co-glycolic acid (PLGA) is often used in drug delivery because its constituent co-polymers have very different degradation rates; poly(glycolic acid) (PGA) degrades more rapidly than PLA [55]. Using this principle, the degradation of the composite polymer can be controlled by varying the ratio of either polymer to achieve the desired degradation rate. The controlled release of drugs can therefore be used to tackle special wound healing conditions, where the drug release profile influences the rate of healing.

4.5.2 Tissue engineering

4.5.2.1 The use of artificial bone marrow fibrous scaffolds to study resistance to anti-leukaemia agents

Tissue-engineering applications benefit from the unique physical characteristics of small-diameter fibres that can be easily controlled by PG. These characteristics include features such as a high surface-area-to-volume ratio and surface features such as roughness and porosity [56]. Furthermore, certain fibrous forms, such as a high degree of uniaxial alignment, can be beneficial for specific tissue engineering applications such as nerve tissue regeneration and wound healing [57, 58]. In tissue engineering, it is important to understand that cells only interact with the surface of a material; therefore, features such as surface roughness, grooves, pits, and pore size can greatly influence the viability of a fibrous biomaterial in any given application.

In 2017, an article showcased PG as a simple and cost-effective way in which to develop artificial bone marrow scaffolds for the study of resistance of anti-leukaemia agents such as the cancer growth-blocker imatinib [59]. Conventional two-dimensional cellular assays have many limitations in predicting longer-term responses to anticancer drugs, since native cell interaction occurs in three dimensions and mechanotransducive cues play an important role in this [60]. Furthermore, there is evidence to suggest that interaction with three-dimensional artificial scaffolds can produce resistance to chemotherapeutic drugs [61]. PG was therefore used to produce a three-dimensional poly(methyl methacrylate) (PMMA)–hydroxyapatite (HA) fibre scaffold which could be used to mimic the bone marrow environment for studies of cancer–therapy interactions. SEM of the prepared PMMA–HA fibres showed that a rough surface was produced that contained the dispersion of HA particles and surface nanopores (figure 4.27). These composite fibres were continuous and were not interrupted by a bead-on-a-string morphology, showing that PG can be used to select optimal operating parameters for this type of fibrous structure.

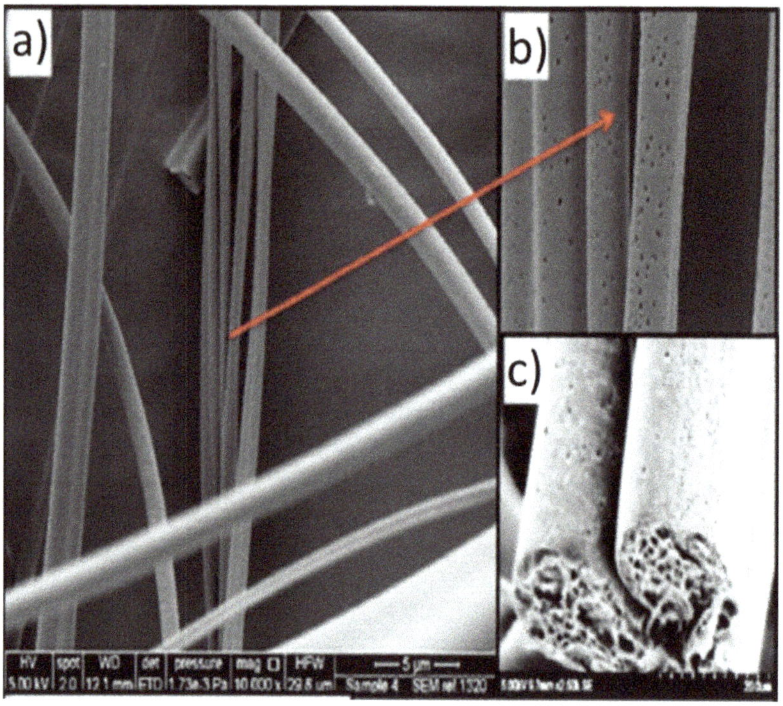

Figure 4.27. SEM micrographs of PMMA–HA fibres: (a) an SEM image of the PMMA–HA fibres, panels (b) and (c) show the surface nanopores and a cross section of the fibres, respectively, at higher magnification [59] John Wiley & Sons. [2018].

The produced PMMA–HA composite fibres were found to be nontoxic under test conditions. Macroscopic analysis revealed cell proliferation on the fibrous scaffold following the culture of cells taken from acute myeloid leukaemia patients. An investigation into the *in vivo* recapitulation abilities of the cell culture found a significant difference between the imatinib-induced inhibition of two-dimensional and three-dimensional cultures. The three-dimensional PMMA–HA cultures were then investigated to assess whether the protective effect of the scaffold was specific against imatinib. More acute myeloid leukaemia-derived cells were found in the three-dimensional culture following treatment with doxorubicin than in the two-dimensional culture, suggesting the PMMA–HA scaffold may have a more protective effect.

The PMMA–HA scaffold was then seeded with a co-culture of HS-5 and K562 cells to further mimic the bone marrow microenvironment. The HS-5 cells appeared to have an affinity for the PMMA–HA scaffold. The scaffold combined with the HS-5 cells reduced the sensitivity of the K562 cells to imatinib when compared to a two-dimensional co-culture with HS-5. As a result of studying multiple bone-marrow-derived cell lines, it was concluded that the fibrous scaffold provided a suitable matrix for the study of leukaemia cells and that the three-dimensional structure of the bone marrow environment protected the cells from chemotherapeutic agents.

4.5.2.2 Bacterial cellulose blended fibrous bandages

One key application of biomaterials and tissue engineering is in medical applications such as wound healing. Wound healing is a complicated multistep process which involves various cells and changes in the wound microenvironment [62]. For these reasons, a bandage needs to be compatible and suitable to facilitate proper wound healing, both physically and biologically. Bacterial cellulose, produced by certain bacteria under specific conditions, has been found to be a source of ultrafine cellulose with highly beneficial wound healing characteristics, such as a high degree of biocompatibility and a high water-holding capacity [63]. The approach of combining bacterial cellulose with other existing polymers to increase its suitability for wound healing has been exploited by electrospinning, which has successfully produced hybrid fibrous structures [64]. However, the use of techniques such as electrospinning limits the maximum amount of bacterial cellulose that can be included in the final fibres. In response, PG has been used to produce blends of polymers and higher concentrations of bacterial cellulose.

As pure bacterial cellulose fibres are extremely difficult to dissolve and reform into fibres, a carrier polymer must be used. Bacterial cellulose:PMMA fibres were produced using a range of different blend ratios and their morphological and chemical features were examined [65]. PMMA is a biocompatible and highly hydrophobic polymer which is chemically suitable for many biomedical applications, but it is let down by its highly brittle nature. By combining PMMA with bacterial cellulose, it may be possible to make a bandage-like fibrous scaffold that leverages the desirable properties of both materials. Eight different weight ratios of bacterial cellulose:PMMA fibres were created, which showed significant differences in their measured physical properties, specifically, their viscosities. The addition of bacterial cellulose to another polymer matrix increases the viscosity exponentially, which further contributes to the additional difficulty in spinning higher loadings of bacterial cellulose. For example, a 5:20 ratio of bacterial cellulose and PMMA had a measured viscosity of 26.8 ± 1.6 mPa s, whereas a 10:40 ratio gave a reading of 5040.4 ± 27.5 mPa s. Highly viscous polymer solutions tend not to produce fibres, even with other spinning techniques such as electrospinning. The polymer solutions were spun with PG at a maximum rotational speed and an applied gas pressure of 3×10^5 Pa under ambient conditions (23 °C, 42% relative humidity). Figure 4.28 shows SEM micrographs of the eight solutions spun into fibres.

The viscosity was seen to increase as the proportion of bacterial cellulose increased, and the same was true for the surface tension of the solution. The viscosity and surface tension are key known factors which affect the morphology of

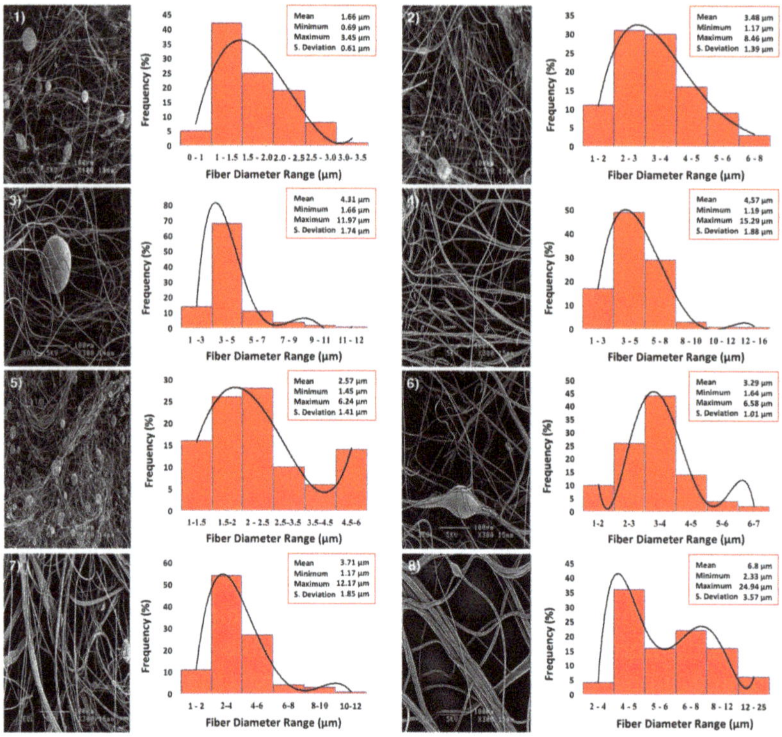

Figure 4.28. SEM images and corresponding fibre diameter distributions of the samples made from (1) 5:20, (2) 5:30, (3) 5:40, (4) 5:50, (5) 10:20, (6) 10:30, (7) 10:40, and (8) 10:50 bacterial cellulose:PMMA solutions [59] John Wiley & Sons. [2018].

the produced fibres. Overall, the fibres did show a prominent bead-on-a-string morphology, and the 10:20 bacterial cellulose:PMMA ratio showed the greatest occurrence of this. The beads are hypothesised to be caused by the addition of bacterial cellulose and the subsequent increases in the bacterial cellulose content; this is possibly due to the processing conditions of bacterial cellulose, which first needs to be solubilised in order to form a fraction of the polymer blend. As the PMMA polymer concentration increased, the overall fibre diameter increased. This study found that at a 5:50 ratio of bacterial cellulose:PMMA, a compromise between fibre diameter and uniformity was reached.

The produced fibres were intended to act as a bandage-like scaffold for the purpose of wound healing. Given that both bacterial cellulose and PMMA are biocompatible in their own right, cellular testing was performed on the scaffolds to discern whether they were nontoxic to the cells of the wound healing response. Saos-2, a human osteosarcoma cell line, was used for the cell viability assays. The cell viability showed no indication of toxicity for all but three of the tested bacterial cellulose:PMMA samples, and at the end of the testing period, the Saos-2 cells on the scaffolds showed a similar behaviour to that of the positive control sample. Polymer blends of bacterial cellulose:PMMA at ratios of 10:20, 0:50, and 10:50

displayed a cell viability of less than the acceptable 85%, which could be caused by the higher proportion of PMMA than that of bacterial cellulose. With the addition of 5 wt% bacterial cellulose to 50 wt% PMMA, the cell viability showed a significant increase, however at 10 wt% of bacterial cellulose, the cell viability did not increase. DAPI (4′,6-diamidino-2-phenylindole) staining and SEM allowed cell migration and proliferation to be observed on the different blended scaffolds. The scaffolds exhibited suitable cell spreading and proliferation and showed increased metabolic activity compared to the control groups upon observation. Samples containing 5 wt% bacterial cellulose demonstrated enhanced proliferation compared to the scaffolds containing 10 wt% bacterial cellulose. Increasing the ratio of bacterial cellulose comes at the cost of increased processing complexity because, as mentioned previously, the insolubility of bacterial cellulose results in a change in bioactive properties. MTT assays performed on the scaffolds gave matching results, in which 5% bacterial cellulose loadings resulted in increased cellular proliferation.

In order for a material to be suitable for use as a wound healing bandage, its mechanical properties must not be compromised by the natural movements of the patient. Mechanical testing of these constructs showed there the bandage-like scaffolds had greater ductility and that the tensile strain at fracture of the 5:50 bacterial cellulose:PMMA structures was about 2.5 times higher than the strain at fracture of structures produced via electrospinning. A suitable wound healing material must be able to absorb a great deal of exudate. The optimal 5:50 scaffold also demonstrated a swelling ratio of approximately four in preliminary water-holding capacity tests. This initial work on bacterial-cellulose-containing fibrous structures showed the feasibility of spinning such fibres into bandage-like structures and demonstrated the benefits of PG. Fibres ranging in size from 690 nm to 25 μm were produced, and it was seen that optimisations were necessary in order to achieve the most suitable end product.

Following on from the first study which produced bacterial-cellulose-containing fibres, a second study was completed to demonstrate the improved production of bacterial cellulose scaffolds with higher yields and antimicrobial capabilities [66]. This subsequent work showcased a detailed investigation into the production of bacterial cellulose:PMMA bandage-like scaffolds that incorporated antimicrobial nanoparticles containing silver and copper (UHNP-1 and AVNP-2). The scaffolds were tested in a co-culture containing both keratinocytes (skin cells) and *Staphylococcus aureus* (pathogenic bacteria), and their cytotoxic performance was examined.

The first study had demonstrated the increased complexity of spinning fibres loaded with higher bacterial cellulose content. To combat this, bacterial cellulose was subjected to high-frequency ultrasonication in order to break down the polymer matrix and increase its solubility. In addition to ultrasonication, dimethylformamide was also used to further solubilise the bacterial cellulose. Micrographs of the produced bandage-like scaffolds are shown in figure 4.29.

This study was the first to truly demonstrate the ability of PG to produce quantities of bandage-like constructs that have a physical form suitable for direct use as a wound-covering material. Unlike fibres produced via other methods such as

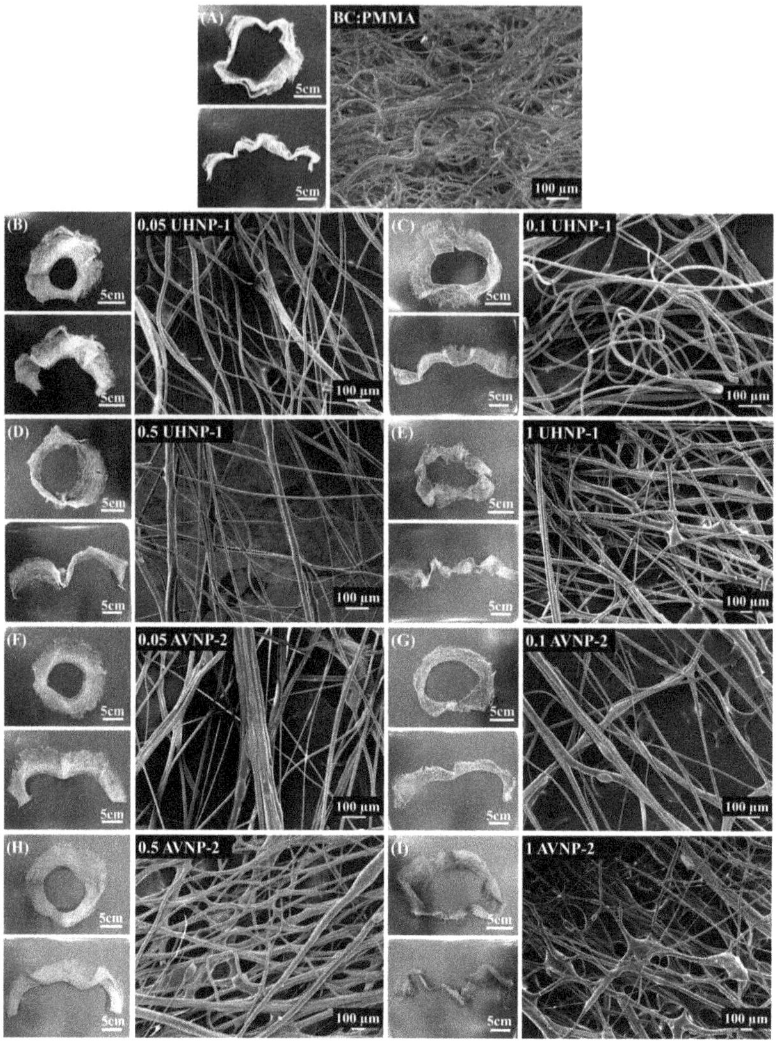

Figure 4.29. Macro photos and SEM images of bandage-like samples: (A) BC:PMMA, (B) 0.05 wt% UHNP-1, (C) 0.1 wt% UHNP-1, (D) 0.5 wt% UHNP-1, (E) 1 wt% UHNP-1, (F) 0.05 wt% AVNP-2, (G) 0.1 wt% AVNP-2, (H) 0.5 wt% AVNP-2, and (I) 1 wt% AVNP-2 [66] John Wiley & Sons. [2018].

electrospinning, the actual mass produced does not directly translate into suitability for use as a bandage. We can see from the photographs in figure 4.29 that by utilising a customised collection unit, large quantities of structurally sound bandage-like constructs were produced in just 15 s. The BC:PMMA fibres displayed a smooth surface topography, whilst the antimicrobial nanoparticle-loaded fibres appeared to have some surface roughness.

Mechanical tensile testing was performed on these bandage-like fibres in order to assess how favourable they would be as wound-dressing materials, since typical fibrous constructs produced by methods such as electrospinning lack structural integrity. All of the samples had sufficient mechanical properties to be used as bandages; the addition of antimicrobial nanoparticles seemed to increase the stiffness and the tensile strength of the fibres. For example, the measured ultimate tensile strength of the bacterial cellulose:PMMA-only fibres was 0.19 ± 0.01 MPa; however, with the addition of 1 wt% UHNP-1, the fibres exhibited a tensile strength of 0.99 ± 0.06 MPa, a fivefold increase. Although bacterial cellulose alone had a stiffness more comparable to that of natural skin, it is beneficial to know that this can be tweaked by adding nanoparticles to achieve the desired properties.

One of the notable benefits of using bacterial cellulose is its ability to provide a good microenvironment for wound healing, in that it facilitates ample absorption of exudate. Therefore, since the capability of a wound healing material to maintain desirable levels of moisture absorption is a highly scrutinised factor, the bandage samples were assessed for their water uptake behaviour in phosphate buffer saline. Compared to using only the bacterial cellulose:PMMA fibres, the addition of antimicrobial nanoparticles greatly altered the water uptake capabilities of the bandage-like scaffolds. The addition of UHNP-1 and AVNP-2 nanoparticles both increased the water uptake of fibres at a pH of 4 but had the effect of decreasing uptake at pH 7.4. This decrease was observed at higher concentrations of antimicrobial nanoparticles at both pH 4 and 7.4, which can be attributed to the binding of the nanoparticles to the electron-rich oxygen atoms of the hydroxyl groups found in bacterial cellulose.

In addition to its water uptake ability, a suitable wound healing mesh should effectively protect the compromised skin, which acts to prevent the invasion of pathogens. The exterior skin (epidermis) is mostly composed of keratinocyte cells. The samples were therefore tested in a co-culture of keratinocytes and *S. aureus* in order to assess their suitability for preventing pathogen invasion and cell cytotoxicity. The cell viability of all the tested fibres showed similar results to those of the control material, confirming that neither the inclusion of bacterial cellulose nor the inclusion of antimicrobial nanoparticles had affected the toxicity of the materials. Following 24 h of co-culture, the viability of the keratinocytes did not negatively deviate by a considerable amount for any of the nanoparticle-loaded samples. The presence of AVNP-2 also led to a significant reduction in the *S. aureus* population. The keratinocyte viability decreased after 48 h post co-culture, but this was also the case for the control samples. Images of the completed co-culture showed that the samples containing 1 wt% UHNP-1 and AVNP were almost devoid of bacterial attachment, indicating strong antibacterial action against these pathogens. This work showed that composite additions to the polymer solution could have multiple beneficial effects, such as improving the mechanical properties of the fibres and giving them antimicrobial properties.

4.5.2.3 Silk fibroin in tissue engineering

Many natural materials have the tendency to exhibit beneficial properties for tissue engineering, such as being highly biocompatible and biodegradable, that are not as commonly found in synthetic polymers. For this reason, the use of silk fibroin (SF) as a biomaterial has garnered much recent interest, especially when formed into small-diameter fibres, in which its physical properties become even more prominent. The formation of SF into fibres also aims to overcome one of its greatest limitations, the fact that initial SF production requires the use of silk cocoons and batch processing, which limits the scale-up of this material to meet the demands of tissue engineering. SF can be formed into fibres using a range of different methods, such as electrospinning, wet spinning, and dry spinning but such techniques often require the use of harsh solvents in their production, which can lead to negative environmental consequences. Even leaving aside the impact of strong solvents, the yields obtained via these techniques are low, and they are difficult to scale up in order to meet demand. PG has been used to manufacture fibres from silk and has the capacity to improve polymer yields when processed via this technology [67].

Hexafluoroisopropanol (HFIP) was used to dissolve SF into a solution that could be spun using PG. It was found that concentrations of less than 6% (w/v) did not have adequate chain entanglement to facilitate fibre production. Three differing concentrations of SF were eventually used to generate fibres: 8%, 10%, and 12% (w/v) at three different applied pressures. It was found that increasing the concentration of SF increased the viscosity as well, leading to the deposition of thicker fibres. Additional pressure also had the effect of reducing the average fibre diameter. Smooth SF fibres were produced in all instances and their average diameters ranged from 2.1 to 29.6 μm. This pivotal study showed that pure silk fibres can be processed using a rapid technology capable of producing a large amount of fibre in less than 30 s (figure 4.30).

Although SF can be spun using PG, the real challenge is the use of cytotoxic, environmentally harmful organic solvents such as HFIP in its processing. A follow-up investigation looked into the dissolution of SF in water and compared it to other processing routes used to generate tissue engineering scaffolds via PG [68]. This work showed the feasibility of generating solvent-free and environmentally friendly SF-based fibres and how they differed in performance from fibres made using harsher organic solvents. Aqueous SF did not spin into fibres on its own, therefore a carrier polymer, PEO, was used to increase the polymer chain entanglements and improve the production quality of the SF. Using a blend of 90% aqueous SF and 10% PEO, fibres were generated with average diameters as low as 710 nm to 1.27 μm, depending on the spinning conditions. The fibres showed excellent unidirectional alignment due to the rotational speed of the PG vessel and they were found to have a particularly smooth surface morphology (figure 4.31). Compared to techniques such as electrospinning, PG can often present an easier method with which to obtain unidirectionally aligned fibres, whereas electrospinning typically deposits the fibres randomly due to the whipping instability of the jet. Newer techniques, such as the use of a rotating collector, allow aligned fibres to be produced in electrospinning, but this comes at the cost of increasing complication and adding further steps during manufacture. Thermogravimetric analysis showed that the SF-containing fibres had different thermal decomposition profiles as compared to pure PEO or pure SF fibres (dissolved in the harsher solvent). The work demonstrated the benefits of adding a biocompatible polymer matrix into an existing material in order to customise its physical properties.

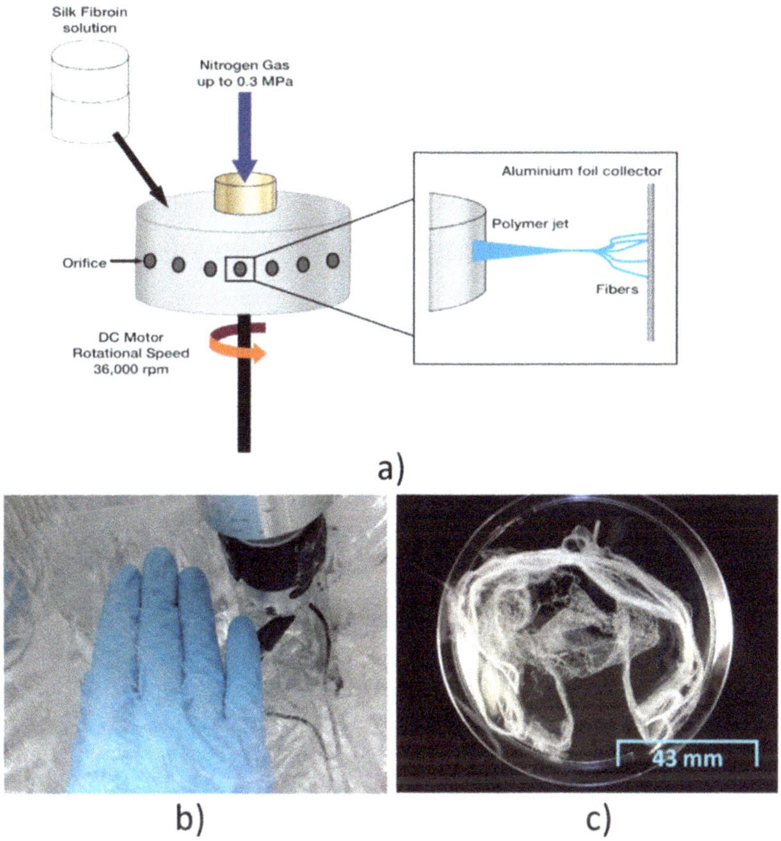

Figure 4.30. (a) A diagram of the PG setup depicting how the silk solution was processed. (b) A photograph of the deposited SF fibres. (c) A photograph showing a large number of 8 w/v% SF fibres produced in less than 30 s [67] John Wiley & Sons. [2018].

It has been established that blended fibres containing SF and PEO have different physical properties compared to pure SF, but an analysis of their cytotoxic properties is required in order to show whether there are any major drawbacks of utilising green solvents. Live/dead cell viability studies and cell proliferation assays were carried out on the fibrous samples using both osteosarcoma SaOS-2 cell lines and human foetal osteoblast (hFob) cells. The number of viable SaOS-2 cells increased with longer incubation times for all of the produced samples, indicating that they all had a low degree of cytotoxicity. The number of cells at the end of the seventh day was found to be higher in SF–PEO fibres for samples spun without the addition of pressure. hFob cell proliferation was found to be significantly higher in the SF–PEO fibres than the control and SF–HFIP sample groups on the fourth and seventh days. Silk fibres produced using environmentally friendly solvents such as water have advantages over harsher solvents when silk fibres are used as tissue engineering scaffolds. Reducing the use of harsher solvents may increase *in vivo* performance as well as having a less detrimental effect on the ecosystem.

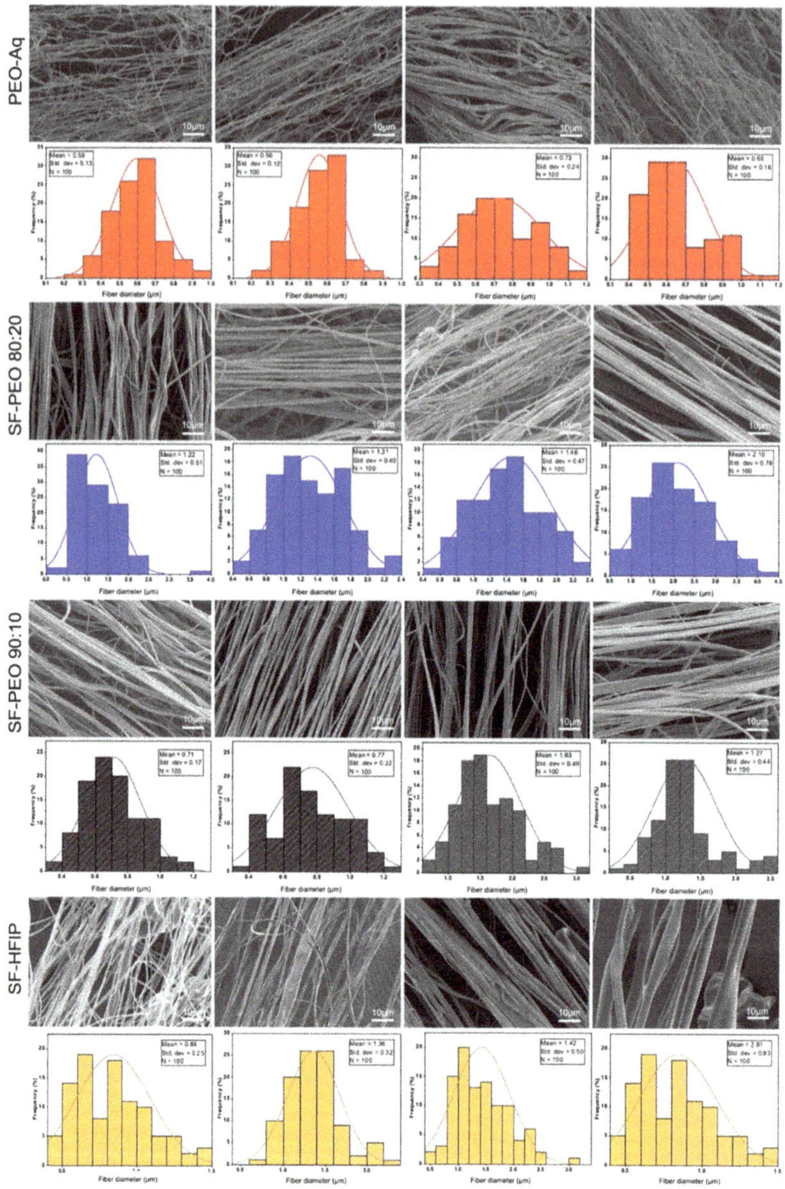

Figure 4.31. SEM micrographs of fibres produced from different polymer blends with their corresponding histogram distribution plots. The fibres were produced at a range of applied pressures and at a rotational speed of 36 000 rpm. Key: PEO-Aq (PEO dissolved in water), SF–PEO (Silk:PEO) and SF–HFIP (silk dissolved in harsh solvent). Reprinted from [68], Copyright (2022), with permission from ACS Publications.

4.5.2.4 Poly(glycerol sebacate) in tissue engineering

Many polymers with excellent physical properties exist which every now and then show promising potential in tissue engineering applications. However, they are usually let down by the difficulty of processing them, which if not overcome can make their adoption unlikely. Polyglycerol sebacate (PGS) is such a polymer which is biocompatible and has elastomeric properties comparable to those of some native tissue niches; it is of particular interest for use in corneal replacement, blood vessel engineering, and nerve tissue engineering [69]. PGS also has difficulties such as low solubility and difficult processing.

By blending PGS with other synthetic polymers such as PVA or poly(hydroxy butyrate), a viscous spinning solution can be made, improving the processability of PGS. Using PG, PGS blended with different molecular weights of PVA was used in order to overcome some of the shortcomings in the solubility and melting of cross-linked PGS [70]. The PGS–PVA solution was spun into fibres using PG; the resulting mesh was cross-linked and the PVA removed via washing. The cytotoxicity of these PGS scaffolds was then assessed to see whether processing via this method would lead to increased levels of toxicity.

Fibres were not obtained through the use of medium and high molecular weights of PVA, as these increased the overall viscosity, resulting in blockages. Even at lower-concentration blends of medium-molecular-weight PVA with PGS, fibre formation with a high bead density occurred; for this reason, lower-molecular-weight (30 000–70 000) PVA was chosen as the optimum polymer for blending. Figure 4.32 shows images of the fibres at different stages, namely straight after the PG process, following thermal cross-linking, and after the PVA had been removed.

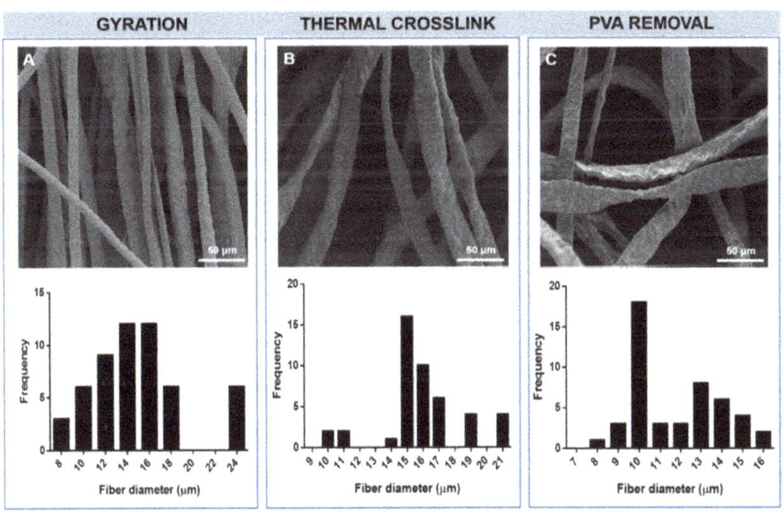

Figure 4.32. SEM micrographs and the size distributions of pressure-spun PGS:PVA fibres after (A) Pressurised gyration (B) thermal cross-linking, and (C) PVA removal. Reprinted from [70], Copyright (2019), with permission from Elsevier.

Fibres collected directly following the PG process yielded a morphology characterised by high unidirectional alignment, an overall smooth topography, and a few small ridges and grooves. The average diameter of these fibres was measured and found to be 15.6 ± 4.2 μm. Following the cross-linking process, the fibres appeared to assume a more ribbon-like flat structure with an overall rougher topography; these fibres had an average diameter of 15.8 ± 3.1 μm. After the removal of the PVA, the PGS fibres had a measured average diameter of 11.8 ± 2.9 μm and the fibre morphology was seen to change to flatter fibrous structures.

MTT cytotoxicity assays preformed on the PGS fibres showed that these scaffolds had a cell viability of 93% ± 13%, demonstrating low toxicity. As PGS is inherently biocompatible and nontoxic, this shows that the processing conditions did not increase toxicity of the fibres. PGS fibres produced using PG also exhibited superior cell viability and spreading, as confirmed by the high levels of adhesion and proliferation of dermal fibroblast cells. This study of the production of PGS scaffolds suitable for tissue engineering demonstrated that alternative and novel approaches in materials science and engineering are required to overcome many of the shortcomings in processability. PG offers such a platform for innovations in materials science and the ability to rapidly produce such fibrous scaffolds, even using difficult materials.

4.5.2.5 Antimicrobial peptides

Wound healing is a significant field of tissue engineering in which the aim is to restore the previous tissue function following physical trauma which has compromised the mechanical and physiological function of the skin and the underlying tissues. The wound healing process is therefore a uniquely complicated series of events that broadly includes haemostasis, inflammation, proliferation, and remodelling [71]. During the process of wound healing, the cellular niche changes to facilitate the dynamic stages of the aforementioned processes. For a wound healing material to be successful, it must be able to meet a few demands, such as the ability to properly manage wound exudate, provide the correct mechanical responses, and provide the essential proteins and nutrients.

The use of synthetic and naturally occurring peptides in tissue engineering and other biological applications had seen a steady increase due to their abilities to facilitate bioactive effects as well as their antimicrobial properties in some cases [72]. Antimicrobial peptides are typically short cationic peptides with an amphipathic effect against many bacteria, fungi, and viruses. Antimicrobial peptides (AMPs) have the ability to modify the membrane permeability of pathogenic cells, causing an antimicrobial effect by destroying the cell membrane [73]. AMPs generally show a high level of biocompatibility and are especially useful due to their effectiveness against multidrug-resistant bacterial strains. Using PG, AMP-loaded nanofibres were prepared using water as the solvent [74]. An engineered AMP known as GLLWHLLHHLLH_GSGGG_K (GH12-M2) was used in the study to assess its antimicrobial action in fibrous form. PEO was used as the carrier polymer to ensure that the polymer was able to form into fibres. Water is a beneficial solvent due to its virtually zero environmental impact and also because of its ability to facilitate the formation of very fine fibres. Nonvolatile solvents such as water allow for greater jet elongation compared to more volatile solvents, meaning that fibres smaller than

1 μm can be obtained. In this work, a range of applied gas pressures was used with the PG apparatus. It was found that at 0.1 MPa of additional pressure, the average fibre diameter was 506 ± 156 nm, which dropped to an average of 395 ± 101 nm at 0.2 MPa of pressure and fell further to 192 ± 55 nm at 0.3 MPa of gas infusion pressure. Although PG is not synonymous with the generation of thin fibres, this study shows that fibre scaffolds with an average fibre diameter of less than 200 nm can be achieved using this process.

Two types of AMP (type I and type II) were used in the study to generate fibres at differing peptide concentrations with a constant concentration of PEO. High-magnification images of the fibres are shown in figure 4.33.

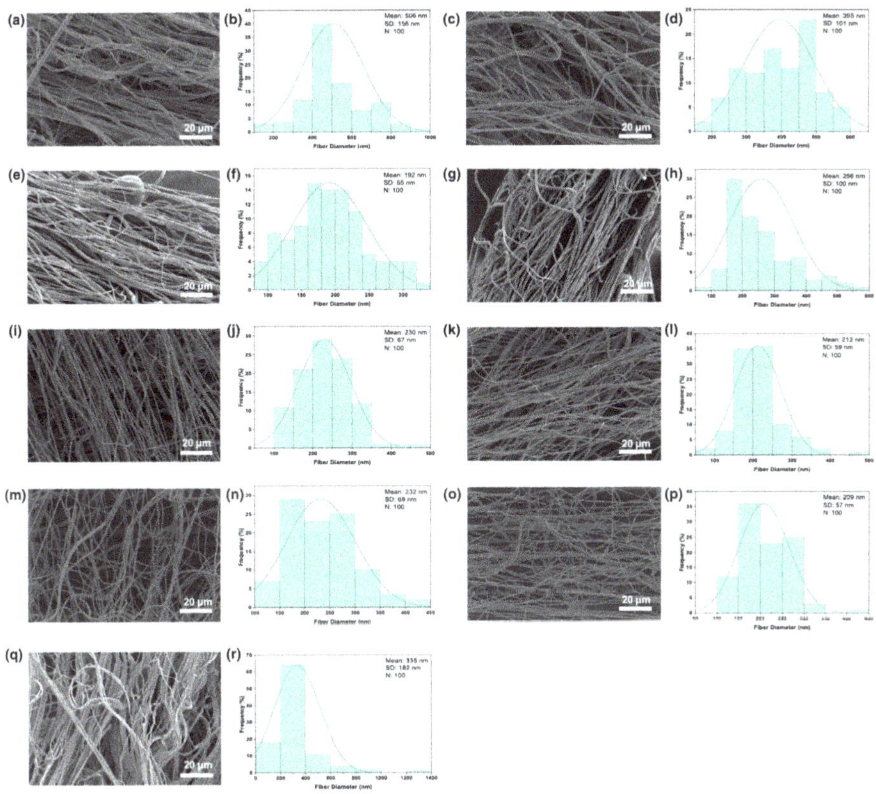

Figure 4.33. SEM micrographs and size distribution graphs of 15 w/v% PEO–water fibres incorporated with: (a, b) type 1 AMP at 35 μg ml^{-1} (0.1 MPa), (c, d) 35 μg ml^{-1} (0.2 MPa), (e, f) 35 μg ml^{-1} (0.3 MPa), (g, h) 70 μg ml^{-1} (0.3 MPa), (i, j) 105 μg ml^{-1} (0.3 MPa), (k, l) 140 μg ml^{-1} (0.3 MPa), (m, n) using type 2 AMP at 105 μg ml^{-1} (0.3 MPa), (o, p) 140 μg ml^{-1} (0.3 MPa), (q, r) 15 w/v% PEO–water control (0.3 MPa). The produced fibres were spun at 36 000 rpm [74] John Wiley & Sons. [2020].

Overall, the produced AMP–PEO fibres had a smooth topography and fibres which were all aligned in a common direction; this makes them suitable for many applications in which a high surface area and common alignment are beneficial.

The average diameter of the M2-AMPs (75 μg ml^{-1}) was 256 ± 100 nm, but an increase in AMP concentration resulted in a decrease in the average to 230 ± 67 nm at 105 μg ml^{-1} of AMP and a further decrease at 140 μg ml^{-1} to 212 ± 59 nm. In certain scenarios, control over the AMP concentration could be crucial in an application-specific basis: higher concentrations may be required in wounds that are more susceptible to pathogenic invasion. A similar trend in the reduction of the average fibre diameter was also observed using the AMP2 peptide. Thinner fibres benefit from a higher surface-area-to-volume ratio, which could increase bioavailability in wound healing environments.

The highest concentrations of the type I and type II AMPs were then tested for their antibacterial viability against *Staphylococcus epidermidis*, which is a common Gram-positive bacterial species which can be found on human skin and can form troublesome biofilms on catheters, amongst other devices [75]. It was found that the viability of *S. epidermidis* reduced with increasing concentrations of type I and II AMP. Compared to virgin PEO fibres and bacteria alone, significantly less bacterial viability was observed in the AMP–PEO scaffolds. This work again demonstrated the effectiveness of incorporating synthetic and naturally derived polymeric additions into composite fibres capable of being used in tissue engineering. The use of AMPs in tissue engineering is still in its early stages but the use of techniques such as electrospinning and PG can improve their processability in order to meet the stringent demands of wound healing.

4.5.2.6 Polyhydroxyalkanoates for hard and soft tissue engineering

One of the fundamental bottlenecks of medicine, which has led to the introduction of tissue engineering, is the lack of available and suitable organ transplants. At its core, tissue engineering aims to overcome this limitation by processing materials into soft tissue which can be used as a replacement for, or an enhancement to native tissue [76]. There is therefore an essential requirement for tissue-engineered constructs to mimic the native cellular niche in terms of both its mechanical properties and its original function—for example, by providing a supportive cellular environment and facilitating cell attachment, migration, and proliferation. Natural polymers tend to have superior biocompatibility and degradation properties compared to their synthetic alternatives. Polyhydroxyalkanoates (PHAs) are a class of natural biopolymers that have a high level of biocompatibility and favourable degradation profiles that make them suitable for use as soft tissue engineering materials. Because of their promising properties, PHAs have been fabricated via several technologies into three-dimensional scaffolds via electrospinning, self-assembly, and soft lithography, amongst many other methods. PG has also been used to fabricate PHA-based fibrous scaffolds for both hard and soft tissue engineering, as it allows such constructs to be made using rapid, economical, and large-scale processes [77].

A short-chain-length PHA (SCL-PHA) P(3HB) and a medium-chain-length PHA (MCL-PHA) P(3HO-co-3HD) were produced using a bacterial culture, purified, and prepared in spinning solutions. PHAs exhibit good solubility in organic solvents such as chloroform, making them much simpler to process than other natural polymers. PG was used with 7.4% (w w^{-1}) solutions of P(3HB) and composite P (3HB)/P(3HO-3HD) to form fibres at an applied gas pressure of 0.3 MPa. The resulting fibres were then assessed for their suitability in both hard tissue engineering (bone tissue engineering) and soft tissue engineering (nerve tissue engineering). PHA containing the bioactive material hydroxyapatite and blends of PHA were spun into fibres, which can be seen in figure 4.34.

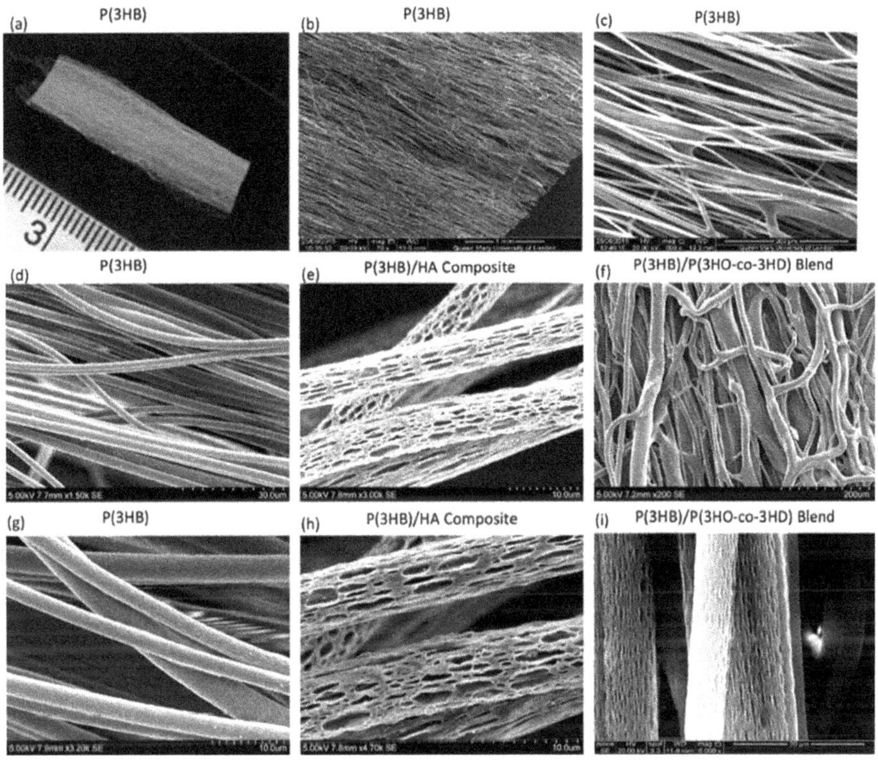

Figure 4.34. (a) An optical image of the pressure-spun P(3HB) fibrous sheet. (b, c) Low-magnification SEM images of the P(3HB) fibrous sheet showing the morphology and alignment of the fibres in the scaffolds. (d, g) High-resolution SEM images of the P(3HB) fibres within the scaffolds. (e, h) P(3HB)/HA composite fibres illustrating the uniform distribution of 200 nm hydroxyapatite particles and the high porosity of the scaffolds. (f) P(3HB)/P(3HO-co-3HD) 80:20 random blend fibres and (i) P(3HB)/P(3HO-co-3HD) 80:20 aligned blend fibres within the pressure-spun scaffolds. Reproduced from [77]. CC BY 4.0.

The produced fibres were seen to be highly aligned and cylindrical in nature, making them suitable for applications in which alignment is beneficial, such as in nerve tissue engineering. It is clearly visible from the photograph in figure 4.34(a) that the entire fibrous scaffold contains fibres with a highly aligned morphology. The fibre topography was shown to be highly porous and to contain surface pores which were the result of using a volatile solvent such as chloroform. When a volatile solvent is used, condensation microdroplets form as a consequence of rapid evaporation; these droplets then evaporate away at a later time, leaving behind surface pores [21]. Surface nanopores can be beneficial in both hard and soft tissue engineering applications by increasing the available surface-area-to-volume ratio for cell attachment and other bioactive features. The P(3HB) fibres had an average diameter of 6.9 ± 1.9 μm, while the P(3HB)/P(3HO-co-3HD) blend had an average diameter of 9.1 ± 3.7 μm and the P(3HB)/HA composite fibres had an average diameter of 2.5 ± 0.7 μm. The blended PHA fibres exhibited the largest average diameter, corresponding to their higher viscosity. Depending on the specific tissue engineering application, a different fibre diameter and morphology could be desirable to mimic the extracellular matrix and other components. For example, in nerve tissue engineering, thicker fibres (~8 μm) have been shown to support the longest neurites, whereas thinner fibres (~1 μm) have been seen to facilitate increased levels of Schwan cell migration and superior neurite outgrowth [78, 79].

The PHA, PHA composite, and PHA-HA fibres were then characterised using tensile strength tests to discern their mechanical properties and suitability for use as hard and soft tissue engineering constructs. In their bulk forms, P(3HB) and P(3HO-co-3HD) have markedly different mechanical properties; therefore, blending them allows an intermediate mechanical performance to be achieved. For example, P(3HB) is significantly stiffer than P(3HO-co-3HD), whilst P(3HO-co-3HD) is much tougher and can withstand much more deformation before failure. By combining P(3HB) with hydroxyapatite, we see that this increases the Young's modulus, making the resulting material more brittle; this is to be expected, as hydroxyapatite is a ceramic. For the combination of P(3HB) and P(3HO-co-3HD), we see that the stiffness decreases and the toughness increases dramatically, being resistant to more strain. When the fibre bundles were tested, it was found that compared to P(3HB) alone, the P(3HB):HA composite fibres showed greater toughness and were resistant to increased levels of strain.

Although bone grafts are the most proven method of bone regeneration, they are limited by donor numbers. Using biomaterials to aid bone regeneration would reduce the number of complicated procedures required and ensure that there would be no shortage of donors. Aligned P(3HB) and P(3HB)/HA composite fibres together with human bone marrow stromal cells (HBMSCs) and enriched skeletal stem-cell populations were assessed to study the suitability of these fibres for bone regeneration. The *in vitro* reaction of these fibres was also assessed to determine the cell viability, differentiation, and mineralisation. The PHA fibrous scaffolds demonstrated an excellent ability to enhance and support bone formation, as evidenced by hydroxyapatite crystal formation on the surface of the implants.

The scaffolds were seeded with Stro-1+ cells and placed on the chorioallantoic membrane of chick embryos. At the end of the implantation period, the survival rate of the chick embryos was 100%. The study showed that both the aligned P(3HB) and P(3HB)–HA scaffolds were able to facilitate vascularisation, i.e. the formation of new blood vessels, which is essential for the regeneration of any tissue. The composite HA fibres demonstrated the highest level of vascularisation, in which the greater number of blood vessels was consistent with the paracrine influence of bone marrow stromal cells. The composite fibres had a higher degree of surface porosity, which possibly led to this increase in vascularisation.

To further assess the potential of these PHA scaffolds for bone regeneration, the scaffolds were subjected to *in vivo* subcutaneous co-implantation in immunodeficient mice. Collagen deposition was observed in both types of scaffolds and a higher level of deposition was realised by the composite P(3HB)–HA fibres. There was also evidence of erythrocyte formation, which confirmed that the scaffolds were able to facilitate vascularisation; higher levels of erythrocyte formation were seen in the composite. These results are extremely promising for bone tissue engineering, particularly because additives such as external growth factors were not added, which would otherwise drive up costs and complications.

Peripheral nerves generally retain the ability to regenerate when a gap of less than 5 mm has been caused by trauma. In cases in which this gap is larger, nerve guidance is usually required for regeneration [80]. The PHA fibrous scaffolds were investigated for their nerve guidance and regenerative properties using NG108-15 neuronal cells. Neuronal cell differentiation was successfully supported by the PHA fibres. The neurite length was found to be the longest on the composite P(3HB)/P(3HO-co-3HD) blend, reaching an average length of 83.9 ± 20.4 μm, and slightly shorter on the P(3HB) scaffold, reaching an average length of 76.9 ± 19.8 μm. A morphological assessment of rat primary Schwann cells tested on the two types of scaffolds showed high cell viability at levels of more than 95%. There is evidence to suggest that Schwann cells preferentially attach and migrate faster on aligned scaffolds as opposed to randomly oriented fibres [81]. The length of the Schwann cells can be a good indicator of their ability to retain their phenotype in cultured conditions. There was no statistical difference between the Schwann cell lengths measured on the P(3HB) fibres (74.4 ± 15.7 μm) and those measured on the blended P(3HB)/P(3HO-co-3HD) fibres (76.1 ± 14.9).

A three-dimensional *ex vivo* physical model can be used to mirror a proximal nerve stump following trauma by utilising the dorsal root ganglion. This tool can then be used to efficiently assess the ability of the scaffolds to promote axon regeneration. The aligned PHA fibres were placed into fabricated polyethylene glycol 5 mm nerve guide conduits. After seven days of culture, both Schwann cells and axons grew from the dorsal root ganglion along the PHA fibres.

The Schwann cells on the P(3HB) fibres were noted to have grown preferentially on one side. In contrast, those grown on the P(3HB)/P(3HO-co-3HD) fibres showed a more consistent outgrowth, which can be seen in figure 4.35.

A longer outgrowth distance was seen on the P(3HB) fibres than on the composite P(3HB)/P(3HO-co-3HD) fibres. For both fibre samples, large outgrowths of Schwann cells and axons were detected; 67% was measured on the P(3HB) fibres and 78% was detected on the composite P(3HB)/P(3HO-co-3HD) fibres. The average axon outgrowth on the P(3HB) sample was 0.6 mm, while the average was 0.5 mm for the blended fibres. The P(3HB) fibres facilitated an average Schwann cell migration of 1.84 mm and the 80:20 P(3HB)/P(3HO-co-3HD) blend promoted an average cell migration of 1.89 mm. Given that the native P(3HB) is stiff and difficult to process, PG offers an easy way to make composite fibres with more

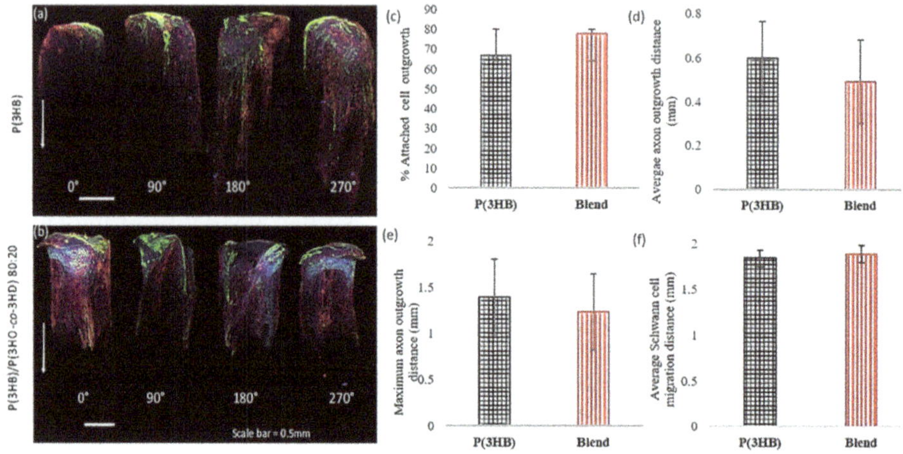

Figure 4.35. Light-sheet microscopy images showing the outgrowth of axons (β-III tubulin, green) and Schwann cells (S100β, red) along aligned (a) P(3HB) fibres and (b) P(3HB)/P(3HO-co-3HD) 80:20 blend pressure-spun fibres inside a 5 mm long polyethylene glycol conduit. Nuclei were labelled with DAPI (blue). Images are shown as maximum projections using multiple views stitched together. The outgrowths were captured at four angles using 90° rotation (0°, 90°, 180°, and 270° from left to right). The arrows indicate the outgrowth direction. Representative images are shown from three independently repeated experiments. Scale bar = 0.5 mm. (c) Percentage attached cell outgrowth on the P(3HB) and P(3HB)/P(3HO-co-3HD) 80:20 blend pressure-spun fibres. (d) Average axon outgrowth distance (mm) on the P(3HB) and P(3HB)/P(3HO-co-3HD) 80:20 blended pressure-spun fibres. (e) Maximum axon outgrowth distance (mm) on the P(3HB) and P(3HB)/P(3HO-co-3HD) 80:20 blended pressure-spun fibres. (f) Average Schwann cell migration distance (mm) on the P(3HB) and P(3HB)/P(3HO-co-3HD) 80:20 blended pressure-spun fibres. Reproduced from [77]. CC BY 4.0.

favourable mechanical profiles for use in nerve tissue engineering as soft tissue replacements.

The cardiovascular system is known to have very limited regenerative capabilities as compared with the skeletal and nervous systems. Cardiomyocytes in particular suffer from little to no regenerative capacity [82]. Following myocardial infarction, scar tissue forms which alters cardiac compliance. The ideal surgical intervention would aim to replace scar tissue with viable myocardial tissue. Three-dimensional scaffolds can be designed and created to act as cardiac regeneration patches, here, P(3HB) and P(3HB)/P(3HO-co-3HD) fibres were assessed as potential cardiovascular regeneration materials.

The effect of the fibre alignment on cardiomyocyte functions such as calcium handling was evaluated. Human-induced pluripotent stem-cell-derived cardiomyocytes were cultured into the PHA fibres. From the detection performed by calcium-sensitive Fluo-4 acetomethoxy (AM) dye, it was seen that these scaffolds displayed a functional level of calcium uptake. For aligned fibres, there was a significant reduction in the time taken to peak and to reach 90% decay compared to the time taken by randomly oriented fibres, indicating that calcium handling was superior on the aligned structures. The results point to the great potential of PG-spun polymeric fibres for soft and hard tissue engineering due to their ability to promote the maturation of key cells required for tissue regeneration.

4.5.2.7 Manufacturing cyclodextrin fibres using water

As discussed previously, the pursuit of materials with desirable bioactive and biocompatible properties for tissue engineering applications often introduces additional issues, such as the requirement for harsh solvents. As we progress further from the industrial revolution, we must find more pathways that can be used to manufacture environmentally friendly materials. Cyclodextrins are a family of extremely water-soluble polymers which show great biocompatibility and have been routinely used in the pharmaceutical industry as agents to increase the water solubility of active substances as well as their bioavailability [83]. Cyclodextrins are potentially useful in tissue engineering applications, as they have a highly specific cavity structure which gives them the ability to capture specific organic molecules. On their outer surface, cyclodextrins contain hydroxyl groups which can form strong covalent bonds with metallic ions, allowing for highly specific adsorption. Given their use as material additions, there has been little work in the field of utilising pure cyclodextrin fibres. PG was used to electrospin pure cyclodextrin dissolved in water alone. The cyclodextrin was spun into a hybrid 'supermat' containing a pressure-spun mechanical support and a fine electrospun surface mesh [84]. Because PG and electrospinning have their own unique strengths and weaknesses, by leveraging both of them, novel structures can be made that provide more biomimetic environments and have the necessary mechanical support. In this work, PG was used to make the initial cyclodextrin base consisting of thicker fibres, which was intended to provide better mechanical support. Electrospinning was then used to print a layer of thinner nanofibres, which acted as the surface of the 'supermat' (figure 4.36).

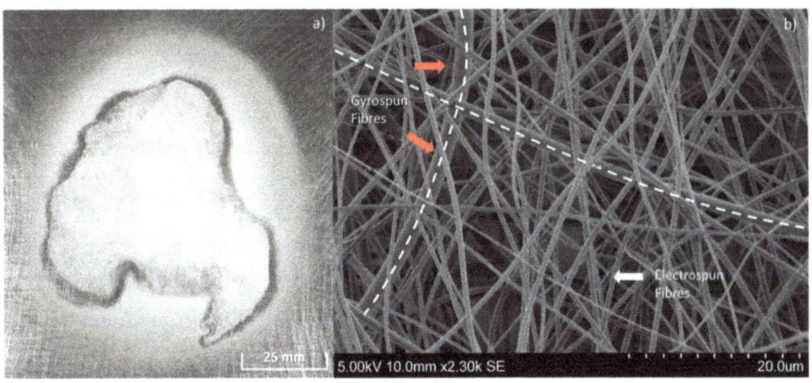

Figure 4.36. An image of the pressure-spun cyclodextrin and the electrospun 'supermat' consisting of a pressure-spun cyclodextrin base and an electrospun exterior, (b) an SEM image of the 'super-mat' under high magnification, showing the interface between the electrospun and the pressure-spun cyclodextrin fibres, thicker gyration fibres have been highlighted with dotted lines [84] John Wiley & Sons. [2022].

The cyclodextrin fibres produced using PG had an average fibre diameter of about 6 μm when an applied gas pressure of 0.3 MPa was used, while the electrospun fibres were able to achieve a diameter as low as 140 nm on average at the lowest tested concentrations. The benefits of having such thin fibres on the surface are that it vastly increases the surface-area-to-volume ratio and can be used to release bioactive or pharmaceutical compounds for tissue engineering or drug delivery applications. Because there are two layers involved, each layer could incorporate a different active ingredient, which makes the scaffold more adaptable to the operation of three-dimensional cell niches. The electrospun fibres demonstrated excellent interconnectivity of the pores between the fibre strands, giving them advantageous properties for use in ultrafiltration applications in which the filtration capability must be effective down to the nanometre range. Visually, the fibres had a smooth surface with no visible surface roughness and they were bead-free at higher concentrations, allowing higher uniformity during production.

4.5.3 Filtration

Due to their high surface area and porosity, small-diameter fibres are especially suited for ultrafiltration applications and are already widely used in facemasks. Filters work by entrapping small particulates whilst allowing the free flow of air or water through them. In order to provide better filtration properties, the netting can be designed to have a smaller mesh size, or it can be made of materials that are inherently antimicrobial. In hospital environments, for example, there is often a higher concentration of pathogenic microbes, therefore producing filters that have antimicrobial properties reduces maintenance costs and increases the quality of the air or water supply. Fibre meshes produced by PG can be used directly as filters for air and water inlets and outlets.

An early study of the production of nylon fibres with embedded silver nanoparticles showed the potential of PG to produce antimicrobial fibrous meshes that could be used for filtration [85]. Nylon is a synthetic polymer consisting of polyamides, developed to meet the requirement for a material which has very high tensile strength and toughness [86]. Silver has long been used as a standard metal in antibacterial applications due to its effectiveness against both Gram-positive and Gram-negative bacteria. Silver nanoparticles were therefore incorporated into nylon fibres, and their antimicrobial activity was assessed against two Gram-negative bacterial species, *Escherichia coli* and *Pseudomonas aeruginosa*. Nylon fibres with a concentration of 10 wt% were able to form fibres with an average fibre diameter of only 75 nm when spun at the maximum rotational speed and an applied gas pressure of 0.3 MPa. Even with the addition of silver nanoparticles, the fibre diameter remained constant at only 84 nm. Higher-concentration (20 wt%) nylon fibres had an average diameter of 113 nm at the maximum speed and pressure, and the addition of silver nanoparticles caused little to no difference, as the average fibre diameter was 125 nm. The fibres exhibited a smooth topography with an overall unidirectional alignment. In antimicrobial tests, 20 wt% nylon fibres with a loading of 1 wt% silver nanoparticles showed an antibacterial rate that was consistently greater than 99% when tested against both *E. coli* and *P. aeruginosa*. The effective bactericidal rate of around 100% shows that highly antibacterial fibrous meshes can easily be produced using PG and can be put to use in many biomedical applications; in particular, filtration performed using the nano-sized fibres provides additional filtration capability.

4.5.3.1 Antimicrobial nanoparticle-loaded fibrous polymeric filters

Following on from the work with silver nanoparticles and nylon fibres, it was clear that there was great potential in incorporating antimicrobial additives which could be used to produce antimicrobial meshes capable of filtering out pathogens. Using PG, two different types of antimicrobial nanoparticles were incorporated into PMMA fibres to produce polymeric filters intended for use in hospital filtration systems [87]. Hospital-acquired infections account for a large mortality and morbidity rate amongst patients. Such infections are often caused by drug-resistant microorganisms and contribute to a colossal economic burden. Modern hospital filtration systems employed at water outlets serve to trap microbes but not kill them; therefore, residual bacteria can form biofilms which become difficult to remove [88].

The proprietary antimicrobial nanoparticles produced by the University of Hertfordshire, named AMNP1 and AMNP2, contained antimicrobial metals such as calcium, aluminium, zinc, nickel, tungsten, and copper. After they were added to a PMMA polymer solution, fibres were generated and deposited onto meshed metallic discs to be tested as filters (figure 4.37).

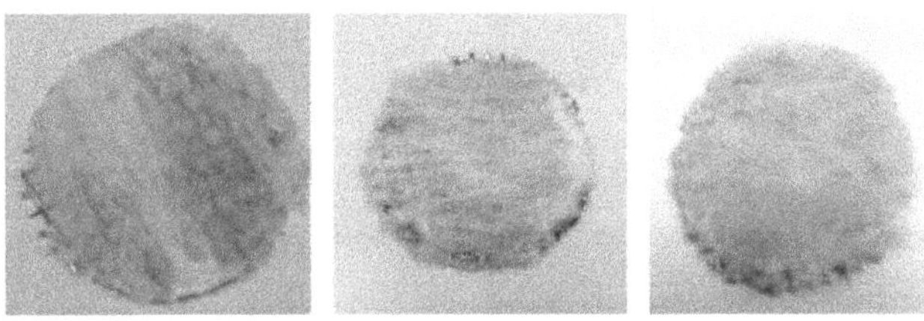

Figure 4.37. Images of PMMA fibre scaffolds deposited onto metal discs, intended for use as 'point of contact' filtration elements. Reprinted from [87], Copyright (2017), with permission from Elsevier.

Various concentrations of PMMA and AMNP were tested, and it was observed that the solution properties influenced the fibre morphology. Fibres were generated at the maximum rotational speed and applied pressure. The fibres showed a continuous bead-free morphology that included surface nanopores, which increased the surface area available for filtration. High-magnification images of these fibres can be seen in figure 4.38. The thickest fibres were produced when PMMA was spun without the addition of AMNP; these fibres had an average fibre diameter of 20 ± 12 μm. Following the addition of 0.5% (w w^{-1}) AMNP1, the average diameter reduced to 6 ± 4 μm, and it reduced to 7 ± 4 μm with the addition of 0.5% (w w^{-1}) AMNP2. As is often the case, the addition of nanoparticles can lead to a reduction in viscosity, which results from an alteration in the polymer matrix such as additional slippage.

The average pore size of the 0.5% (w w^{-1}) AMNP1-PMMA fibres was measured and found to be 36 ± 18 nm, while the average pore size of the 0.5% (w w^{-1})

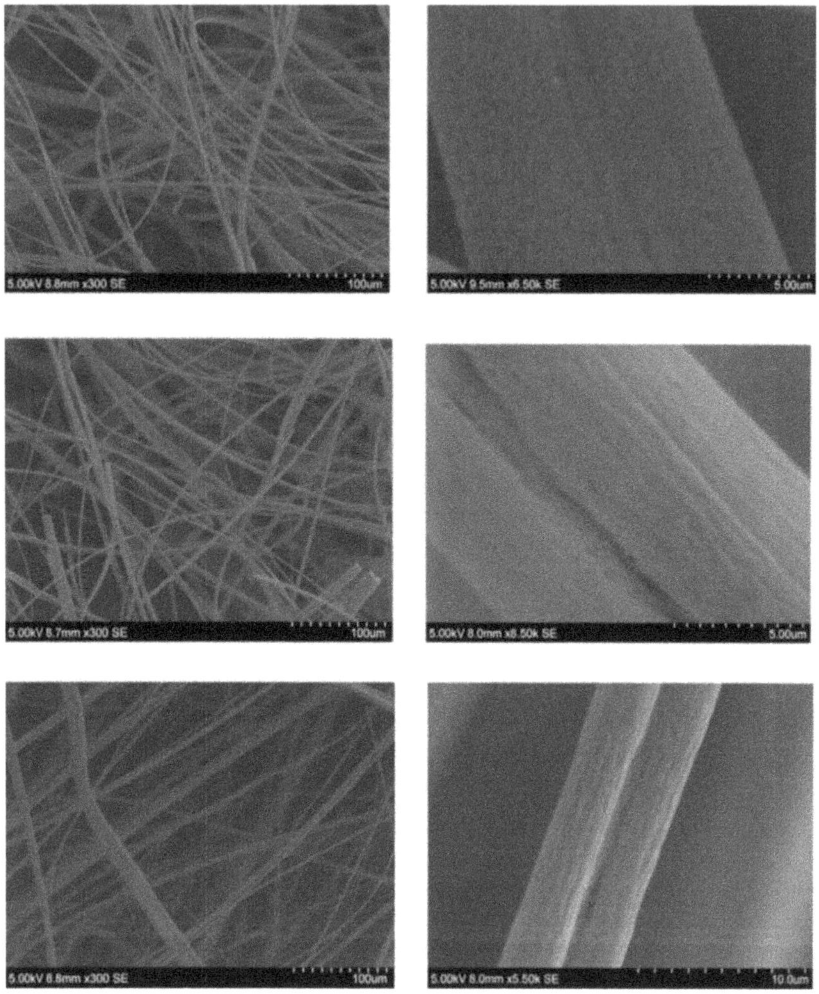

Figure 4.38. SEM images of the PMMA and AMNP nanoparticles incorporated into PMMA fibres obtained at a rotational speed of 36 000 rpm and a working pressure of 0.3 MPa. Reprinted from [87], Copyright (2017), with permission from Elsevier.

AMNP2-PMMA fibres was found to be 300 ± 38 nm. These findings suggest that pore size does not depend on the polymer concentration but is possibly influenced more by factors such as humidity and the formation of condensation droplets on the fibre surface [89].

The fibrous meshes were also tested for their ability to reduce the numbers of *P. aeruginosa* cells. PMMA fibres without the addition of AMNP reduced the bacterial count by around 35%, indicating that the filters may be inherently antimicrobial, possibly due to their porosity or the brittle, glassy nature of PMMA. AMNP1- and AMNP2-loaded fibres both reduced bacteria by more than 70%, demonstrating significant killing power. The metallic ions of metals such as copper and silver can contribute to bacterial reduction by inhibiting the growth of bacteria and by breaking down important lipids, proteins, and DNA via reactive oxygen species [90].

4.5.3.2 The antimicrobial action of tellurium-loaded polymeric fibrous meshes

Many antimicrobial agents have potent bactericidal properties; however, their overuse can lead to the formation of bactericide-resistant strains and can cause toxicity if not used in suitable amounts. Antimicrobial nanoparticles such as AMNPs present a new approach that can be used to tackle infections without the fear of rapid resistance that is so prevalent with chemical-based solutions. Tellurium (Te) was first discovered in 1782 and has many different ionic states, giving it antibacterial properties via the release of reactive oxygen species. Typical metallic antimicrobial nanoparticles usually contain a form of copper or silver which has some known toxicity. Te nanoparticles have recently come into fashion as potential antibacterial agents due to their ability to eradicate biofilms of bacterial species such as *E. coli, P. aeruginosa*, and *S. aureus* [91]. PG has been used to generate fibre meshes made of tellurium-loaded PMMA [92].

Fibres made at a range of Te loadings from 0 to 4 wt% were produced at the maximum rotational speed and an applied gas pressure of 0.1 MPa. Unlike antimicrobial nanoparticles, it was found that the addition of Te led to an increase in the average fibre diameter from 7 ± 4 to 14 ± 7 μm. The reason for this may be that the Te was obtained in powder form and not as nanoparticles. All the fibres demonstrated a smooth and continuous bead-free morphology. Energy-dispersive x-ray spectroscopy (EDX) was utilised to confirm the presence of Te on the fibres. The EDX data and images of the fibres can be seen in figure 4.39.

Agar diffusion Gram-positive (*S. aureus*) and Gram-negative (*E. coli* and *P. aeruginosa*) bacteria were used to assess the antimicrobial capabilities of the Te-loaded fibres. Testing all the samples from 0 wt% to 4 wt% allowed the effect of increasing the concentration of Te to be measured. The control sample (0 wt% Te, PMMA) showed low cytotoxicity and resulted in an average log reduction of about 0.03. When the tellurium concentration was increased to just 1 wt%, a significant increase in log reduction in bacterial numbers was seen. This trend continued exponentially from 1 wt% to 4 wt%, at which point there was a log reduction of about 1.16. Yet again, the work here showed the feasibility of using PG to produce functional fibrous meshes for antimicrobial activities—these fibres showed great potential as point-of-contact antimicrobial filters.

4.5.3.3 The antimicrobial effect of tungsten on hospital filters

Healthcare-acquired infections are prominent in healthcare settings during healthcare interventions and as a result of interacting with the healthcare environment, these infections can then be spread to the public by employees. Healthcare-acquired infections include a wide range of pathogens, such as *E. coli*, *S. aureus*, *P. aeruginosa*, and adenoviruses, which cause thousands of deaths annually [93]. Tungsten is a rare metal and the heaviest metal known to have a biological role; certain bacteria contain enzymes which consume tungsten to reduce carboxylic acids to aldehydes [94]. There has also been recent exploration of the antibacterial and

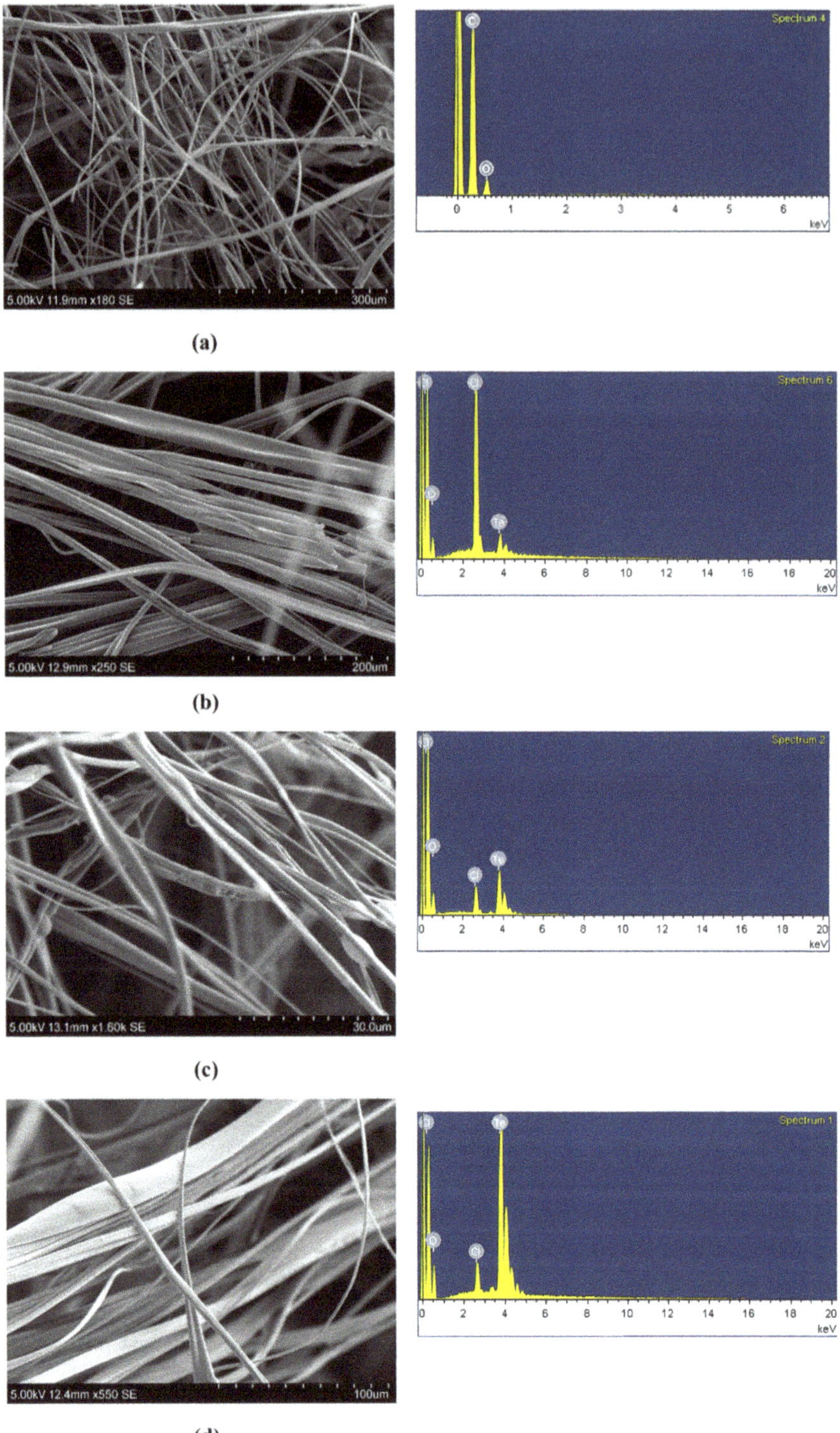

Figure 4.39. SEM images and EDX spectra of (a) pure PMMA fibres, (b) PMMA fibres with 1.0 wt% tellurium, (c) PMMA fibres with 2.0 wt% tellurium, and (d) PMMA fibres with 4.0 wt% tellurium [92] John Wiley & Sons. [2018].

antiviral properties of this metal in conjunction with other metallic nanoparticles, as mentioned earlier. The antimicrobial activities of tungsten, tungsten oxide, and tungsten carbide against *E. coli, S. aureus*, and the adenovirus bacteriophage T4 were compared after PG was used to form tungsten-loaded PMMA fibres intended for use as a hospital filter material [95].

The minimum inhibitory concentrations of the tungsten, tungsten oxide and tungsten carbide powders were first determined using 0–4 wt% loadings of each sample. This revealed when antibacterial activity came into play. Even at only 0.5 wt % loading, all the tested tungsten materials exhibited moderate antibacterial activity against both *E. coli* and *S. aureus*, and tungsten oxide displayed the greatest bactericidal potency. At a tungsten concentration of 2 wt%, the tungsten oxide powder exhibited a large bactericidal potency and significantly higher antibacterial activity than those of the tungsten and the tungsten carbide. When tested against the bacteriophage T4, all tungsten derivatives showed significant virucidal capabilities even at 0.5 wt%. As in the test carried out using the two bacterial species, tungsten oxide particles showed higher overall antiviral ability and were therefore chosen as the selected tungsten derivative to be made into composite PMMA fibres for filtration.

For the rest of the study, tungsten oxide/PMAA nanocomposite fibres were produced by PG at tungsten concentrations of 2 wt%, 4 wt%, and 8 wt%. EDX was used to confirm the presence of tungsten oxide on the surface of the nanofibres, an essential prerequisite to achieving the maximum antimicrobial activity. For the tested concentrations, the overall appearance of the fibres was smooth, continuous, and relatively bead-free. The average fibre diameter depended greatly on the tungsten oxide concentration, and a positive correlation between them was observed. The fibres at 2 wt% of tungsten oxide to PMMA had an average diameter of 2.9 ± 2.1 μm, 4 wt% fibres had an average diameter of 3.3 ± 2.0 μm, and 8 wt% fibres had an average diameter of 6.6 ± 4.4 μm. The tungsten oxide particles had a measured average particle size of 1.7 ± 0.9 μm, showing that these were not nanoparticles and indicating that the addition of microparticles can lead to an increase in solution viscosity.

The tungsten oxide/PMMA fibres at the abovementioned concentrations were then tested for their antimicrobial strength against *S. aureus* and the bacteriophage T4. The 2 wt% and 4 wt% tungsten oxide/PMMA fibres showed no antibacterial activity, and more than 96% of the bacterial population was still alive following the tests. The 8 wt% tungsten oxide/PMMA fibres showed moderate antibacterial activity and were able to kill 29% of the bacterial population. However, all the tested tungsten oxide/PMMA fibres demonstrated robust antiviral activity; the 8 wt% tungsten oxide loading demonstrated the most prominent virucidal potency and reduced the viral population by 93%. Florescence microscopy was used to visualise the surface of the 8 wt% tungsten-oxide-loaded fibres to verify the death of bacterial cells, as shown in figure 4.40. This study showed that tungsten oxide is a viable polymeric addition for the production of highly antiviral structures suitable for use in preventing the spread of common healthcare-acquired infections.

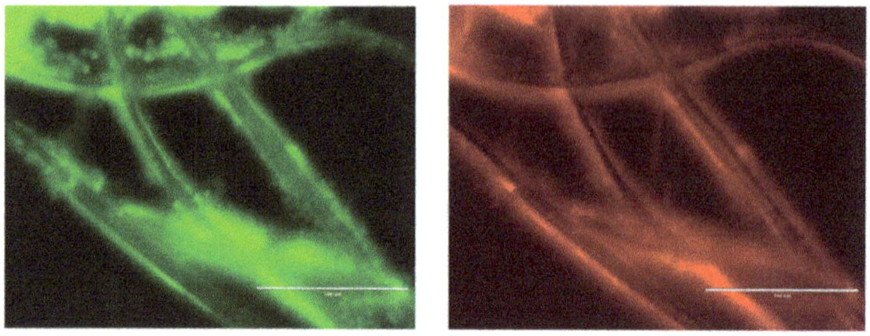

Figure 4.40. Images showing the antibacterial activity of the 8 wt% tungsten oxide/PMMA fibres against *S. aureus* after 24 h of incubation. (a) Green, SYTO®9, corresponds to viable cells and (b) red, propidium iodide, corresponds to nonviable cells. Reproduced from [95]. CC BY 4.0.

4.5.3.4 Viral filtration using carbon-based materials.

The work with tungsten microparticles showed the benefit of adding materials to polymeric solutions to produce meshes for filtration. It is well-known that viruses are not killed by antibiotics, therefore great efforts are being made to develop more antivirals. Despite the use of chemical antiviral approaches, such as attacks on the outer viral membrane and the utilisation of metallic nanoparticles, viruses have been found to survive in aerosols on copper and other surfaces for several hours [96]. Recently, carbon-based materials such as graphene and its derivatives have been investigated for their antibacterial properties but until recently, their antiviral properties have been unknown. PG was used to create polymeric fibrous filters that incorporated graphene nanoplatelets and graphene oxide, and the inhibitory effects of these filters on the *E. coli* T4 bacteriophage were investigated [97]. PMMA was used as the carrier polymer for these filters, which contained 2 wt% of either graphene nanoplatelets or graphene oxide nanosheets. One way in which graphene-based nanomaterials differ in their antiviral activity is that they exhibit a unique morphological structure which leads to the physical disruption of the viral membrane, causing the leakage of its contents [98]. Physical virucidal properties are more desirable, as it is significantly more difficult to evolve a physical defence than a chemical defence such as with the use of antiviral drugs. Graphene-based nanomaterials can also have antiviral effects due to their direct electrostatic and hydrophobic interactions with viruses [99].

To assess the antiviral ability of graphene derivates, both graphene nanoplatelets and graphene oxide were loaded into PMMA polymer solutions at concentrations of 0 wt%, 2 wt%, 4 wt%, and 8 wt%, and the effect of the concentration was evaluated. At the highest graphene loading of 8 wt%, the fibres formed had a smooth surface topography. The PMMA fibres containing both graphene nanoplatelets and graphene oxide showed antiviral properties across all the test conditions. These tests were performed at 3 h following treatment and at 24 h following treatment. Even at only 3 h, there was sufficient antiviral activity in the fibres, which increased linearly with the concentrations of both graphene oxide and graphene nanoplatelets.

Compared to the three-hour period, the 24-hour period showed higher viral reduction, suggesting that the antiviral properties became stronger over time. After 24 h of treatment, 2 wt% fibres achieved viral reductions of 21% and 23% for graphene nanoplatelets and graphene oxide, respectively. The 8 wt% graphene nanoplatelets and graphene-oxide-containing fibres showed the greatest antiviral potencies, achieving viral reductions of 33% and 39%, respectively. The increase in graphene concentration seems to correspond to better antiviral properties, suggesting that a physical antiviral action may result from the use of additional graphene content. Although further work must be done to fully understand the antimicrobial mechanisms of action of graphene-based materials, this work has shown the feasibility of making graphene–polymer composite fibres for antiviral filtration applications.

4.6 Materials exploited by pressurised gyration

We have established that the choice of material to process is absolutely essential in the translation of biomaterials for healthcare and biomedical applications. The ease of use of the PG setup (along with its ability to incorporate a wide range of materials, irrespective of whether they carry a charge or not) makes PG a formidable contender in the production of functional biomaterials for a wide range of healthcare-related fields. A biomaterial must have several desired properties before it can be used in healthcare. The ultimate goal for biomaterials in medicine is to mimic or replace the function of native tissue organs for the purpose of treating, improving, or enhancing their original purpose [99]. All manner of materials ranging from synthetic to natural polymers have inherent characteristics which could be exploited by biomaterials. Therefore, there are several key properties of potential materials which are especially relevant to materials scientists. These include, but are not limited to: biocompatibility, host response, toxicity, mechanical properties, wear and fatigue responses, corrosion properties, and considerations related to design and manufacturability.

4.6.1 Natural materials for wound healing

As alluded to previously, many natural materials have desirable bioactive properties which could make them especially useful in healthcare. Natural materials, such as those used in plant-based approaches, show better biocompatibility than artificial alternatives and are often less harmful to the environment in the long run. The main problem with the use of natural materials is that they need to be created by natural methods, which are often very difficult to scale up. By incorporating natural materials and plant-based extracts in fibrous form, we can ensure that there is a greater supply of functional biomaterials that can satisfy the needs of healthcare applications.

Even before the advent of modern medicine and antibiotics, natural remedies based on natural ingredients were used due to their numerous health benefits. Many commonly consumed foods have inherent bioactive properties, such as antimicrobial, anticancer, anti-inflammatory, and even wound healing properties. Today, these methods are still used sporadically, although they have mostly been superseded by modern scientific approaches which aim to quantify and synthetise the key components of naturally derived materials. In isolating the individual principal compounds, however, the intended biological effect may often be compromised, as these plants and spices have evolved to contain combinations of many different chemical compounds. This section will present the use of raw natural materials combined with a polymer matrix to form fibres and will describe how they can be used in medicine for the purpose of improving wound healing.

4.6.1.1 Cinnamon fibres for wound healing

Cinnamon is a spice native to southern Asia, famous for its characteristic sweet aroma. It is used industrially to make perfumes and to add flavour to dishes all around the world. The use of cinnamon for its medicinal properties dates back thousands of years, and references to it can be found in the Bible [100]. The use of plant or food products is very rare in modern medicine, mainly because useful compounds are isolated as extracts from such sources and used as required. However, the isolation of single compounds may often not have the cumulative beneficial effect of using the entire plant or spice in its natural form. The two most common types of cinnamon are known as *Cinnamomum verum* (Ceylon) and *Cinnamomum cassia* (cassia). The former has a higher trade value due to its lower abundance but the latter can be obtained in large quantities [101]. However, the lower-cost and more abundant cassia form of cinnamon contains a higher concentration of its principal chemical component, which is thought to be responsible for its medicinal properties, cinnamaldehyde. There are many available reports of the beneficial properties of cinnamon that are relevant to wound healing, including its anti-inflammatory, antithrombotic, antimicrobial, and antifungal properties [102].

Extracts of cinnamon in its raw form can be created which contain a concoction of active compounds that work together to provide potential health benefits. PG was used to create bandage-like fibrous mats from extracts of cinnamon to produce an antifungal covering which would protect against the formation of fungi, in particular *Candida albicans* [103]. The fungal growths prevalent in wound environments can cause infections and form a protective biofilm which can support other pathogenic bacterial species. Polycaprolactone (PCL) was therefore used to produce four sets of bandages at different concentrations of cinnamon extract and their antifungal activities against *C. albicans* were observed. The average fibre diameter of the PCL bandages without cinnamon extract was 6.0 ± 2.6 μm, and this number reduced with the addition of cinnamon extract, proving a higher surface area for the release of key antimicrobial ingredients. The fibres also showed a high degree of porosity, which is desirable to support the movement of exudate in and out of the wound microenvironment.

Figure 4.41 shows images of the fibres during their testing in culture. Raw cinnamon powder showed a potent antifungal effect, as seen by the exclusion zone sounding its perimeter. An inhibition zone is formed when a fungal colony cannot populate a certain area in the Petri dish due to an antifungal force that either repels or kills it. Virgin PCL fibres showed no apparent inhibition zone, signalling that they

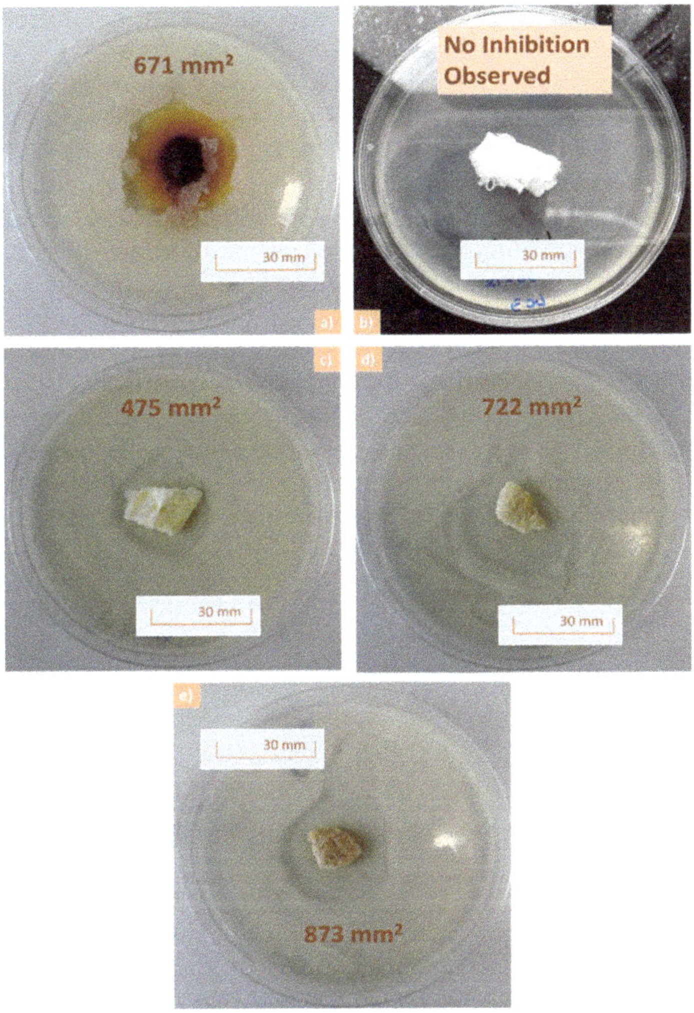

Figure 4.41. Images of fibre samples following 48 h of incubation showing plates containing: (a) ground cinnamon powder, (b) virgin PCL fibres, showing the absence of an inhibition area, (c) C1 cinnamon-extract fibres, (d), C2 cinnamon-extract fibres, (e), C3 cinnamon-extract fibres. In each case, 100 mg of sample was investigated. For each plate, the size of the inhibition area is given [103] John Wiley & Sons. [2019].

were devoid of antifungal properties on their own. Raw cinnamon has already been established as a potent antifungal material; however, the extraction process allows the concentration in fibre form to be controlled. Cinnamon-extract–PCL fibres were produced at three concentrations (C1, C2, and C3), which corresponded to a low concentration (250 mg ml^{-1}), a medium concentration (375 mg ml^{-1}), and a high concentration (500 mg ml^{-1}). We can see that increasing the extract concentration scales up the antifungal effect of the bandage-like fibres, as evidenced by a larger inhibition area. This work demonstrated the possibility of using crude unpurified extracts of natural materials in wound care and other antimicrobial filtering applications.

Using such a technique, high-yield bandage-like biodegradable fibres can be produced with a potent antifungal ability. These fibres are suitable for use as wound healing bandages. Because the cinnamon extract concentration can easily be altered, this approach provides the ability to tailor-make bandages for different wound healing applications in which different levels of antifungal action are required. What was perhaps more fascinating was that the cinnamon-extract fibres had a longer-lasting antifungal effect than the raw cinnamon powder itself.

Three weeks after incubation, it was found that the dish containing raw cinnamon powder showed extensive fungal growth characterised by the robust formation of spores (figure 4.42). It is evident that the cinnamon powder facilitated a regrowth of fungal colonies, indicating that the antifungal effect of the ground cinnamon powder was only temporary. All the extracted cinnamon fibres were shown to still retain their original inhibition zones intact, demonstrating that their antifungal effect was long-term and that the fungi were likely killed instead of repelled.

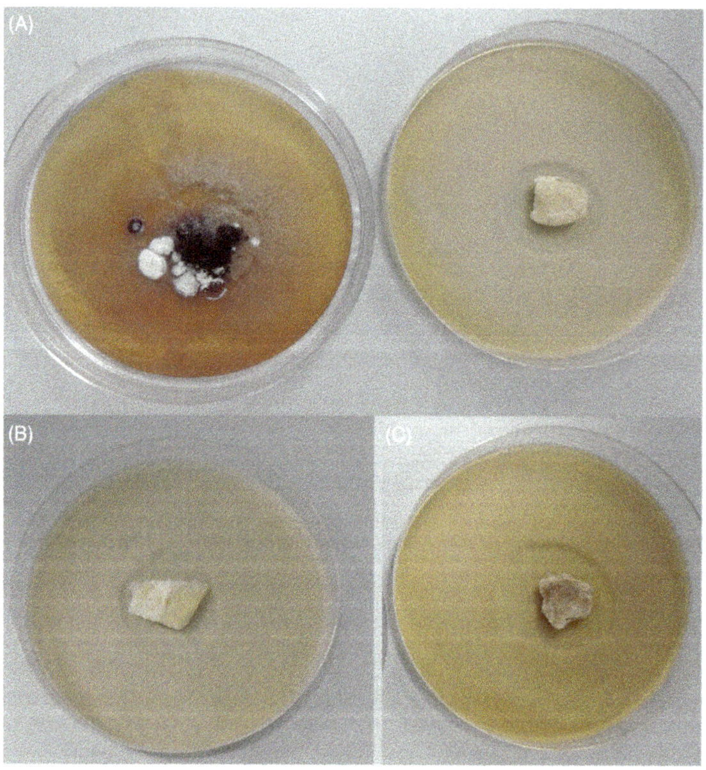

Figure 4.42. Images taken 504 h after initial incubation comparing: (a), fibres containing C1 extracted cinnamon (right-hand side) with raw cinnamon powder (left-hand side) (b), fibres containing C2 extracted cinnamon (c), fibres containing C3 extracted cinnamon. All Petri dishes shown are 90 mm in diameter [103] John Wiley & Sons. [2019].

The high concentration of cinnamon in the bandage-like fibres raises concerns about possible cytotoxicity to the native cells of the wound healing response. In order to put those concerns to the test, the produced cinnamon-extract fibres (C1, C2, and C3) were subjected to cytotoxicity and viability assays and also tested to see whether they were effective against bacterial species [104]. High-magnification images of these fibres can be seen in figure 4.43. As the concentration of cinnamon extract in the fibres increased, the average diameter reduced. The fibres demonstrated a good degree of interconnective porosity, supporting their suitability for use as a wound-dressing material.

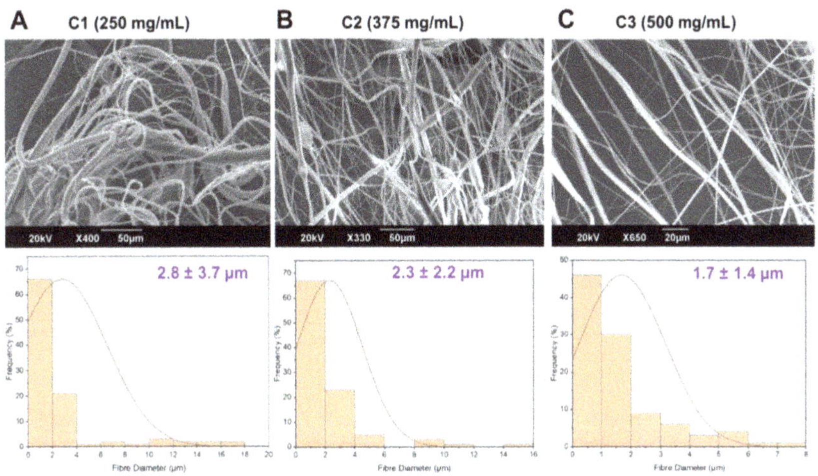

Figure 4.43. SEM micrographs of: (A) C1, (B) C2, (C) C3 cinnamon-extract-containing fibres and the corresponding diameter distributions for these fibrous constructs [104] John Wiley & Sons. [2019].

Cell viability studies using an indirect MTT assay measured the viability of mouse fibroblast cells in the presence of the bandage-like fibres. Fibroblasts are crucial cells of the wound healing response which synthesise collagen, an essential protein for tissue regeneration and the elasticity of the healed skin. As a biocompatible polymer, PCL is widely used as a biomaterial, therefore it is no surprise that it retains a cell viability of over 80%, as evidenced by the testing (figure 4.44). As the concentration of cinnamon in the PCL fibres increased, however, so did the viability of the fibroblast cells. In fact, at the highest tested concentration of 500 mg ml^{-1} (C3), the cell viability was significantly higher and even exceeded that of the control material (Dulbecco's Modified Eagle Medium). The cytotoxicity results therefore give a very positive outlook to the potential of these cinnamon-loaded bandage-like fibres, showing that they have minimal cytotoxicity and could potentially be used in a wound healing environment to provide antimicrobial aid.

In addition to their effectiveness against fungal species such as *C. albicans*, the fibres were tested against a few key pathogenic bacterial species, namely *E. coli, S. aureus,* Methicillin-resistant *S. aureus* (MRSA), and *Enterococcus faecalis.* The cinnamon-containing fibres were most effective against *E. coli*, a gram-negative

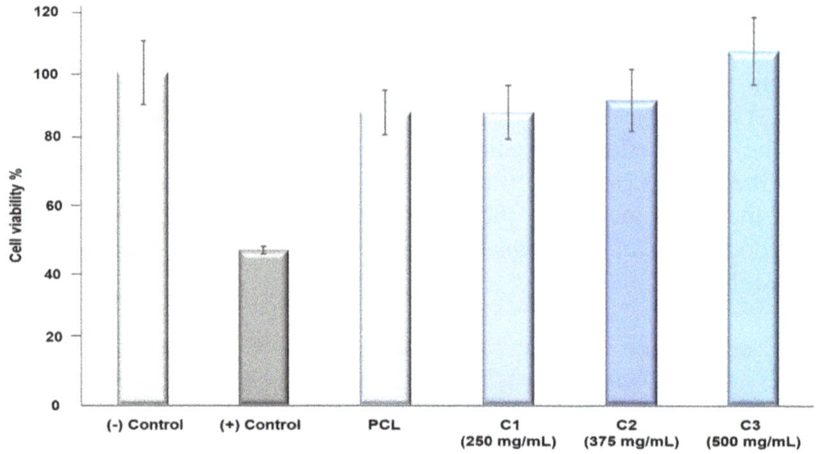

Figure 4.44. Cell cytotoxicity test results for PCL–cinnamon-extract polymeric fibres at concentrations C1, C2, and C3 [104] John Wiley & Sons. [2019].

bacterium which is a common cause of infection in surgical wounds. As the cinnamon concentration increased, the reduction in the bacterial population also increased. The cinnamon fibres were less effective against *S. aureus* compared to *E. coli*; however, all the fibres showed a significant reduction in the log number of bacteria. For some tests, for example with MRSA, an increase in cinnamon concentration did not affect the antimicrobial performance, suggesting that a lower minimum inhibitory concentration of cinnamon extract is required to produce the intended effect. The results shown here again highlight the excellent ability of these fibres to sustain a high degree of antimicrobial protection, which is highly desirable in a wound healing dressing. High-magnification images of the tested fibres were taken following the bacterial testing to show the effectiveness of the cinnamon extract within the fibres, as shown in figure 4.45.

As evidenced by figure 4.45, the PCL fibres with no cinnamon extract showed a large degree of bacterial growth for every tested bacterial species. Since PCL is a biocompatible polymer, it provides ideal attachment sites for these bacterial cells without having any inherent antimicrobial properties itself. With the inclusion of even a low concentration of cinnamon extract, it can be seen that the fibre strands have visibly fewer attachments of bacterial cells for all the tested species. At higher concentrations, the bacterial cell attachments mostly disappear; any remaining cell is likely to be nonviable due to the antimicrobial potency of the cinnamon-loaded bandage-like fibres.

4.6.1.2 Honey fibres for wound healing

Given that cinnamon-loaded fibres showed the benefits of using natural materials for wound healing applications, the further utilisation of other such substances could advance the field of low-toxicity, bioactive wound healing bandages. Honey has long been used as a remedy and a treatment for infected wounds, in which it is seen to

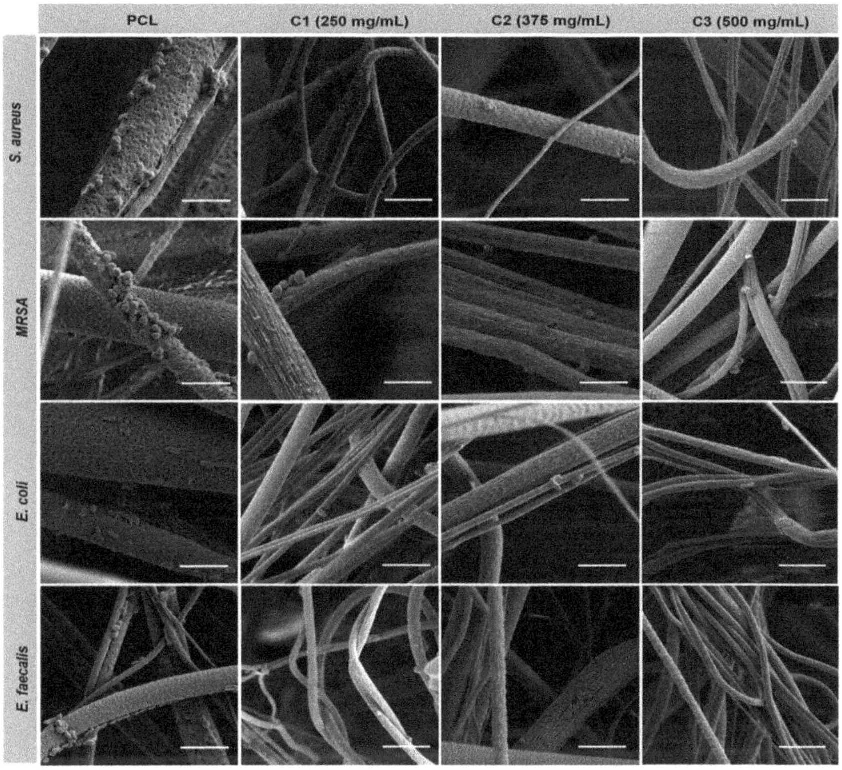

Figure 4.45. SEM images of antibacterial test results for the tested PCL fibres. (The scale bar denotes 5 μm.) [104] John Wiley & Sons. [2019].

accelerate wound healing, especially for burns [105]. Honey is also a potent antibacterial agent, consistently demonstrating effectiveness against pathogens such as *E. coli, Enterobacter aerogenes, Salmonella typhimurium,* and *S. aureus* [106]. Compared to standard honey, manuka honey is thought to have more potent antimicrobial and wound healing properties, making it especially beneficial for wounds. Using PG, manuka honey was loaded onto biodegradable and flexible PCL fibres intended for use in wound healing, and their antimicrobial properties in bandage form were assessed [107]. The aim of this work was to achieve the highest honey content in fibre form to obtain the most beneficial properties for wound healing; for this reason, PCL was used as the carrier polymer, as it provides a mechanically suitable support for the bandage-like fibres. Three concentrations of honey–PCL fibres were produced using PG at an applied gas pressure of 0.1 MPa (10 v/v%, 20 v/v% and 30 v/v%). These fibres were subsequently characterised in terms of their morphology, chemical characteristics, and antibacterial properties. Figure 4.46 shows high-magnification images of the manuka-honey-loaded fibres.

PCL fibres without any honey loading had an average fibre diameter of 7.5 ± 2.4 μm and the fibre surface showed the presence of surface porosity due to the use of a highly volatile solvent. The addition of manuka honey to the PCL solutions

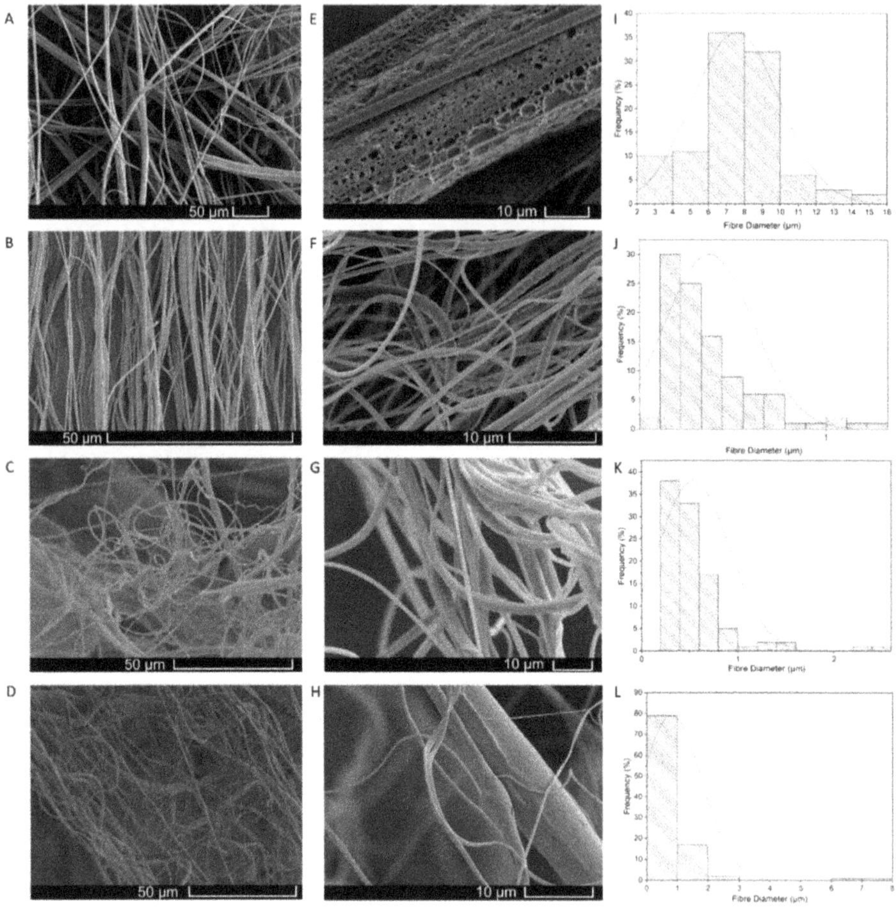

Figure 4.46. Electron micrographs of: (A) virgin PCL fibres, (B) 10% honey-composite fibres, (C) 20% honey-composite fibres, (D) 30% honey-composite fibres. High-magnification images of (E) virgin PCL fibres, (F) 10% honey-composite fibres, (G) 20% honey-composite fibres, (H) 30% honey-composite fibres, along with corresponding fibre diameter distribution histograms (I-L). Reproduced from [107]. CC BY 4.0.

resulted in a substantial increase in viscosity; for example, with the addition of only 10% honey, the viscosity of the solution increased from 7638 to 44 091 mPa s. Typically, an increase in viscosity results in the formation of thicker fibres; however, this was not the case for the manuka-honey-loaded fibres, which showed an average fibre diameter of 437 ± 21 nm at 10% loading. This behaviour of fibre size reduction may be attributed to the fact that the highly viscous honey–PCL solution works to reduce the effective size of the gyration orifice, leading to thinner fibre production. The fibres produced at this concentration were also highly unidirectionally aligned and very uniform in thickness. At a concentration of 20%, the honey–PCL fibres had an average diameter of 543 ± 374 nm, and at the highest tested concentration of 30% they had an average fibre diameter of 815 ± 98 nm. It should be noted that the honey concentrations were recorded in volume ratios. Given that honey has a higher density than PCL, the actual loading of honey was very high. As a result, concentrations higher than 30 (v/v%) were difficult to achieve and would have resulted in a loss of mechanical integrity, making them unsuitable for use as wound healing bandages.

The manuka-honey–PCL composite fibrous meshes were then tested for their antibacterial activity against the Gram-negative *E. coli* and the Gram-positive *S. epidermidis*; the results can be seen in figure 4.47. The control material, PCL, had no antibacterial effect and thus did not result in a significant number of dead cells. The manuka honey fibres were effective against *E. coli*, as evidenced by the proportion of dead cells. As the concentration of manuka honey in the fibres increased, so did their bactericidal efficacy. Comparatively, however, the manuka-honey–PCL fibres were significantly more effective against *S. epidermidis*, a bacterium commonly found on the skin, which can cause infection in immunocompromised patients with wounds.

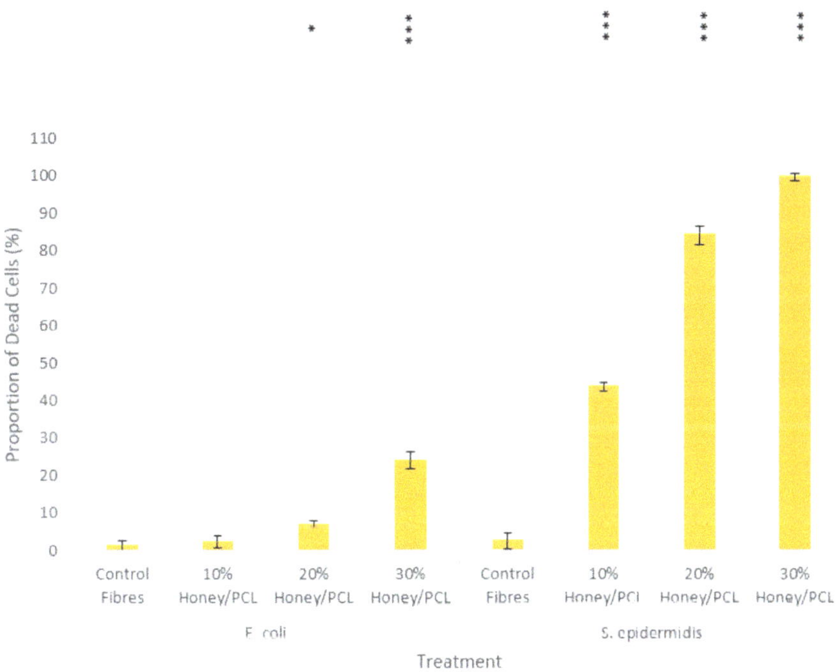

Figure 4.47. The antibacterial activities of 10 v/v%, 20 v/v%, and 30 v/v% manuka–PCL composite fibrous meshes compared to the negative control of virgin PCL fibres; antibacterial effectiveness is expressed as the percentage bacterial reduction. The post-hoc Tukey honestly significant difference (HSD) results of the treatments compared to the control are shown on the graph as p values of <0.05 (*) and <0.001 (***). Reproduced from [107]. CC BY 4.0.

This work shows that bandage-like composite fibres that have a very high loading of honey can be made into viable materials for wound healing. The bandages are highly effective at killing *S. epidermidis* and potentially many other hospital-acquired infections. By continuing to make the most of natural materials, one can adopt highly biocompatible approaches to wound healing, which have the combined effect of being antibacterial, pro wound healing, and less harmful to the environment upon disposal.

4.6.2 Graphene

In 2004, Geim and Novoselov rediscovered a material derived from graphite, a widely available form of carbon, which has since been hailed as a potential miracle material [108]. By isolating a single-atom-thick layer of graphite, graphene can be created. It consists of sp^2-bonded carbon atoms, which are responsible for many of its extraordinary feats such as its mechanical, optical, thermal, and electrical properties [109]. Graphene also has plenty of uses in biomedical applications. Graphene oxide (GO), produced by treating graphene with strong oxidisers via the Hummers method, can be used as a nanocarrier for gene and drug delivery [110]. GO can also be used for cancer therapy, as polyethylene glycol (PEG) ylated GO can be utilised for highly targeted tumour destruction [111]. Graphene and its many derivate materials can also be used as biosensor components due to their numerous beneficial properties. Novel GO-based biosensors which utilise the electrochemical principle have been produced which take advantage of the material's great electrical conductivity, high surface area, and its ability to load various biomolecules through physical and chemical interactions [112]. Naturally, because of its numerous advantages, graphene and its derivates have limitless applications in many different fields. One downside to the use of graphene is the difficulty of processing it into secondary materials, due to its single-atom nature. The use of graphene in fibre form is a viable means to leverage its properties whilst also maximising scalability. Methods such as electrospinning have been used to process graphene into fibre form. Whilst these have been successful, they are still far from scaling to large quantities, as they are often bottlenecked by slower manufacturing processes. PG has therefore been explored as a technique that can be used in the production of graphene–polymer composite fibres. These developments are presented in the following section.

4.6.2.1 Graphene nanoplatelet-loaded polyurethane fibres

Significant interest in hybrid polymer composites has been seen in materials science and engineering in the last few decades, as the use of hybrid polymer composites remains an attractive approach for enhancing the properties of the individual material components. The inclusion of a polymer matrix can lead to improved stiffness, higher strength, and better scalability. In order to manufacture graphene-based polymeric composites, a suitable blending method must be utilised, such as melt blending, solution compounding, or *in situ* polymerisation [113]. These methods can often be energy-intensive and damaging to the environment. Graphene nanoplatelets (GNPs) are a form of graphene produced through plasma exfoliation; the use of this method to create nanoparticles can reduce their cost and increase scalability [114]. PG has been used to make thermoplastic polyurethane (TPU) and phenolic resin fibres loaded with graphene nanoplatelets [115]. In this work, several different concentrations of TPU and phenolic resin polymer solutions

(15 wt%, 20 wt%, and 25 wt%) were prepared with and without a loading of 5 wt% of GNPS. The composite fibres consisting of TPU, phenolic resin, and GNPs had an average fibre diameter of about 8 μm and a bead-on-a-string morphology when spun at low applied gas pressures (figure 4.48). At higher applied gas pressures, the average diameter of these fibres dropped to about 8 μm and the bead density reduced significantly.

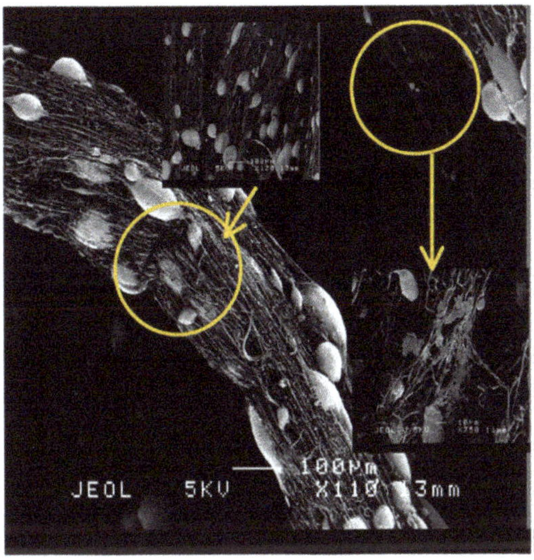

Figure 4.48. A micrograph showing the dispersion of graphene nanoparticles in the GNP-loaded composite fibres. Reprinted from [115], Copyright (2016), with permission from Elsevier.

This work was the first to demonstrate that PG could be used to produce graphene-loaded composite fibres from polymers such as phenolic resin and TPU. The uptake of GNPs was confirmed using techniques such as FTIR and Raman spectroscopy as well as by surface imaging obtained using focused ion beam milling and electron microscopy. Using such an approach, strongly adhered graphene in a hybrid polymer matrix can be exploited for several biomedical applications while benefiting from low cost and scalability [116]. As graphene and its derivative materials can be quite difficult to process into secondary structures, studies that use PG and other methods such as electrospinning are pivotal for its long-term success.

4.6.2.2 Polyacrylonitrile-based carbon nanofibre–graphene nanoplatelet materials

Carbon nanofibres (CNFs) are cylindrical nanomaterials consisting of stacked layers of graphene arranged in conical structures. CNFs display extraordinary properties and can thus be used in many different applications, such as sensor components, batteries, catalysis, electrical devices, and selective adsorption devices [117]. Polyacrylonitrile (PAN) is a synthetic polymer used as a precursor in the production of CNFs due to its high carbon yield and relative affordability [118]. PG has been used to produce nanofibres consisting of PAN with GNPs [119].

The produced fibres were then treated using postprocessing techniques including pyrolysis and spark plasma sintering (SPS) to remove any polymer and improve the carbonisation.

PAN fibres without any GNP loading had an average fibre diameter of about 3.2 μm. Following the addition of GNP into the polymer solution, there was an instant reduction in the observed diameter to about 1.1 μm. The behaviour of nanoparticles is markedly different from, microparticles. It is often observed that the addition of nanomaterials such as graphene can lead to a reduction in polymer viscosity and the production of thinner fibres. At 8 wt% GNP loading, a very high concentration, the average fibre diameter increases to about 1.9 μm. The pyrolysis process also leads to a reduction in the fibre diameter; for example, PAN-only fibres had an average fibre diameter of about 2.4 μm. Following pyrolysis, the 1 wt% PAN–GNP fibres reduced in diameter to about 730 nm. Following SPS treatment, the fibres saw a further reduction in overall diameter: PAN-only fibres had an average fibre diameter of 1.5 μm, 1 wt% PAN–GNP fibres had an average diameter of 720 nm, and 8 wt% PAN–GNP fibres had an average diameter of 1.3 μm. SEM micrographs of these fibres can be seen in figure 4.49.

Virgin PAN fibres exhibited a smooth morphology that had no observable roughness and an absence of beads. Following the addition of GNPs, the surface

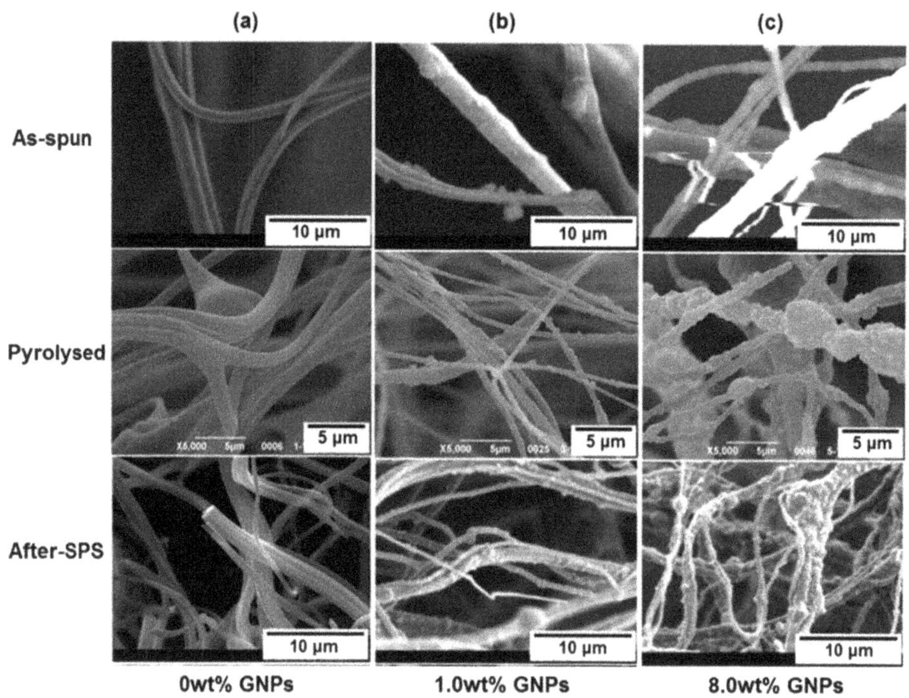

Figure 4.49. SEM micrographs of PAN-based fibres made using various concentrations of GNPs: (a) 0 wt%, (b) 1.0 wt%, and (c) 8.0 wt% and under different conditions (as spun, pyrolyzed, and post SPS). Reprinted from [119], Copyright (2016), with permission from Elsevier.

became rough, and protrusions formed of GNPs could be clearly seen, confirming the successful uptake of GNPs. At higher loadings of GNPs, the surface became significantly rougher and beads started to form. Following pyrolysis and SPS treatment, there did not seem to be a significant change in the fibre morphology.

One of the benefits of utilising GNPs and CNFs is their great electrical conductivity. Using polymeric solutions and fibre manufacturing techniques, high-surface-area fibrous components can be produced that display superior electrical properties. The electrical conductivities of the produced GNP-loaded and CNF-containing nanofibres were assessed. It was found that an increase in the GNP concentration also increased the electrical conductivity of the CNFs. This was true for all the different samples regardless of the method of preparation. The electrical conductivity of the PAN-based fibres increased from ~4 to ~46 × 10^3 S m^{-1} when the GNP loading increased from 0 wt% to 8.0 wt%. Pyrolyzed and SPS-treated fibres showed the greatest electrical conductivity readings, which were significantly higher than even those of commercially available carbon fibre (figure 4.50(a)). The study also showed that the produced fibres were capable of being used as wires, as they

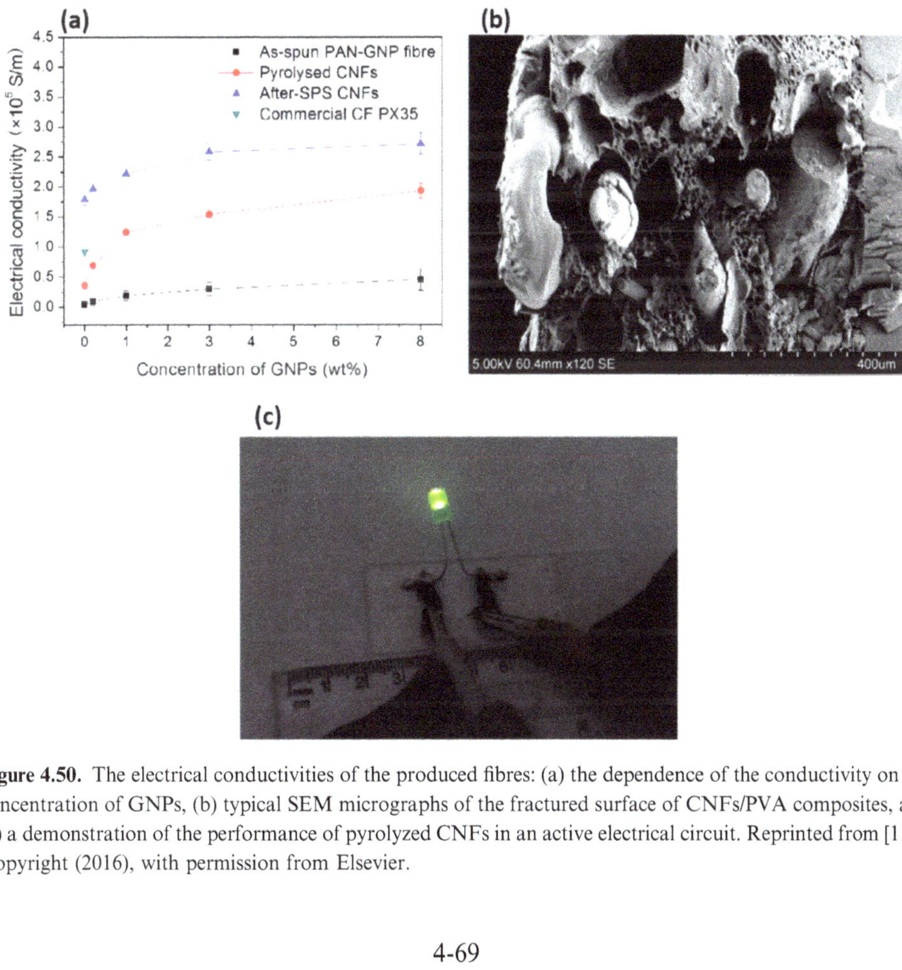

Figure 4.50. The electrical conductivities of the produced fibres: (a) the dependence of the conductivity on the concentration of GNPs, (b) typical SEM micrographs of the fractured surface of CNFs/PVA composites, and (c) a demonstration of the performance of pyrolyzed CNFs in an active electrical circuit. Reprinted from [119], Copyright (2016), with permission from Elsevier.

were able to directly conduct enough electricity to light up a light-emitting diode (figure 4.50(c)).

In this study, carbon nanofibres were produced by the simple PG process and subjected to two different high-temperature processing methods. Using PG, the diameter of the fibres as well as the loading of GNPs can easily be changed. This work highlights the potential of fibre manufacturing techniques to use graphene-based derivates to create high-surface-area secondary materials which can be used in a number of electrical engineering and healthcare applications.

4.6.2.3 The effect of graphene fibres on microbial growth

In addition to the many abovementioned benefits and properties of GNPs which make them suitable for a number of biomedical applications, it has also been reported that under certain conditions, GNPs also have antimicrobial properties. The antimicrobial properties of GNPs can be attributed to the production of reactive oxygen species and microbial encapsulation but also, more interestingly, to the direct physical rupture of microbial membranes by GNPs [120]. The benefit of a physical antimicrobial mechanism is that it is significantly more difficult for these microbes to evade or become resistant to. PG was therefore used to produce PMMA fibres made with various loadings of GNP in order to assess the conditions under which antimicrobial capabilities are present [121]. The fibres thus produced were then tested against Gram-negative *E. coli* and *P. aeruginosa*, two commonly found pathogenic microbial species. Images of the fibres can be seen in figure 4.51.

Without any GNP loading, the produced PMMA fibres showed a generally aligned, tubular, and continuous morphology that included surface pores and a slight bead-on-a-string structure. At a 2 wt% loading of GNPs or more, the alignment and the bead-on-a-string morphology start to become less apparent. Virgin PMMA fibres have an average fibre diameter of about 0.7 μm. Following the addition of GNP loading, this value went up to about 1 μm for both 2 wt% and 4 wt% concentrations and then grew to about 2.7 μm at a GNP concentration of 8 wt%. During the bacterial growth testing, interesting results were observed when the concentration of GNPs within the fibre was altered, as summarised in figure 4.52.

PMMA-only fibres depicted moderate bactericidal properties, as evidenced by the reduction in bacterial growth observed for both the tested *E. coli* and *P. aeruginosa* colonies. This effect could likely be attributed to the hydrophobic interactions between the polymer and the bacterial cell walls in addition to the sharp nature of PMMA nanofibres which could potentially penetrate bacterial cell walls. At concentrations of 2 wt% and 4 wt%, the fibres had no bactericidal effect and both the bacterial species were able to freely proliferate, as shown by the high levels of bacterial growth. It is well documented that the viability of microbial growth can depend on the carbon content available in the environment [122]. At a high GNP concentration of 8 wt%, a sudden change in the bacterial growth is observed. At this concentration, it can be seen that a significant reduction in bacterial growth occurs, indicating that a potent antibacterial mechanism has been activated. The reason for this sudden antibacterial effect could be that at higher loadings of GNPs, a larger number of GNP protrusions can be seen on the fibre

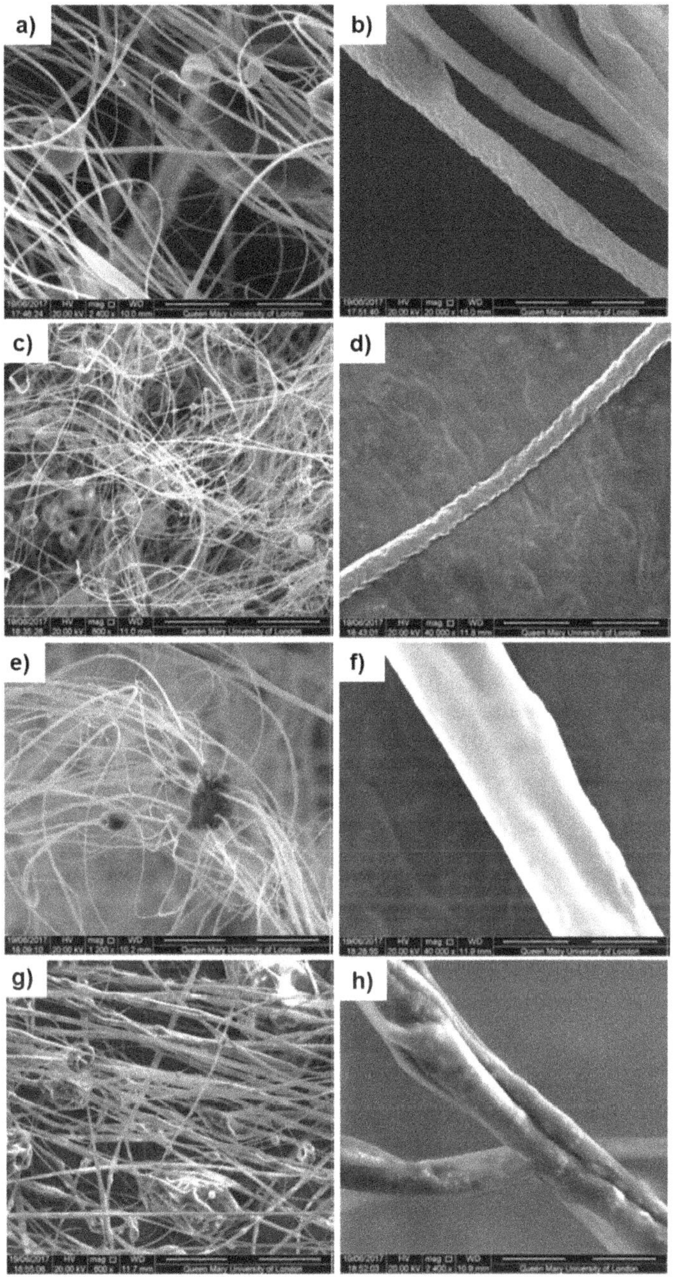

Figure 4.51. SEM images of PG fibres formed at: 0.2 MPa and 36 000 rpm. (a) A low-magnification image illustrating the fibre morphology of pure PMMA fibres, (b) a high-magnification image illustrating the pore morphology of pure PMMA fibres; (c) a low-magnification SEM image of 2 wt% GNP-loaded PMMA fibres; (d) a high-magnification SEM image of 2 wt% GNP-loaded PMMA fibres; (e) a low-magnification SEM image of 4 wt% GNP-loaded PMMA fibres; (f) a high-magnification SEM image illustrating the surface topography of 4 wt% GNP-loaded PMMA fibres; (g) a low-magnification SEM image of 8 wt% GNP-loaded PMMA fibres; (h) a high-magnification SEM image of 8 wt% GNP-loaded PMMA fibres. Reproduced from [121]. CC BY 4.0.

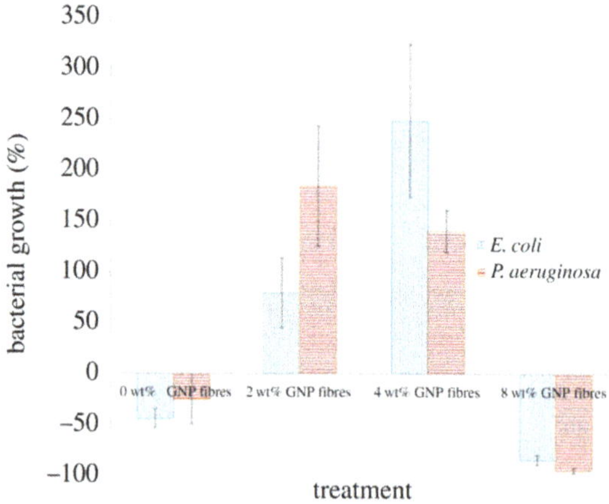

Figure 4.52. The microbial properties of 0 wt%, 2 wt%, 4 wt%, and 8 wt% GNP-loaded fibres against *E. coli* and *P. aeruginosa*. Reproduced from [121]. CC BY 4.0.

surfaces; these protrusions act as daggers, penetrating microbial cell walls and causing rapid death. This phenomenon can also be seen in figure 4.49, in which a higher concentration of GNPs leads to dagger-like protrusions on the fibre surface. This work supports the viability of creating antibacterial fibrous scaffolds with a long-lasting bactericidal effect.

4.6.2.4 Polyacrylonitrile–graphene oxide composite fibres

The use of GO can be a viable way to reduce the costs associated with producing the more expensive single-layered graphene. GO has many of the same physical properties as graphene and is therefore a very extensively explored material. As PG can be used to generate fibres as a rapid rate, by incorporating GO into polymer solutions, we can produce structures with superior mechanical and electrical properties. GO–PAN composite fibres were produced by PG at several different GO concentrations, pyrolyzed, and subsequently analysed [123]. The PG operational parameters such as the rotational speed and applied gas pressure had a discernible effect on the fibre morphology. Images of 7 wt% GO–PAN fibres produced using different processing conditions can be seen in figure 4.53.

In this study, six different weight loadings of GO were used with PAN (1 wt%, 2 wt%, 3 wt%, 5 wt%, 7 wt%, and 10 wt%) in order to observe the differences when the GO loading is increased. Generally speaking, higher rotational speeds and applied gas pressures resulted in the production of thinner fibres. The fibres produced were the thinnest at 3 wt% GO. The fibres appeared to have some unidirectional alignment but also contained beads due to the addition of GO to the polymer solution. In electrical conductivity testing, only the 1 wt% and 2 wt% GO–PAN fibres were able to conduct enough electricity to light up a diode; their conductivities were 973 S m^{-1} and 459 S m^{-1}, respectively. At higher loadings of GO, the thickness increases, decreasing the electrical conductivity of the material and changing its behaviour to that of an insulator. This work demonstrates the

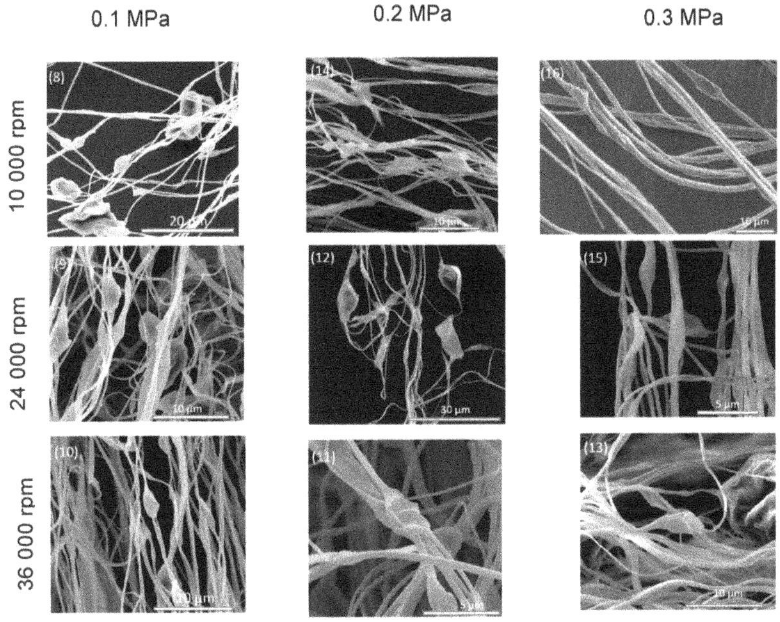

Figure 4.53. SEM images of 7 wt% GO–PAN fibres produced at different pressures and speeds. Reprinted from [123], Copyright (2020), with permission from Elsevier.

complexity of utilising graphene and its derivate materials: on the one hand, low concentrations could allow a thin layer of graphene or GO to be deposited, which would benefit its electrical properties, but on the other hand, higher loadings can be beneficial for other biomedical applications such as antimicrobial filters. The following section therefore focusses on the antibacterial efficacy of GO composite fibres.

4.6.2.5 The microstructure and antibacterial efficacy of graphene oxide nanocomposite fibres

Given that GNPs successfully displayed antibacterial properties, GO was also investigated to determine whether it too had viable bactericidal effects. PG was used to create fibres from GO nanosheets imported into a PMMA polymeric structure. The antibacterial performance of the fibrous meshes against *E. coli* was then measured [124]. As in the previous tests involving GNPs, GO loadings of 0 wt%, 2 wt%, 4 wt%, and 8 wt% were prepared. Images of the resulting fibres can be seen in figure 4.54.

Pure PMMA fibres devoid of GO had an average fibre diameter of 3.9 ± 2.0 μm; these fibres appeared to be tubular and continuous with low overall unidirectionality. Following the addition of 2 wt% GO, the average fibre diameter reduced to 1.4 ± 0.9 μm and thinner and more uniform fibres were produced. The addition of material at the nanometre scale often leads to a reduction in viscosity. In this case, the addition of graphene oxide caused slippage within the polymer matrix,

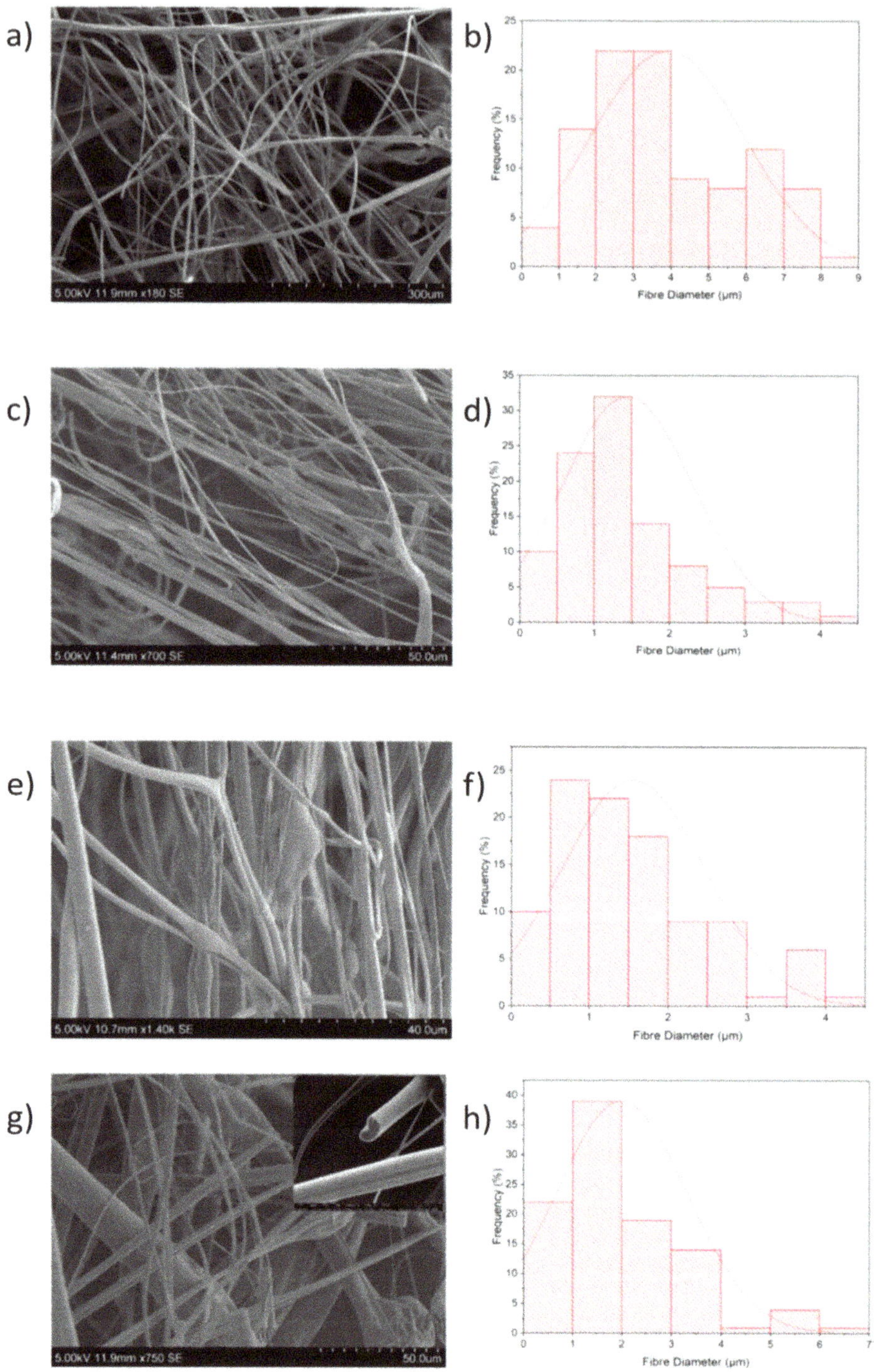

Figure 4.54. Electron micrographs and fibre diameter distributions of GO-loaded PMMA fibres: (a) and (b) pure PMMA fibres, (c) and (d) 2 wt% GO fibres, (e) and (f) 4 wt% GO fibres, (g) and (h) 8 wt% GO fibres. In (g), the inset micrograph shows the fibres to have smooth surfaces. Reprinted from [124], Copyright (2020), with permission from Elsevier.

producing finer fibres. Further increases in GO loading did not contribute to an additional fibre diameter reduction but rather produced a small incremental increase. At a GO concentration of 4 wt%, the fibres show high uniformity and have an average fibre diameter of 1.6 ± 0.9 μm; at 8 wt%, they have an average diameter of 2.0 ± 1.3 μm. Images of the surface of the fibres depict a smooth surface, although it is possible that surface nanopores could be present on other fibre strands due to the use of a volatile solvent (chloroform). The antibacterial activity of these PMMA–GO fibres was then investigated using *E. coli* K12; the results can be seen in figure 4.55.

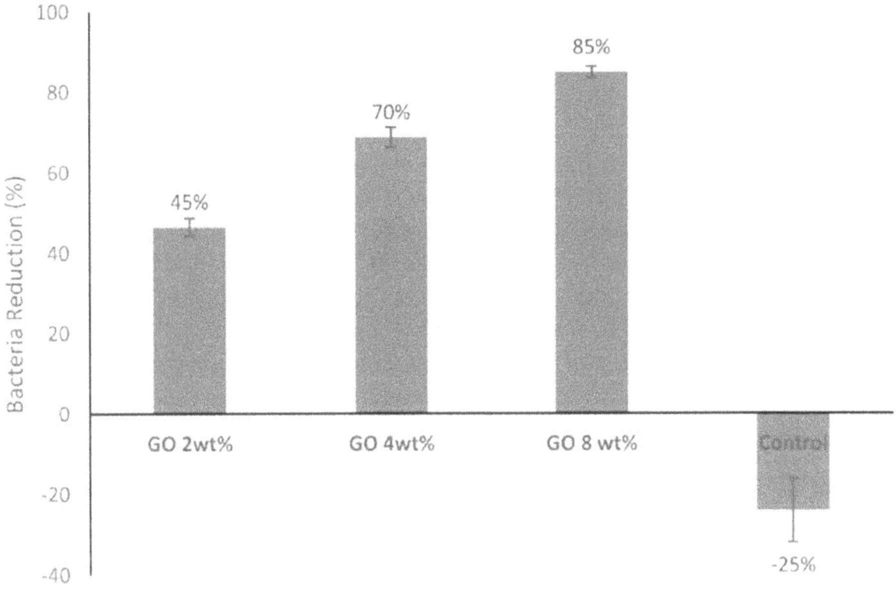

Figure 4.55. Bacterial reductions observed after the incubation of 0 wt%, 2 wt%, 4 wt%, and 8 wt% GO–PMMA fibres with *E. coli* K12 for 24 h. Pure PMMA fibres with no GO were used as a control group. The error bars represent standard deviation (n = 3). Reprinted from [124], Copyright (2020), with permission from Elsevier.

Pure PMMA fibres devoid of GO loadings showed no bacterial reduction, indicating that the fibres themselves were not inherently antibacterial. At GO loadings of 2 wt% and above, the fibres proficiently reduced the bacterial numbers, and the bactericidal action increased significantly with the concentration of GO. However, compared to the GO nanosheets alone, which showed a bacterial reduction of over 90% during testing, the fibrous meshes showed lower antibacterial efficacy. The effect of higher GO concentrations within the fibres was to expose more GO nanosheets on the fibres, leading to a greater bactericidal effect. The GO nanosheets within the fibres produce their antibacterial effect using different mechanisms of action. One mechanism is the production of reactive oxygen species. In this work, the 8 wt% PMMA–GO fibres were shown to release a high quantity of dichloro-dihydro-fluorescein diacetate, which is a quantitative way of assessing oxidative stress [125]. In addition, the sharp features of the GO nanosheets act as physical disruptors of the bacterial membrane, causing death by penetration and subsequent leakage of vital cellular material. This research showcased the antibacterial activity of PMMA–GO nanocomposite fibres, which have immense potential for use in filtration applications, especially for hospital systems.

4.6.2.6 Porous graphene composite polymer fibres

The use of graphene and its derivative materials is widespread in the fields of biomaterials and biomedical engineering. Many techniques have been utilised to produce graphene-based materials which have the added benefits of being cheaper to make and mass-produce. Porous graphene, which consists of highly porous graphene nanosheets, has recently been discovered to possess refined properties compared to graphene, such as great optical transparency, super hydrophobicity, chemical stability, a high surface area, and resistance to oxidation [126]. For this reason, PG has been explored as a means of producing porous graphene composite fibres from a PCL polymeric backbone [127]. As graphene is difficult to bulk process into functional nanomaterials, its incorporation within a polymeric carrier allows for a composite graphene-based solution, which is far easier to upscale and can meet the soaring demands. Using a material such as PCL, PG can produce over 1 g of graphene-loaded fibres in under 10 s. PCL was used to produce fibres with porous graphene loadings of 3 wt%, 4 wt%, and 5 wt% (figure 4.56).

As the rheological properties of the prepared polymer solution play a large role in the final fibre production via PG, the measured values can tell us a lot about the morphological outcome. PCL without porous graphene and with 3 wt% loadings showed very similar viscosity readings; as such, the two fibres had comparable average fibre diameters of 7.5 ± 2.5 μm without graphene and 7.6 ± 5.2 μm with graphene. However, at a graphene concentration of 4 wt%, the viscosity of the PCL solution dropped from 7625 ± 86 mPa.S to 3679 ± 78 mPa.S. This reduction in viscosity was caused by the interaction of the porous graphene with the polymer chains, which consequently led to the deposition of thinner fibres that had an average diameter of 2.6 ± 2.6 μm. At a concentration of 5 wt% of porous graphene, the diameter-reducing effect was muted, and the average fibre diameter was 3.5 ± 4.1 μm. Analysis by Raman spectroscopy showed that the 3 wt% and 4 wt% fibres were encased within a single layer of graphene, which is beneficial in maximising graphene's unique properties. At 5 wt%, the layers begin to double up, reaffirming the importance of optimising the operational and solution parameters used in fibre manufacture. This study marked the first successful production of porous graphene composite fibres that also benefited from a high production rate.

4.6.3 Self-healing materials

Elastomeric materials have various uses in many sectors such as sealing, textiles, car tyres, and medical devices. The development of this class of materials can therefore lead to great technological strides that have direct applicability to several biomedical devices. Recently, there has been a focus on elastomers which display desirable

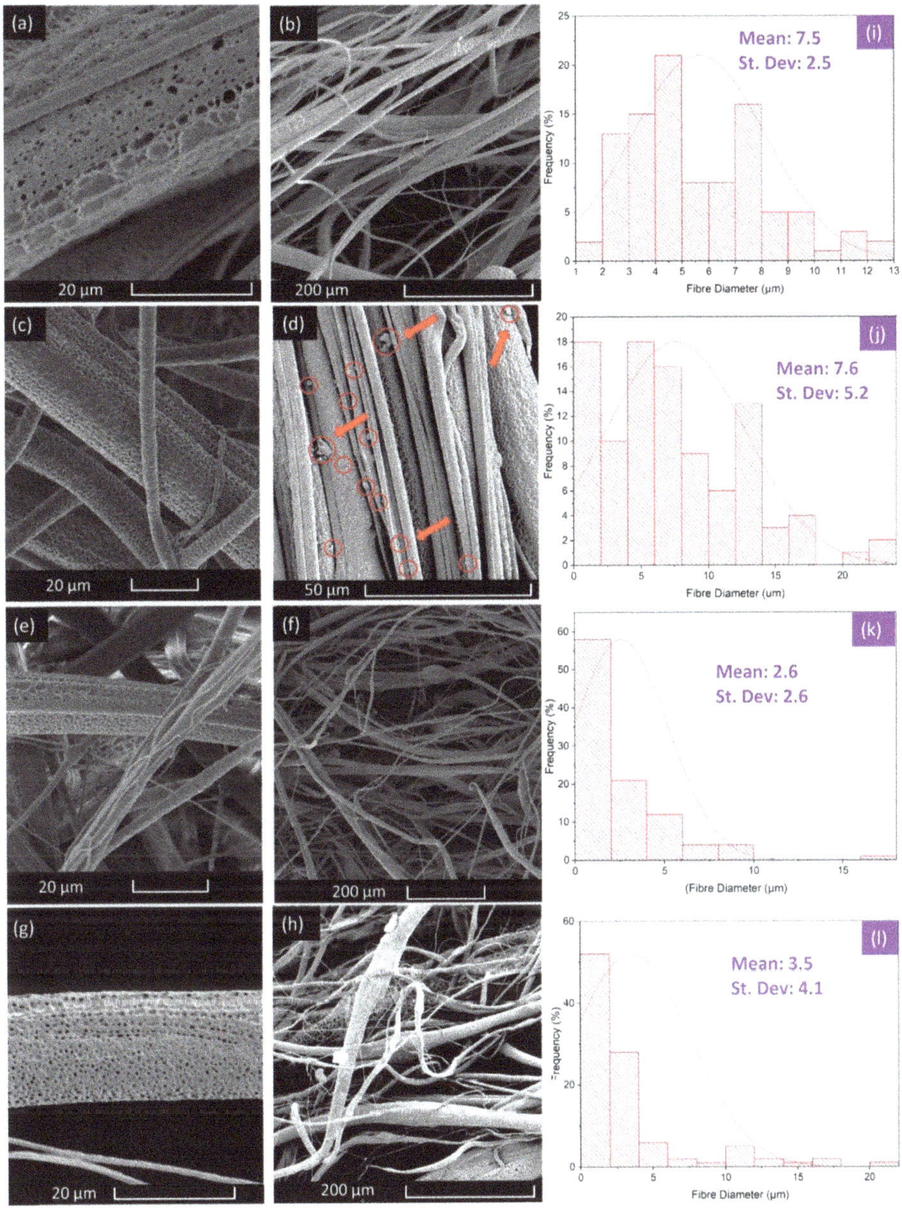

Figure 4.56. SEM micrographs of: (a,b) 15% virgin PCL fibres without porous graphene; (c,d) fibres incorporating 3 wt% porous graphene; red circles and arrows indicate the presence of surface particles; (e,f) fibres incorporating 4 wt% porous graphene; (g,h) fibres incorporating 5 wt% porous graphene including a surface view and a full view; all images are accompanied by diameter distribution graphs (i–l). For each graph, 100 fibre strands were measured at random. Reproduced from [127]. CC BY 4.0.

properties, such as extremely high stretchability and self-healing properties. These materials have attracted much attention for use in biomedical devices for soft robotics, wearable devices, biosensors, and smart flexible electronics [128–130]. The self-healing capabilities of these elastomers are provided by dynamic covalent bonds between the monomers, which allow the polymer to heal itself without the need for external intervention. A novel and completely bio-based autonomous self-healing elastomer (PA36,36) was developed which benefited from zero water uptake, high self-healing efficiency and melt processability and was processed using PG to produce fibre yarns [131]. Water contact angle and water uptake testing showed that PA36,36 did not display any water absorption due to its high content of nonpolar hydrocarbons. This feature provides great suitability for use in anticorrosive coating products and is especially beneficial for usage in salty environments. To assess the anticorrosive properties of the novel polymer, a stainless steel razor was coated with a sheet of PA36,36 and submerged into a sodium chloride–water solution for seven days. The coated razor did not show any signs of corrosion, whilst an uncoated razor showed corrosion products (figure 4.57). In addition, the self-healing nature of the elastomer further contributes to its protective effects.

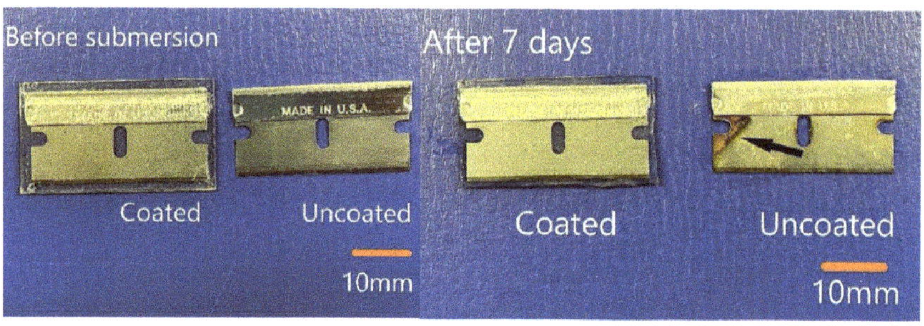

Figure 4.57. Photographs of stainless steel razor blades with and without a PA36,36 (24 h) coating before and after immersion in a NaCl–water solution. Reprinted from [131], Copyright (2021), with permission from ACS Publications.

By dissolving the PA36,36 in chloroform, a polymer solution of 10 wt% was obtained and spun into fibres using PG; the resulting fibres can be seen in figure 4.58(a). The produced fibres were continuous; they had a unidirectional alignment and an average fibre diameter of 14.2 ± 1.4 μm. The fibres in the form of yarns were then subjected to tensile testing to evaluate their stretchability (figure 4.58(b)).

Tensile tests showed that the PG-spun fibres had outstanding stretchability, demonstrated by an elongation at breaking of 950% ± 74%, which is higher than those of commercially available spandex (650%–700%) and natural rubber (600%–700%). The tensile strength of these fibres was measured to be 1.02 ± 0.50 MPa. The exceptional properties demonstrated by these fibres allows them to be explored for a range of applications ranging from textile manufacture and fibre-based wearable devices to soft robotic components.

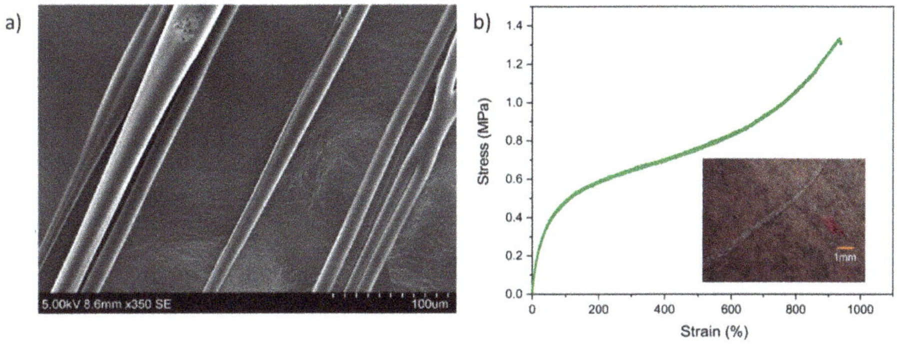

Figure 4.58. (a) An SEM micrograph of PA36,36 fibres produced using PG and (b) the tensile stress–strain curve of the PG-spun fibre yarn (inset: optical micrograph of the yarn showing approximately 25 fibres). Reprinted from [131], Copyright (2021), with permission from ACS Publications.

4.6.4 Composite materials

Although there is a plethora of materials that have desirable properties which still need to be developed, composites are a class of materials which aims to combine the advantageous properties of two or more different constituent materials. The advantage of using hybrid or composite materials is that one can often merge the desirable properties whilst simultaneously bypassing some of the inherent weaknesses. This approach to materials science and engineering has radically shifted the landscape of what is possible in terms of functional materials and their various applications. This section presents composite strategies which have been explored in conjunction with PG.

4.6.4.1 Starch-loaded poly(ethylene oxide)

Work with composite materials began shortly after the initial discovery of PG, when starch-loaded PEO fibres were produced [132]. Starch is one of the most abundant naturally occurring polysaccharides and shows excellent biodegradability. Starch alone is too brittle to be spun into fibres; however, combining it with another highly biodegradable polymer such as PEO allows the mechanical properties of the composite material to be improved whilst retaining its desirable properties. In this study, starch derived from potato was added to polymer solutions containing varying ratios of PEO, and the operating parameters of PG were varied to determine the effect that this had on the fibre morphology. The resulting fibres can be seen in figure 4.59.

The fibres were produced at a fixed applied gas pressure of 0.1 MPa, and it became apparent that changing the rotational speed and the mixture of the composite polymer solution could alter the morphology of the resulting fibres. PEO fibres alone showed strong unidirectional alignment and had an average fibre diameter of about 650 nm at a rotational speed of 24 000 rpm; a rotational speed of 36 000 rpm resulted in thinner fibres of about 500 nm. The addition of starch to the polymer solution contributed to a drastic change in fibre morphology. The 90:10

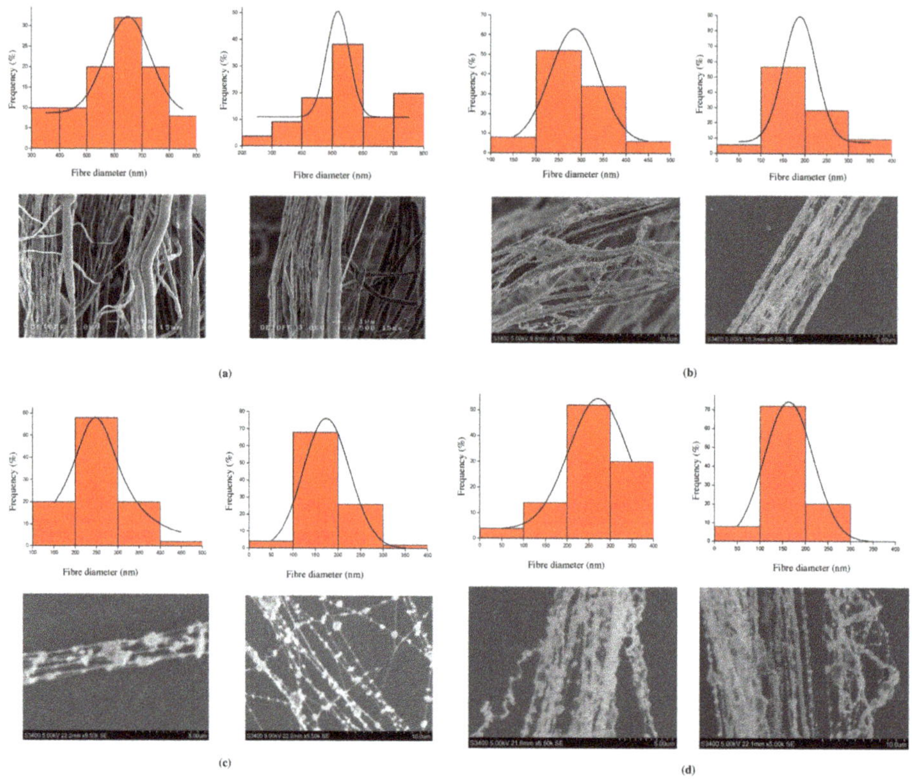

Figure 4.59. Diameter distributions and SEM images of the starch-loaded PEO system at low (24 000 rpm, left-hand side) and high (36 000 rpm, right-hand side) rotational speeds: (a) PEO only, (b) 90:10 PEO–starch, (c) 70:30 PEO–starch, (d) 50:50 PEO–starch. Reprinted from [132], Copyright (2014), with permission from Elsevier.

PEO–starch fibres started to assume a bead-on-a-string morphology and the average fibre diameter reduced from about 650 nm to 290 nm at a rotational speed of 24 000 rpm and an average fibre diameter of about 180 nm at the higher rotational speed of 36 000 rpm. As the ratio of starch increased in the polymer solution, the average fibre diameter reduced to a minimum of 160 nm at the highest recorded starch concentration of 50:50 PEO–starch at the maximum rotational speed of 36 000 rpm. It was also noted that the higher starch concentrations were characterised by the bead-on-a-string morphology.

This work was one of the earliest to demonstrate the spinnability of a composite of two different materials into fibres via PG. The use of composite materials as a strategy plays an important role in advancing the fields of materials science and engineering and the many different healthcare applications that could stem from them. The mechanism of PG, i.e. one that utilises a polymer solution which does not necessarily need to display complete solubility, allows for the endless exploration of composite binary, ternary, and even multicomponent composite fibre production.

4.6.4.2 Bacterial cellulose binary and ternary polymer fibres

Composite polymers offer great advantages compared to the use of just a single polymer. Whilst binary composites (i.e. composites consisting of a blend of two different polymers) are the most common, it is possible to incorporate more than two polymers into a single material. As alluded to above, bacterial cellulose is an extraordinary material which has many advantageous properties for wound healing; however, the difficulty of its processing makes it tough to form into functional constructs. A study examined binary and ternary compositions of bacterial cellulose, PCL, and PLA spun into fibres using PG and gathered various results based on mechanical properties and production yields [133].

This study initially prepared three types of binary polymer solutions and spun them into fibres containing varying ratios of PLA–bacterial cellulose, PCL–bacterial cellulose and a mixture of PLA and PCL. PLA and PCL share solubility with many organic polymers but have slightly different mechanical properties. For example, PLA is the more brittle of the two, whilst PCL is tougher and more flexible. Spinning just PLA and PCL alone typically results in yields of over 90%. No system can deliver the maximum theoretical yield of 100%, which is calculated by dividing the mass of the fibres by the mass of polymer in the original polymer solution. Production yield is lost due to various factors such as solvent evaporation and the loss of polymer solution during the spinning up phase of the high-speed motor. With the binary systems of PLA and PCL, the yields of all the various ratios of the two polymers remain higher than 80% but slight dips are observed at PLA–PCL ratios of 70:30, 60:40 and 50:50. This result could be due to the imperfect solubility of the polymer matrices of the two polymers. Binary systems of 30:70 PLA:PCL showed the highest production yields of over 96%, which are higher than those obtained using just PLA or PCL alone. The results show the potential of optimising composite polymers not only to improve their mechanical properties but also (in some cases) yields using two different polymers.

The addition of even a small amount of bacterial cellulose leads to a reduction in the yield to less than 60%. This phenomenon results from the high crystallinity of bacterial cellulose, which gives it extremely low solubility in most solvents. For progressively higher loadings of bacterial cellulose, the production yield deteriorates drastically, leading to fibres that are unsuitable for applications in wound healing. Therefore, a compromise must be found between the bacterial cellulose content and the resulting mechanical properties. An overview of the mass yields for all the tested binary composite polymer systems can be seen in figure 4.60.

The 30:70 PLA:PCL fibres optimised the production yield and the mixture of the two differing polymers. Therefore, this was taken as a basis from which to find a good compromise between this composite and bacterial cellulose, i.e. to create a ternary system consisting of all three polymers. The fibre diameter can often play an important role in contributing to the performance of wound healing structures, as it provides additional surface area for cellular interactions. Pure (100%) PLA fibres had an average fibre diameter of about 18 μm, whilst 100% PCL fibres had an average fibre diameter of about 5 μm. It was decided that the optimal ternary composition for the two polymers was 70:30 (PLA–BC optimised

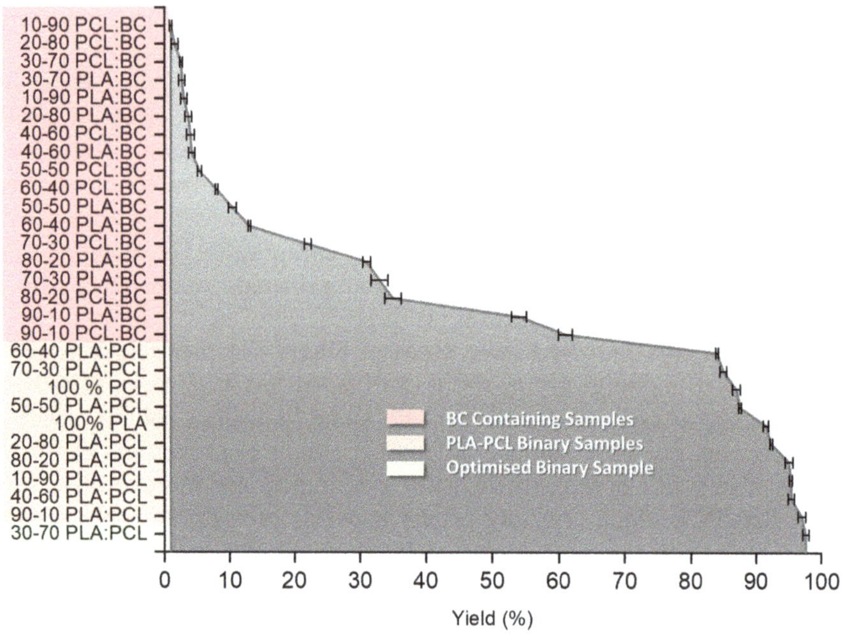

Figure 4.60. Graph showing the mass yield values and percentages for all the tested binary composite fibres, BC = (bacterial cellulose). Reproduced from [133]. CC BY 4.0.

binary:bacterial cellulose). The resulting ternary composite contained 30% bacterial cellulose; this represented a high loading which took into consideration the production yield. The optimised ternary fibres had an average fibre diameter of 11 μm, which was considerably lower than the diameter achieved by spinning 100% PLA fibres.

The optimised ternary fibres consisting of bacterial cellulose, PLA, and PCL were then subjected to mechanical testing in order to observe how the changes in their polymer chains would affect their performance as a wound healing material. Pure (100%) PLA and 100% PCL both displayed a tensile strength of about 2.3 MPa. The addition of bacterial cellulose to the matrix resulted in higher tensile strengths being recorded up to a maximum recorded at 30% loading of bacterial cellulose. At loadings of bacterial cellulose greater than 30%, the fibre yield became poor, which subsequently affected its mechanical properties. An overview of these results can be seen in figure 4.61. The ultimate tensile strength of the optimised ternary composite was measured and found to be about 9 MPa, which was considerably higher than the tensile strengths of any of the tested binary systems, demonstrating the performance increases that can be achieved by utilising a ternary polymer system. Wound healing materials must have an adequate tensile strength to ensure that the fibres can withstand some stretching due to movement, especially around joints.

The stiffnesses of the samples were also recorded in terms of their Young's modulus values. The addition of bacterial cellulose to the polymer solution resulted

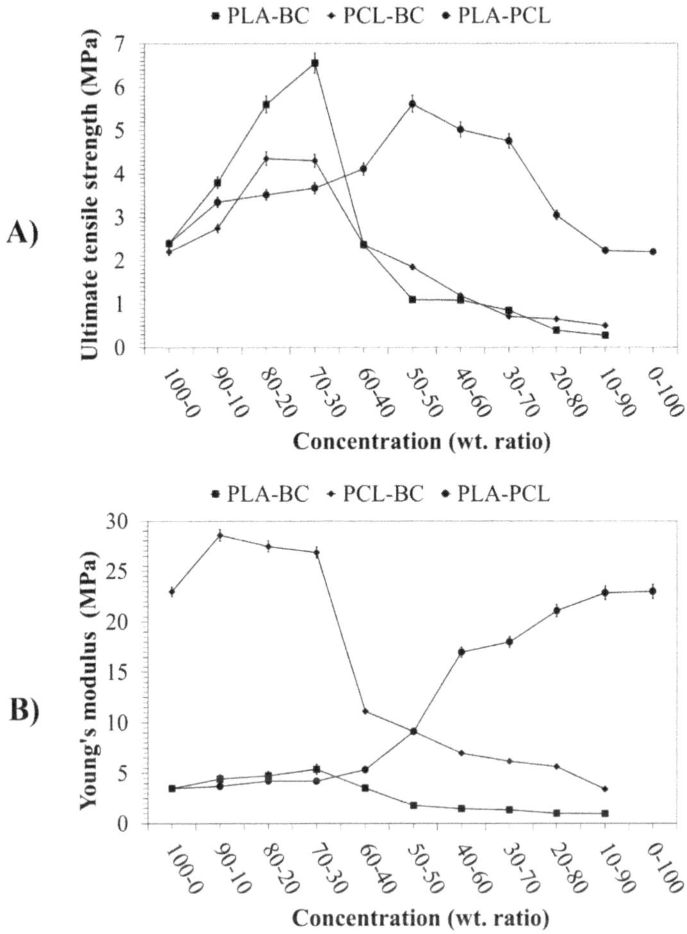

C)

Sample name	Ultimate tensile strength (MPa)	Young's modulus (MPa)
70:30 (PLA-PCL)-BC	9.05 ± 0.04	19.61 ± 0.10

Figure 4.61. Mechanical properties including: (a) the ultimate tensile strength readings of the tested binary systems, (b) the stiffness values (Young's modulus) of the tested binary systems and (c) the ultimate tensile strength and Young's modulus of the optimised ternary sample. Reproduced from [133]. CC BY 4.0.

in the production of fibres with elevated levels of stiffness at bacterial cellulose concentrations of up to 30%. The optimised ternary fibrous sample had a Young's modulus of about 20 MPa, which is less than the maximum achieved using one polymer alone. This shows that by optimising binary and ternary polymeric systems in the production of fibres, more control can be gained over the mechanical and morphological features of fibrous constructs that have use cases in many different biomedical applications.

4.7 The morphologies produced using pressurised gyration

As the PG setup provides a number of operating parameters which can dictate the final morphology of the products, it is important to know how certain morphologies can be achieved and what can be done to achieve the desired structures. This section will detail the studies carried out on different polymeric morphologies produced using PG and the parameters which can be changed to obtain them.

4.7.1 The effect of the solvent on the morphology

In addition to the physical operating parameters offered by PG, as with electrospinning, the technique is first and foremost dependent on the properties of the polymer solution. The selected solvent can have a marked effect on the final fibre morphology and must therefore be carefully chosen to ensure viable fibre production. Solution properties such as viscosity, surface tension, and the molecular weight of the chosen polymer can significantly affect the morphology of the produced fibres. With each individual polymer, solvent mixture, and polymer concentration, a critical minimum polymer chain entanglement exists that results in optimal fibre production; below this critical minimum, beads may form, and above this threshold, other morphologies may arise. The solubility and spinnability of polyethylene (terephthalate) (PET) was investigated using 23 solvents to study the effects of utilising a range of different solvents to solubilise and spin a polymer solution into fibres using PG [14]. The resulting data was mapped onto a Teas graph to identify the regions of solubility and spinnability, which can be seen in figure 4.62.

Polymer solutions which were able to facilitate the generation of continuous fibres with a uniform morphology were considered to have good spinnability; these would also typically have fewer beads and a consistent tubular structure. Solubility plays a major role in producing a polymer solution with adequate polymer chain entanglement. The entangled polymer chains behave similarly to entangled string: given sufficient entanglement, individual string segments will behave as one, forming a longer tubular structure. This is the basis of fibre production and explains why beads are formed when the critical minimum polymer chain entanglement for fibre production is not met [45]. Partially or poorly dissolved polymers seldom produce continuous fibres. When assessing how well a solvent can dissolve a polymer, several parameters can be measured, including the hydrogen bonding, the dispersion forces, and the polar forces. Of the 23 solvents tested, many demonstrated no ability to dissolve PET. The Teas diagram (figure 4.62) can be used to choose a binary solvent system based on the solubility–spinnability region, which allows for a more simplified approach to using solvents with PG.

The inherent properties of the solvent itself, such as its volatility, surface tension, and vapour pressure can greatly affect the morphology of fibres produced from its polymer solution. During the PG spinning process, a polymer jet exits the vessel orifices and is extended by the centrifugal force and the momentum of its exit velocity. This in turn causes a thinning effect on the jet, which results in the production of finer fibres. If a highly volatile solvent is used, this thinning effect can

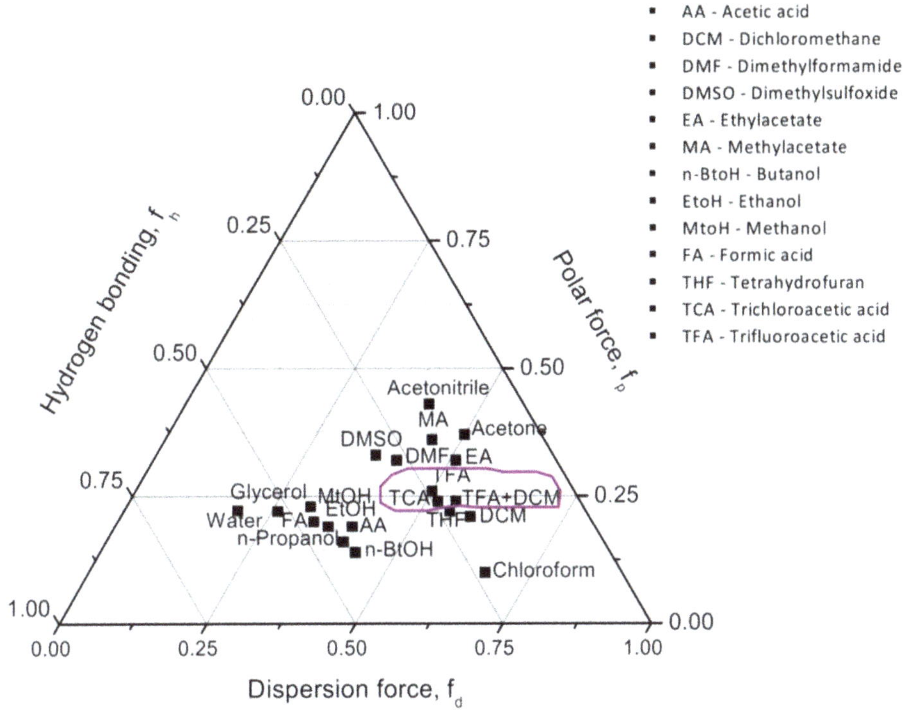

Figure 4.62. A solubility–spinnability map of PET based on the ternary fractional parameter solubility diagram. A 20 wt% PET concentration was used. The conditions used consisted of atmospheric pressure, 20 °C, and a relative humidity of ~ 40%. The map also indicates how the binary solvent systems were selected for nanofibre spinning by PG. Reprinted from [14], Copyright (2015), with permission from Elsevier.

be altered, as rapid evaporation results in reduced jet stretching. The addition of the applied gas pressure in the PG process is also a factor which can greatly influence the final fibre morphology. In order to investigate the effects of using solvents with different physical properties, five solvents were used to dissolve PCL and the impact of increasing the additional gas pressure was analysed [134].

Five solvents, namely dimethylformamide (DMF), tetrahydrofuran (THF), toluene, dichloromethane (DCM), and chloroform were used, as they demonstrated good solubility for PCL at a concentration of 15% (w/v). The Hildebrand solubility parameter (δ) can be used to empirically determine the compatibility of dissolution between a solvent and a polymer using existing values found in the scientific literature; if the difference between the values is small, this indicates good dissolution compatibility [135]. Initially, fibres were formed with the five different solvents with no applied gas pressure to examine the effect of the solvent on the morphology of the polymeric structures produced by PG; the results can be seen in figure 4.63.

Even at the same polymer concentration, we see that the different solvents produce structures that differ greatly in their morphologies. For example, when DMF is used as the solvent, we can see that the structure is highly beaded and has

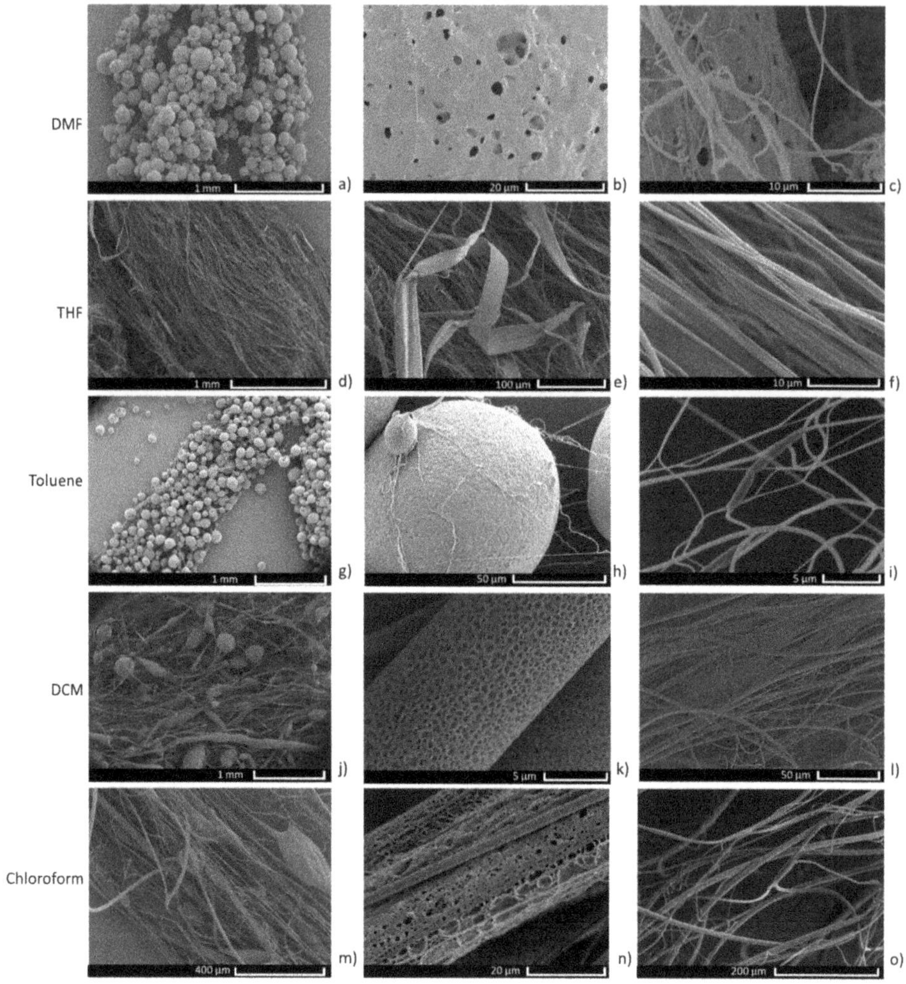

Figure 4.63. SEM images of PCL fibres produced using different solvents: (macroscopic views) (a) DMF, (d) THF, (g) toluene, (j) DCM, (m) chloroform; (surface views) (b) DMF, (e) THF, (h) toluene, (k) DCM, (n) chloroform; (close-up fibre views) (c) DMF, (f) THF, (i) toluene, (l) DCM, (o) chloroform. Reprinted from [134], Copyright (2022), with permission from Elsevier.

very few fibres, resembling more of a collection of particles. We know that a transition between beads and fibres occurs due to polymer chain entanglement, indicating that the solvent itself can impact the chain entanglement and subsequent fibre production. Of all the solvents tested, DMF had the largest difference in its solubility parameter from that of PCL, which could suggest that dissolution was less complete, leading to fewer chain entanglements. However, toluene also produced beads when spun with PG, resulting in more of a bead-on-a-string morphology, even though the difference in the solubility parameters was much smaller for this solvent.

Fibres produced by THF showed a bead-free morphology and a highly unidirectional alignment due to the rotation of the gyration pot. The surface appeared to be relatively smooth with only a few ridges and grooves caused by small irregularities of the gyration pot caused by vibrations. Interestingly, images of THF-based fibres also depicted the inclusion of a flat ribbon-like structure, which is likely caused by a non-axisymmetric change in the polymer jet due irregular motions observed in the gyration pot. THF is significantly more volatile than THF and toluene and thus gave rise to highly beaded structures.

DCM and chloroform are chemically similar and also happen to produce fibres with very similar morphologies when compared side by side. Although DCM is more volatile and has a boiling point of about 40 °C compared to a boiling point of about 62 °C for chloroform, both solvents produce fibres that include some beads. Similarly, both solvents produce fibre strands that have a high density of nanopore formation. As discussed above, the utilisation of a volatile solvent causes rapid evaporation, creating condensation droplets which subsequently dry, leaving behind surface nanopores [21].

The same five solvent systems were also used to spin fibres at different applied pressure values to investigate the impact that this additional driving force has on the final morphology of the products. The resulting images can be seen in figure 4.64.

Polymers dissolved by DMF did not form fibres when the additional pressure applied was more than 0.1 MPa. Without pressure, DMF produced an average fibre diameter of 300 ± 101 nm. For nonvolatile solvents such as DMF, increasing the applied pressure usually leads to a reduction in the fibre diameter due to additional jet thinning; consequently DMF-dissolved PCL resulted in an average fibre diameter of 225 ± 39 nm at 0.1 MPa of additional gas pressure.

The use of THF produced tubular fibres with an average diameter of 515 ± 206 nm without any additional pressure. At 0.1 MPa of additional pressure, this value decreased to 481 ± 248 nm. When a volatile solvent such as THF is used, beyond a certain point, additional pressure does not always yield a smaller fibre diameter. At 0.2 and 0.3 MPa of applied pressure, the average diameters increased to 563 ± 359 and 663 ± 401 nm, respectively. This phenomenon can be explained by the fact that the rapid evaporation rate (exaggerated by increasing pressure levels) of the volatile solvent leads to reduced jet thinning and a scattering influence on the emerging polymer jet, leading to thicker and less uniform fibre production.

Chloroform and DCM had certain similarities. Increasing the additional pressure by 0.1 MPa led to a reduction in the average fibre diameter from 2.17 ± 1.09 μm to 1.01 ± 0.64 μm for DCM and from 6.48 ± 3.30 to 0.75 ± 0.20 μm for chloroform-dissolved PCL. Further increases in the applied gas pressure did not yield additional reductions in the fibre diameters due to the volatile nature of these two solvents. It was also noted that at the higher gas pressure applied to these solvents, the unidirectional alignment suffered due to the instability caused by the applied gas pressure to the drying behaviour of the polymer jet.

Perhaps the most interesting finding was that the application of pressure leads to a reduction in the formation of beads, as evidenced by DMF but more notably by the samples containing toluene. Without pressure, the toluene samples consisted almost

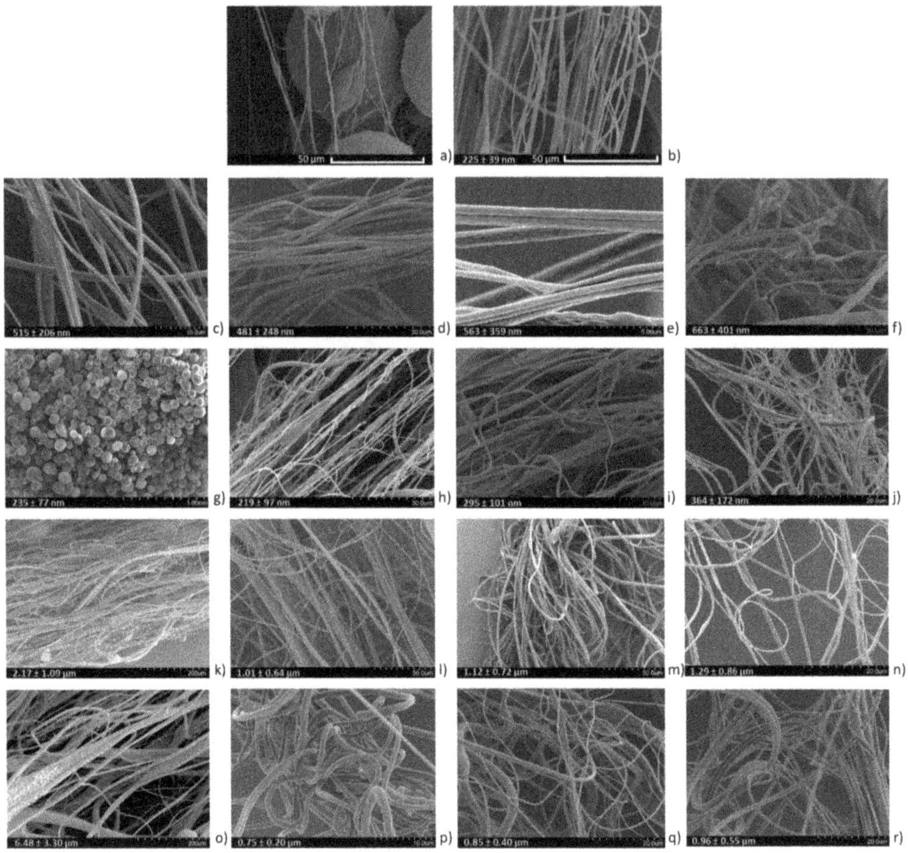

Figure 4.64. SEM images of PCL fibres produced using different solvents; (a), (b) DMF at pressures of 0 and 0.1 MPa, (c)–(f) THF at pressures of 0 to 0.3 MPa, (g)–(j) toluene at pressures of 0 to 0.3 MPa, (k)–(n) DCM at pressures of 0 to 0.3 MPa, and (o)–(r) chloroform at pressures of 0 to 0.3 MPa. In all instances, n = 100. Reprinted from [134], Copyright (2022), with permission from Elsevier.

completely of beads and infrequent fibres were seen between them with an average fibre diameter of about 235 ± 77 nm. Even at just 0.1 MPa of additional pressure, the production converted almost exclusively to fibres, and no observable beads were present at applied gas pressures of 0.2 and 0.3 MPa. It is therefore vital to consider the use of the solvent and solution properties as well as the working conditions used for the production of fibres and other polymeric structures.

4.7.2 Beaded fibres

Although tubular and continuous fibre production is usually preferred, the presence of beads and a bead-on-a-string morphology can often be advantageous. For example, in the context of drug delivery systems, the occurrence of beads can lead to a higher available surface area and a higher encapsulation efficiency for the drug, leading to a more sustained release profile [136]. Using PG, both the solution and operational parameters can be controlled to tailor the morphology of beaded fibres

[137]. Six polymer solutions containing PCL at different concentrations (5–30 wt%) dissolved in acetone were used in a study to assess the effect of concentration on morphology.

The critical minimum polymer concentration is a prerequisite for the successful formation of fibres and is related to the critical minimum polymer chain entanglement. An increase in the physical polymer chain interlocking results in an increase the apparent viscosity of the polymer solution. When the viscosity of the polymer solution is low, the surface tension acts as the main factor that affects fibre morphology, and solutions of higher surface tension give rise to a higher bead density. At 30 wt%, the concentration is too high, and fibres cannot be produced because gelation of the solution occurs. Examples of some of the bead-on-a-string fibres produced using the PCL–acetone polymer system can be seen in figure 4.65.

The study found that average bead width was greatest at the lowest and highest tested concentrations of 5 wt% and 25 wt%, respectively. The smallest beads were formed by the 10 wt% PCL solution. It was also found that increases in applied gas pressure seemed to increase the average bead width but reduce the average interbead width. Increases in rotational speed seemed to have the opposite effect from that of increasing the additional gas pressure, as the average interbead distance became larger at higher speeds. The data obtained showed that the density and distribution of the bead-on-a-string morphology can be controlled by varying the operational and solution parameters. A chart was created using all the combined data to map out the regions in which transitions occur between the production of droplets, beads, and fibres (figure 4.66).

From the chart, we can clearly see that first and foremost, the critical minimum concentration must be met in order to produce any sort of polymeric structure. At lower concentrations (5–15 wt%), bead-on-a-string is the dominant morphology, likely due to various reasons pertaining to polymer chain entanglement and the effect of surface tension at lower viscosities. We can also identify a transition point between 20 wt% and 25 wt% where the bead-on-a-string morphology converts into a morphology that resembles beads with short fibres or 'tails'. This region is unique to every polymer and solvent system, and changes to the molecular weight, temperature, and even the solvent cause shifts in these observed patterns. Above 25 wt% and using acetone as the solvent, PCL forms fibres which show fewer beads. The effect of no pressure, increasing pressure, and increasing rotational speed can also be seen on the map. This work demonstrates that a variety of beaded and fibrous structures can be formed using PG and by altering the solution properties. Changes in the working parameters substantially alter the geometry and morphology of the produced structures.

4.7.3 The surface features of PG fibres

In many biomedical applications, especially in scenarios that involve cellular interactions, the implant surface becomes an important factor in the bioactivity of a scaffold, as cells can drastically change their behaviour based on the topography

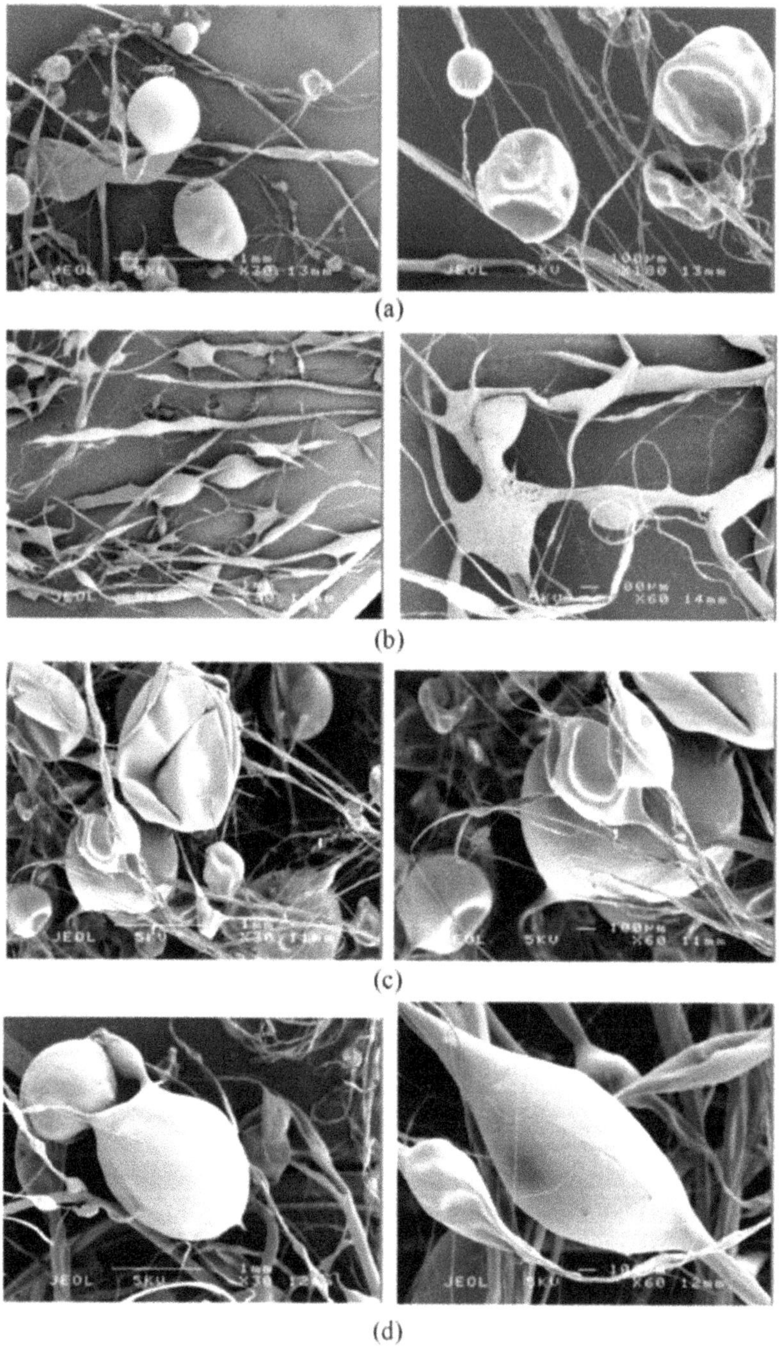

Figure 4.65. SEM images of products showing beaded-morphology fibres: (a) 10 wt% solution at an applied pressure of 0.1 MPa; (b) 15 wt% solution at an applied pressure of 0.1 MPa; (c) 15 wt% solution at an applied pressure of 0.2 MPa, and (d) 15 wt% solution at an applied pressure of 0.1 MPa. Reprinted from [137], Copyright (2016), with permission from Elsevier.

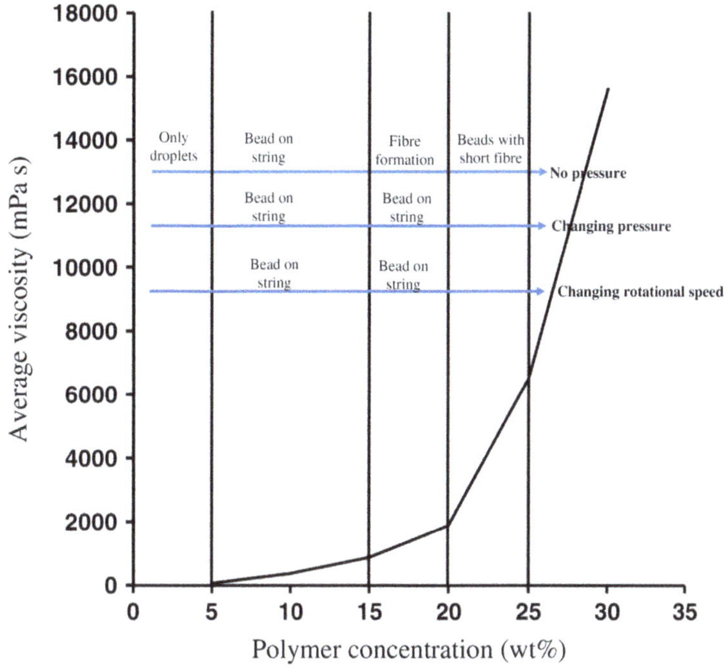

Figure 4.66. A chart that maps the product and condition zones of the gyratory formation of PCL solutions dissolved in acetone. Reprinted from [137], Copyright (2016), with permission from Elsevier.

and roughness of materials they come into contact with [138]. Using the operating and solution parameters available, the surface of polymeric fibres can be functionalised to meet a desired level of activity. Many topological features exist that can be seen on the surfaces of fibres at high magnification, such as pores, grooves, ridges, and dimples. Such surface features can often increase the available surface area and provide a suitable niche for cellular attachment and migration [139]. Research studies have tailored the surfaces of the fibres produced by PG by altering the solution and working parameters; one example is the production of PAN and PMMA fibres using DMF as a solvent [140]. By changing the polymer solution properties and the working parameters, it is possible to obtain different surface features, illustrations of which can be seen in figure 4.67.

We can see the presence of ridges in figure 4.67(a) resulting from the use of 8 wt% PAN in DMF. DMF has a high boiling point, and its slow evaporation could be the reason for the observed topography. Ridges can be useful in applications such as bone tissue engineering, in which this topography can mimic the native cellular environment [141].

Changing the polymer whilst keeping the solvent constant can also lead to the differences observed in the fibre topography. For example, in figure 4.67(b), we can see that the fibre surface is covered in grooves and indentations as a result of spinning 30 wt% PMMA in DMF. The formation of these grooves can be attributed to the mode of solvent evaporation; even whilst using a solvent with low volatility

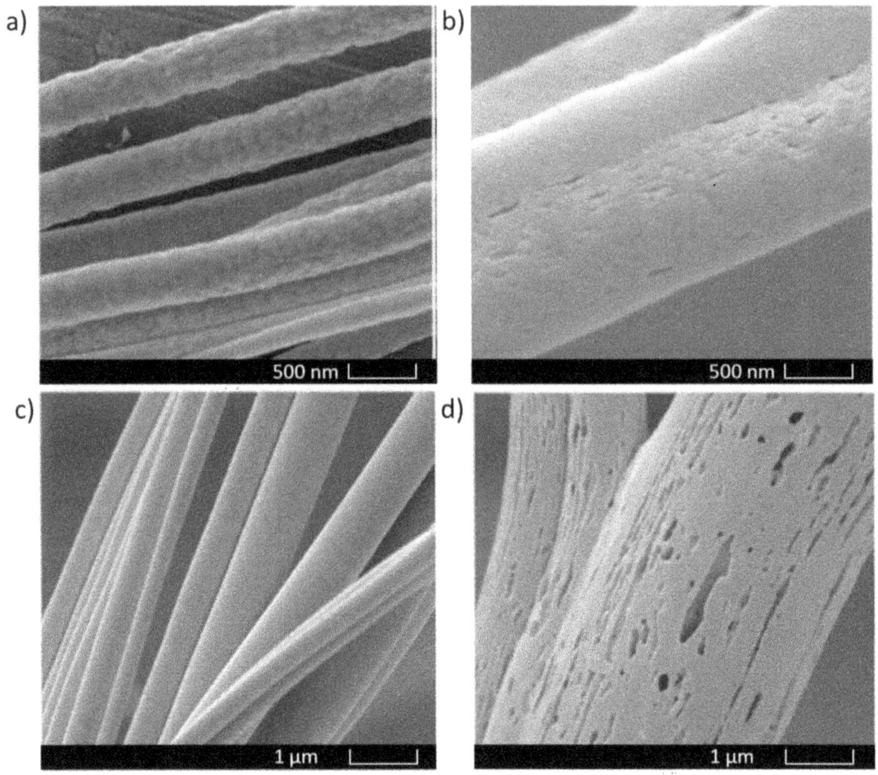

Figure 4.67. SEM micrographs showing the surface features of fibres produced via PG: (a) fibres with ridges, (b) fibres with surface indentations, (c) fibres with deep grooves, and (d) smooth surface fibres. Reprinted from [140], Copyright (2016), with permission from ICE Publishing.

such as DMF, an increase in the added gas pressure can lead to more rapid solvent evaporation. Grooves can also be particularly beneficial for cellular attachment and can provide fibres with a higher surface-area-to-volume ratio.

The application of additional gas pressure can have a marked effect on the topography of certain fibres. In figure 4.67(c), we can see that the fibre has a very smooth surface devoid of features. This can often be achieved by utilising a balance between the applied gas pressure, the rotational speed, and the polymer solution. This balance is unique for each system, while altering the polymer solution properties would require a change in the operating parameters. Smooth fibres can often be beneficial in drug delivery applications in which there needs to be a high degree of control over the dosage.

Surface features can also be created or exaggerated through the use of post-processing techniques on the fibres. The fibre morphology and surface topography can be altered by creating a polymer blend of two different polymers. Figure 4.67(d) shows the surface features of fibres produced using a mixture of PAN and PMMA in DMF. It appears that the fibres formed a topography with deep indentations which resembles valleys and troughs that penetrate the fibre itself. These surface features can lead to an increase in the available surface-area-to-volume ratio whilst also providing attachment sites for cellular activity. These surface indentations were created using a blend of both PAN and PMMA followed by heat-treatment postprocessing. At temperatures between 225 °C and 300 °C and between 300 °C and 475 °C, two distinct weight-loss phases can be observed. The first is due to the cyclisation of the nitrile group in PAN and the second is due to the decomposition of PMMA. When the PMMA portion decomposes, volatile degradation products are released which allow the residual solvent at the surface to penetrate the PAN shell; the solvent subsequently evaporates at the surface of the PAN fibres, leaving behind indentations.

Polymeric fibres with a range of topographies such as smooth, rough, and porous surfaces can be obtained via PG for use in a range of biomedical applications. Studies of these procedures have shown that the applied pressure that PG is able to facilitate plays a significant role in determining both the morphology and the surface features of the produced polymeric fibres.

The choice of solvent furthermore plays a crucial role in determining the surface features of the spun polymer solution, even when the same polymer is used. A study of the spinning of fibres using PG examined the effects of dissolving PMMA in five different solvents (acetone, chloroform, DMF, ethyl acetate, and DCM) [21]. Strong polymer–solvent interactions occur when a polymer is highly soluble in the selected solvent because this ensures that the polymer chains swell and expand during dissolution to maximise the intermolecular interactions between the chains. Although solubility parameters can often be a good indicator of how well the polymer solution may spin, there are other physical parameters to consider, such as the viscosity of the solvent, surface tension, boiling point, and vapour pressure, as mentioned previously. Figure 4.68 shows high-magnification images of the fibre surfaces producing using the different solvents.

From a close look at the surface of the fibres, we can see that the use of different solvents leads to the production of different topographies. Acetone and DMF produced fibres with a smooth surface devoid of porosity. Although acetone has a similar boiling point to those of DCM, chloroform, and ethyl acetate, unlike them, it does not produce surface nanopores. This observation confirms that solvent volatility alone is not responsible for the formation of a porous topography. When we compare the polymer solvent interactions of PMMA acetone and PMMA–chloroform, there is no significant difference in the solubility parameters. This shows that there are other unobserved factors which cause solvents to behave differently when used in polymer solutions. DCM, ethyl acetate, and chloroform all produce fibres with surfaces that contain nanopores. The shape of the pores does seem to change according to the solvent used; for example, DCM produces pores which seem to penetrate deeper into the fibre strand, while ethyl acetate and chloroform seem to produce shallower pores. Undoubtedly, small changes in the microclimate, such as changes in humidity and wind speed (even within controlled environments), lead to differences in pore morphology.

It is apparent that each solvent behaves differently with respect to PMMA, depending on its interactions and solubility parameters. During dissolution, the swelling of the polymer chains and subsequent chain engagement can often be

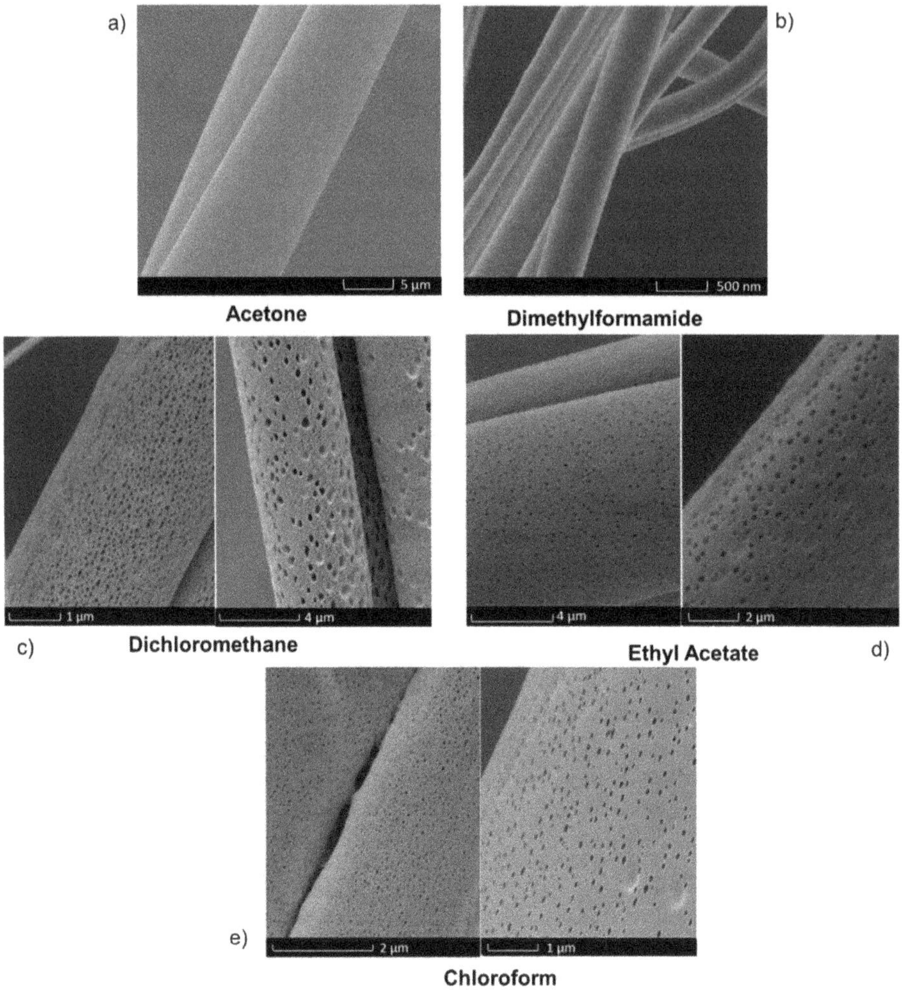

Figure 4.68. SEM images showing the surface topographies of PMMA fibres made from solutions dissolved in: (a) acetone, (b) DMF, (c) DCM, (d) ethyl acetate and (e) chloroform. Reproduced from [21]. CC BY 4.0.

predicted, and there are significant differences between the polymer–solvent interactions. This study showed that the topography of PG-spun fibres can be altered by careful selection of the solvent used to create the polymer solution. Surface porosity can be beneficial in applications in which a higher surface area is required, or, in some cases, it can increase bioactivity.

4.7.4 Microbubbles for diagnostics

Although the focus of PG has been the generation of fibres, it is capable of producing other polymeric structures as well. Due to the utilisation of an applied gas pressure, PG has been found to be able to produce polymeric bubbles with a gas core. As discussed earlier, microbubbles have many interesting applications in biomedical engineering, such as medical imaging and drug delivery. Lysozyme microbubbles with a nitrogen core has been successfully produced by PG and loaded with gold nanoparticles to improve their stability [142]. Compared to other microbubble manufacturing techniques, PG benefits from a rapid production rate due to its use of a high-speed motor.

Bubble formation ensues when the destabilising centrifugal force provided by the gyration vessel overcomes the stabilising surface tension of the protein solution. The protein solution rotates about its vertical symmetry axis whilst an applied gas pressure is blown into the gyration vessel; external forces then create a vortex that leads to free surface deformation. As the rotational speed increases, the nitrogen-filled core penetrates deeper and passes through several states: a stable state, an unstable bubbling state, and then the formation of microbubbles resulting from the rapid fluid flow from the tip of the vortex. The bubbling mechanism of PG is summarised in figure 4.69.

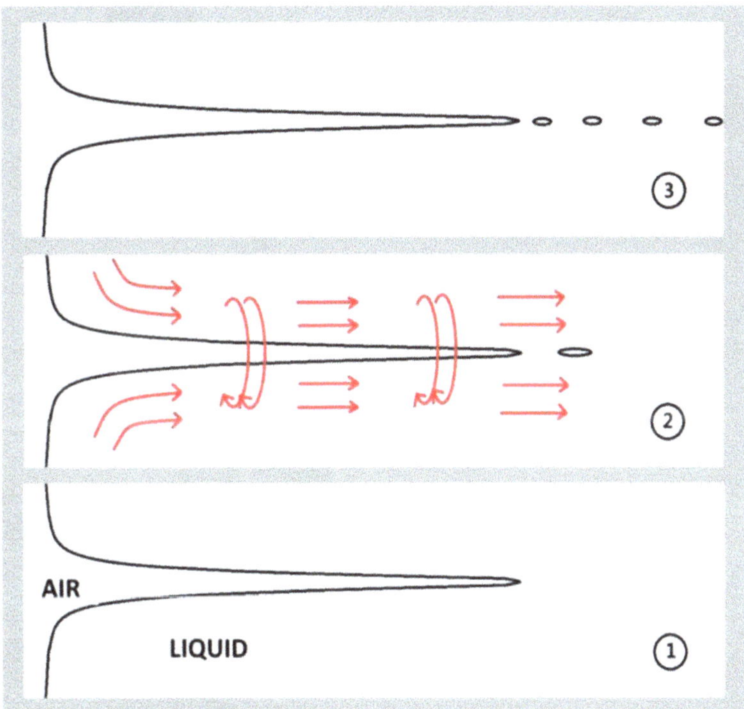

Figure 4.69. A schematic diagram illustrating the physical mechanism of microbubble formation by PG. In this graphic, (1), air-filled core penetration, (2) is the unstable bubbling state and (3) is the periodic formation of microbubbles. Reproduced from [142]. CC BY 4.0.

The morphology of the microbubbles produced by PG can be controlled by its available working parameters, for example, by increasing the rotational speed and applied gas pressure. Higher rotational speeds lead to an increase in the rate at which bubbles are 'cut off' as they leave the gyration orifices via a 'pinch off' process. The pinch off process can be described as follows: when the polymer escapes the orifice as a slug, gas pressure penetrates the inside of the slug and the emerging polymer, including a gas core, is pinched off into a microbubble [143]. At higher rotational speeds, it is expected that the microbubble size will decrease, due to a more rapid breakup of the same volume of solution. The same effect can also be observed due to an increase in the applied gas pressure; higher pressure causes a more rapid pinch off process, leading to smaller microbubbles. In this study, PVA–lysozyme and various ratios of gold nanoparticles were subjected to PG, and the average bubble diameters of the resulting microbubbles were assessed; the findings are illustrated in figure 4.70.

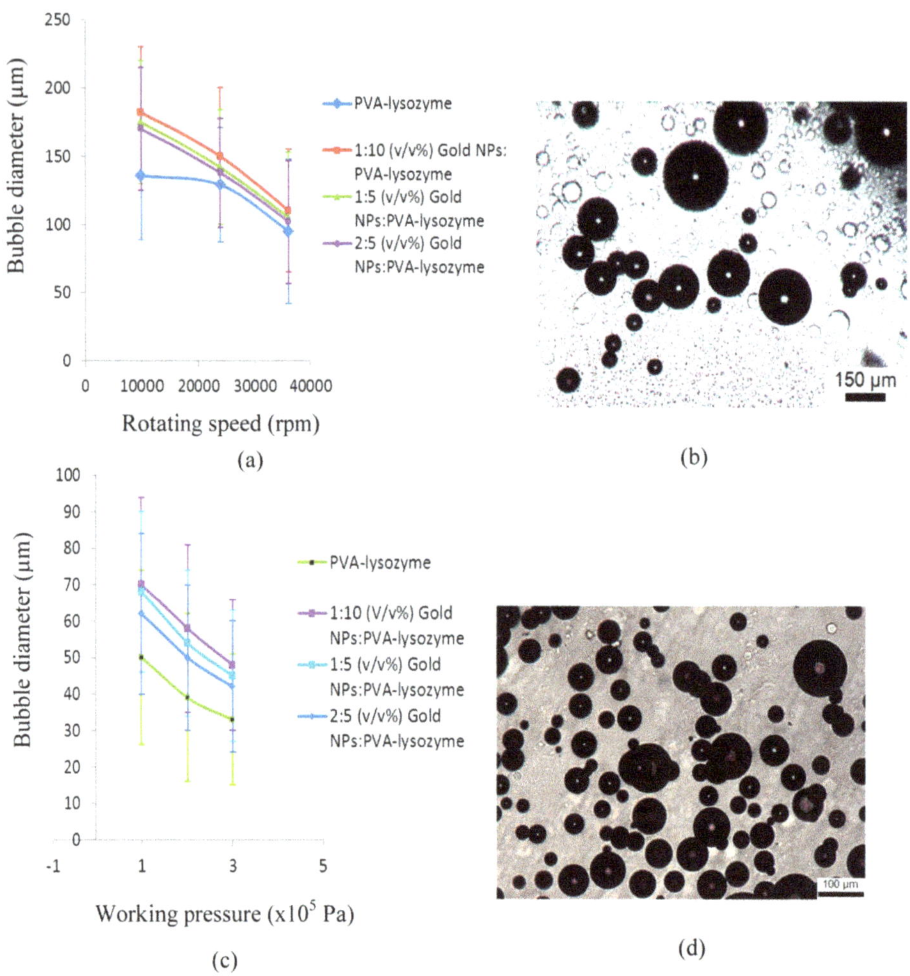

Figure 4.70. (a) A graph showing the effect of the rotational speed on the bubble diameter at a constant working pressure of 0.02 MPa. (b) An optical micrograph of microbubbles generated at 10 000 rpm and 0.02 MPa. (c) A graph showing the effect of the working pressure on bubble diameter at a rotational speed of 36 000 rpm. (d) An optical micrograph of microbubbles processed at 36 000 rpm and 0.1 MPa. NP denotes nanoparticle. Reproduced from [142]. CC BY 4.0.

It is evident from the experimental data that increasing the rotational speed reduces the average diameter of the bubbles. The addition of gold nanoparticles slightly reduces the average fibre diameter compared to the use of PVA and lysozyme only; however, this could be accompanied by the additional benefit of improved microbubble stability. We also see that the applied gas pressure has a strong effect on the size of the produced microbubbles: higher working pressures lead to a reduction in the observed bubble diameter.

Following initial work carried out on microbubbles with PG, the technology has since been used to produce PVA–lysozyme microbubbles with antibacterial and biosensing abilities [144]. In this study, bubbles of up to 250 μm were produced with and without gold nanoparticle loading. The mean microbubble diameter was reduced when the rotational speed and applied gas pressure were increased. Figure 4.71 shows an overview of the produced microbubbles, including a stability analysis performed over a period of 4 h.

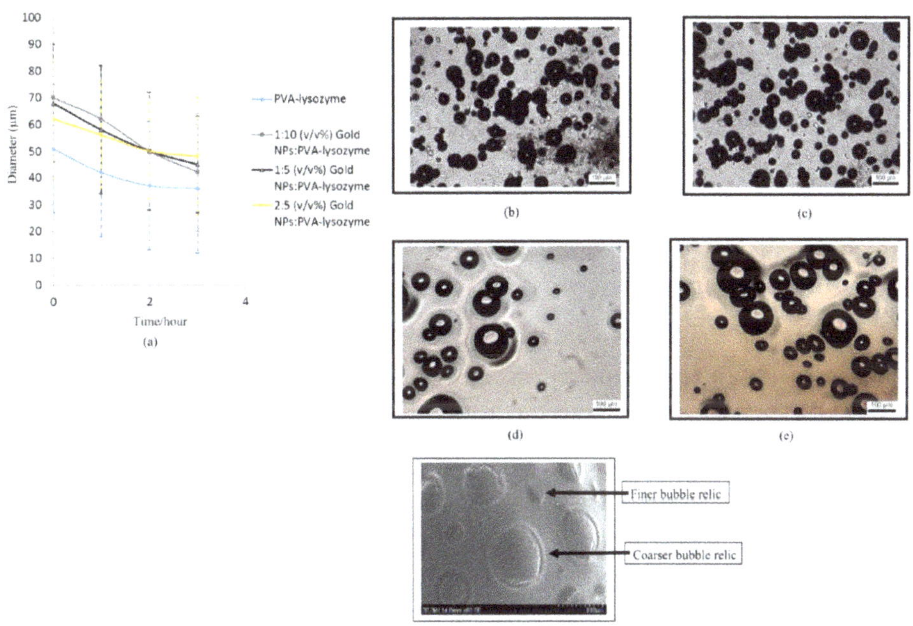

Figure 4.71. (a) A stability analysis of PVA–lysozyme microbubbles. (b)–(e) Optical micrographs of the PVA–lysozyme microbubbles at different times (hours): (b) 0, (c) 1, (d) 2, and (e) 3. (f) Field emission SEM images of PVA–lysozyme microbubble relics. Reproduced from [144]. CC BY 4.0.

The microbubble stability increased when gold nanoparticles were loaded with the protein–polymer solution. The antibacterial activity of the microbubbles was assessed using the Gram-negative bacterium *E. coli*, which showed that the bactericidal effect increased in the samples containing gold nanoparticles compared to that of bare protein. For microbubbles that contained gold nanoparticles, the average antibacterial activity was calculated to be about 73%, while bare protein microbubbles showed an antibacterial activity of 59%. As the lysozyme microbubbles were positively charged, the proposed mechanism of antibacterial action resulted from the interaction between the microbubbles and the negatively charged bacterial cell wall, which caused high stress and subsequent cell lysis [145].

In order to assess the biosensing capabilities of these produced microbubbles, they were assessed by the conjugation of malemide-functionalised alkaline phosphatase to the surface of the microbubbles and the subsequent detection of paraoxon analyte. Paraoxon acts an inhibitor of cholinesterase, an essential enzyme which is part of normal nervous system functions [146]. The produced microbubbles were successfully able to detect paraoxon in conditions with concentrations as low as 0.5 ppm (parts per million). These results demonstrate that highly sensitive biosensing components can be made by using PG to produce microbubbles. PG provides additional working parameters which could offer greater control in producing microbubbles for a wide range of biomedical applications.

4.8 Variants of pressurised gyration

Although many studies have produced biomaterials using the conventional laboratory setup for PG, other versions exist due its simple design. In this section, we discuss the iterations of PG which have been developed to provide extra control over the morphology of the fibres produced by this technology.

4.8.1 Infusion gyration

Following the success of the conventional PG laboratory setup, other approaches were quickly developed which utilised the PG setup but introduced additional control over the final fibre morphology. One of the earliest of these was called 'infusion gyration'; it made use of the basic centrifugal spinning setup but integrated polymer feed infusion into the device [147]. Infusion gyration provides a variable polymer flowrate into the gyration vessel where centrifugal spinning takes place; the polymer flowrate therefore plays a key role in tailoring the fibre geometry and morphology. A diagrammatic overview of the infusion gyration apparatus can be seen in figure 4.72.

In order to test the infusion gyration technology, polyethylene oxide fibres were loaded with genetically engineered proteins (DsRed-AuBP2-engineered protein) and gold nanoparticles. Nanofibres with diameters as low 117 nm were produced using this technique, which allowed the polymer flowrate to be adjusted in a range from 600 $\mu l\ min^{-1}$ to 5000 $\mu l\ min^{-1}$. The fineness of these fibres was comparable to the quality of those obtained using electrospinning but they offered the benefits of improved scalability and an increased production rate. The produced fibres can be seen in figure 4.73.

Analyses of fibres produced using infusion gyration show a general pattern. If the flowrate into the gyration pot can be reduced, this can have a diameter-reducing effect on the produced fibres. As the polymer mass flow is an important consideration during the spinning process, manipulation of this flow can provide additional

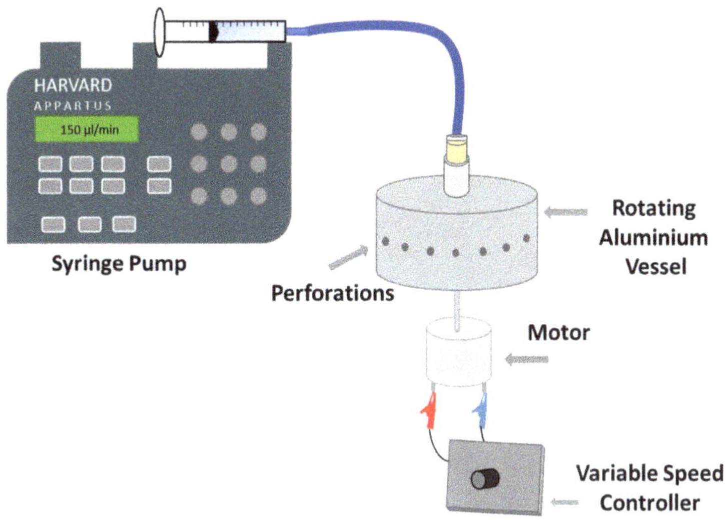

Figure 4.72. A diagram showing the components of the infusion gyration setup.

control over the final morphology. Within the PG vessel, if the volume of the polymer is too high, the result is that the internal gas has a smaller volume in which to manipulate the solution, requiring greater external forces to produce the polymer jet. At a lower polymer flowrate, the air within the vessel can be fully replaced, further increasing the effect of centrifugal force on the polymer, which in turn produces finer fibres. However, at higher flowrates, even though the fibres were minimally thicker, they did show a greater yield due to the increase in polymer mass flow. Therefore, a compromise is always required between the production speed and the fibre morphology. A gold-binding peptide tag which is genetically conjugated to red fluorescent protein was used to confirm the integration of the gold nanoparticles with the genetically engineered protein in the nanofibre complex. These results can be seen in the fluorescent micrographs shown in figure 4.73.

Infusion gyration and the work it has carried out have shown how this technology can be used to produce functional nanofibres that can integrate important biological materials such as genetically engineered proteins and gold nanoparticles. Because this technology and its other derivatives offer additional control over fibre production, they increase our ability to produce the required morphology for each intended application.

Although infusion gyration introduced a new element into the gyration setup, it lacked the ability to provide an applied gas pressure, something which differentiated PG from ordinary centrifugal spinning. To rectify this, pressure-coupled infusion gyration (PCIG) was later created; this combined both PG and infusion gyration [148]. The PCIG setup consists of the standard gyration vessel and high-speed motor, but also includes a nitrogen gas supply (up to 0.3 MPa) and a polymer infuser capable of a flowrate of up to 5000 µl min^{-1} based on a T-junction. Therefore, the PCIG setup is able to offer three major operational parameters that can be used in

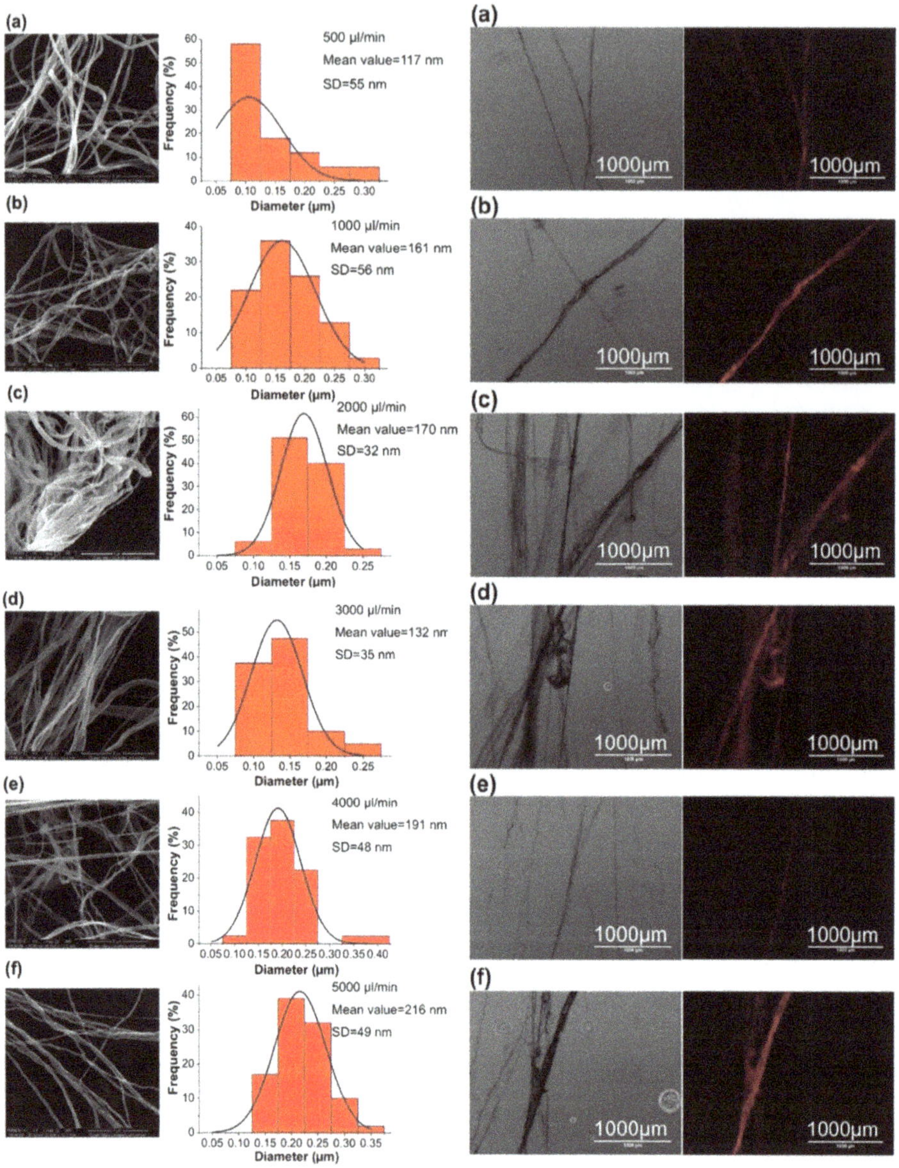

Figure 4.73. SEM images, diameter distributions, and fluorescence micrographs of protein-integrated fibres produced at flowrates of (a) 500 μl min^{-1}, (b) 1000 μl min^{-1}, (c) 2000 μl min^{-1}, (d) 3000 μl 1^{-1}, (e) 4000 μl min^{-1}, and (f) 5000 μl min^{-1} at a fixed maximum rotational speed [147] John Wiley & Sons. [2015].

the generation of fibres, namely the rotational speed, the applied gas pressure, and the polymer flowrate. The setup is illustrated in figure 4.74.

To test the effect of the operational parameters on fibre production, PCIG was used to generate PEO fibres using a range of different concentrations from 3 wt% to 21 wt% dissolved in water. In the standard PG process, the centrifugal force and

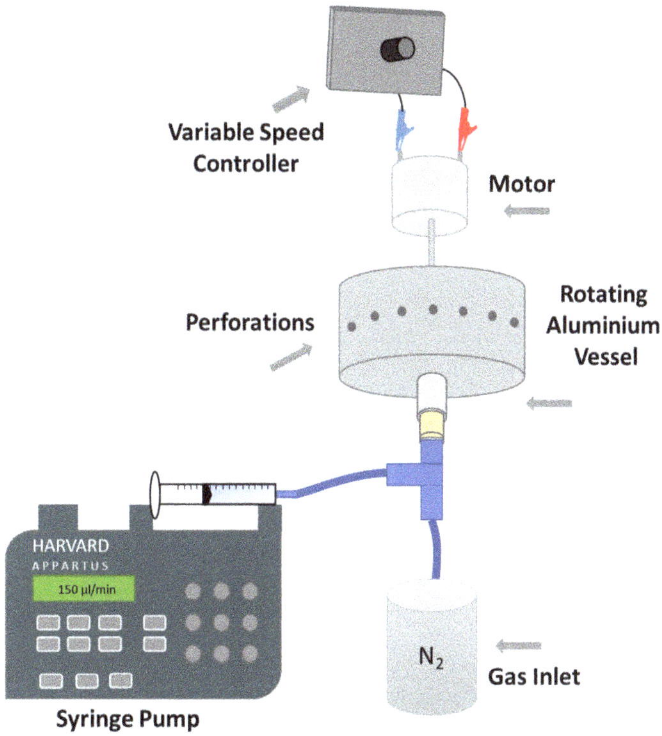

Figure 4.74. Diagram illustrating PCIG equipment.

applied gas pressure create the driving force for polymer jet formation. The addition of polymer infusion provides a further driving force in the form of hydrostatic pressure applied to the rotating chamber. An overview of PEO fibres produced using this technology can be seen in figure 4.75.

Whenever additional operating parameters are available, there is always an optimal balance between them that produces the optimal product morphology. As we have seen above, an increase in the polymer flowrate generally leads to the production of thicker fibres, but an increase in the applied gas pressure and rotational speed may help to offset that. Out of all the tested solutions, 10 wt% PEO was deemed the most optimal in achieving the thinnest fibres. Fibres produced from PCIG show highly unidirectional alignment due to the combination of both the unidirectional rotation of the motor and the applied gas pressure.

Utilising a high working pressure and rotational speed in conjunction with polymer infusion, fibres with an average diameter of less than 100 nm were achieved. PEO at 10 wt%, at the maximum rotation speed and applied pressure, and at a polymer infusion rate of 3000 µl min^{-1} formed fibres that had diameters as low as 92 nm. The fineness of these fibres rivalled even that of electrospinning, but PCIG was able to produce them at a much more rapid rate. Mathematical modelling has also been used with experimental data to develop and optimise a framework for the selection of optimal conditions that can be used to tailor the desired morphology of

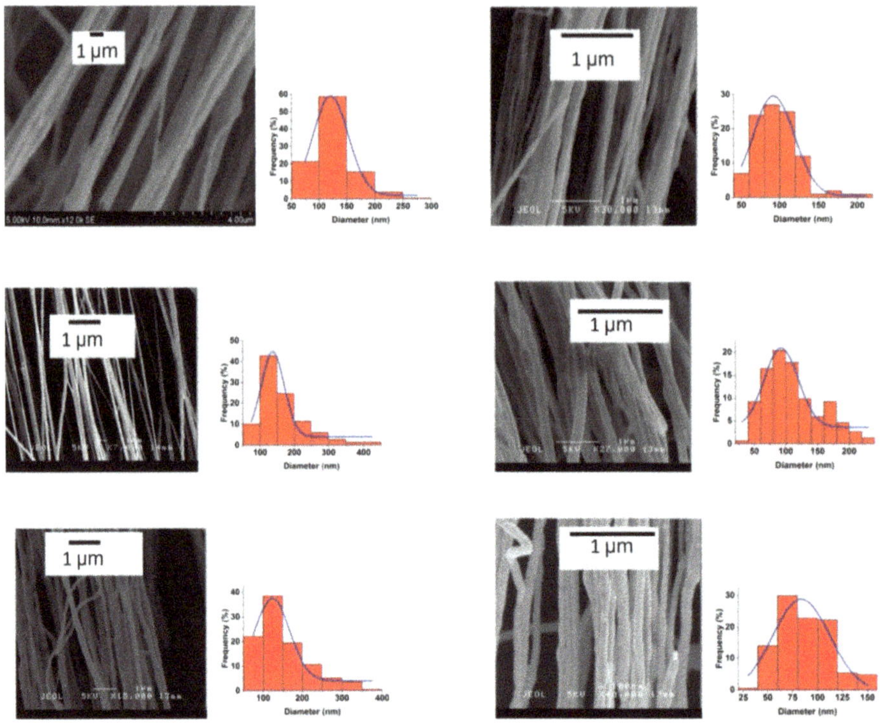

Figure 4.75. SEM images and diameter distributions of 10 wt% PEO fibres produced by PCIG at: (a–c) 1×10^5 and (d–f) 3×10^5 Pa for flowrates of 1000, 2000, and 3000 μl min^{-1}, at 36 000 rpm [148] John Wiley & Sons. [2017].

PEO fibres [149]. Figure 4.76 shows the output of these empirical models, which demonstrates the effect of the operational parameters on the morphology of the fibres produced using PCIG.

The data further supports the notion that additional operating parameters offer greater control over the final fibre morphology and that there are multiple regions that can be found when adjusting these, requiring the need for advanced modelling and experimental work. The PCIG setup therefore offers simple, low cost, and continuous production of fine fibres that may be suitable for a range of biomedical applications.

4.8.2 Melt-pressurised gyration

Typically, in PG, a polymer solution is used which consists of a polymer dissolved within a solvent. Many hydrophobic polymers require the use of harsh solvents which can pose a risk to health and the environment. Melt-PG is a method by which the standard PG setup can be utilised to produce fibres without the need for any solvents. Because of the versatility and ease of setup afforded by PG, the melt-PG equipment consists of the standard setup but with the application of a direct heat source which is able to form a melt within the vessel prior to spinning. The melt-PG equipment is diagrammatically shown in figure 4.77.

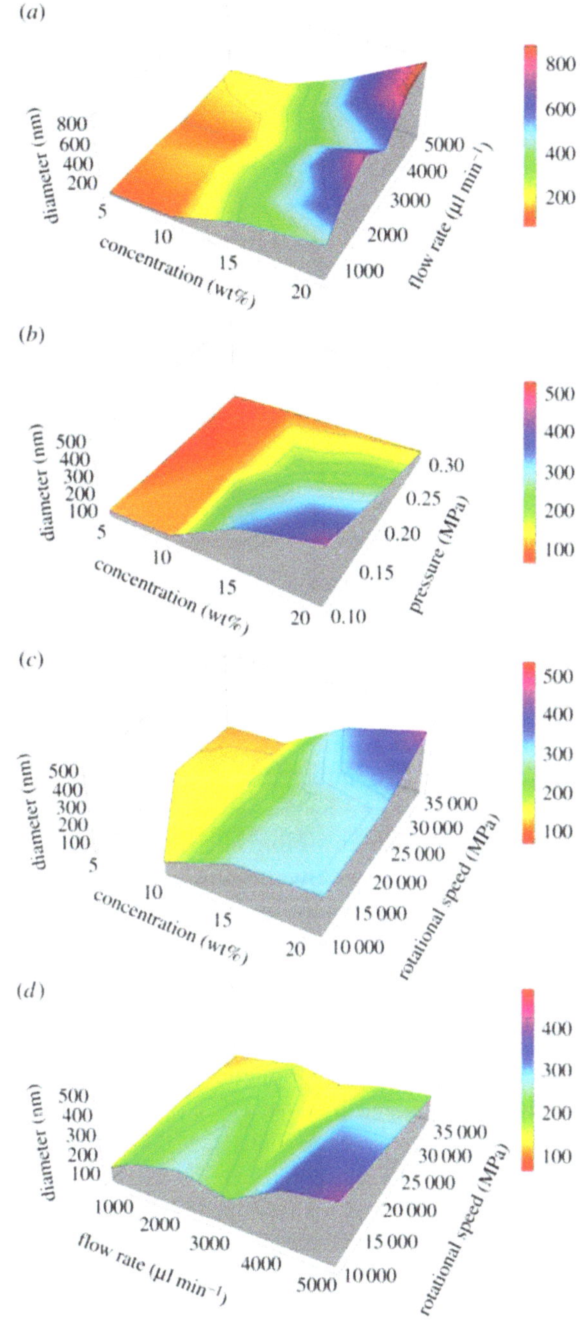

Figure 4.76. Response surface plots showing the effect on fibre diameter as a function of: (a) flowrate and concentration, (b) concentration and pressure, (c) concentration and rotational speed and (d) flowrate and rotational speed. All plots relate to the use of PCIG. Reproduced from [149], Copyright (2019) with permission from The Royal Society.

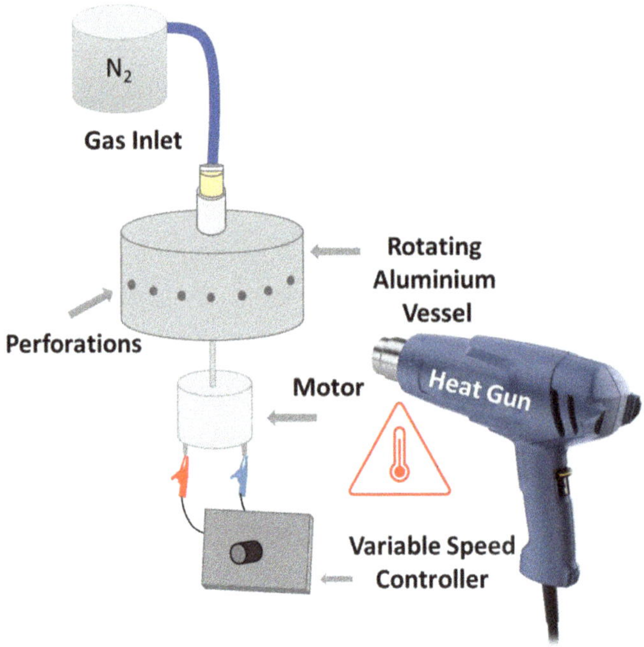

Figure 4.77. Diagram of the experimental setup used for the melt-PG process.

The first study of melt-PG was conducted to determine the effects of temperature on the morphology of fibres produced by the technique [150]. PCL is commonly used as a biodegradable polymer for many biomedical applications and was a strong candidate for this technique due to its low melting point. PCL fibres were produced for tissue engineering applications; therefore, they were doped with silver nanoparticles to elicit antibacterial activity that was later assessed.

The PCL polymer pellets were placed within the gyration vessel, where a temperature of up to 600 °C could be applied via a heat gun. The temperature was recorded via a thermocouple. Fibres were then produced using different operating parameters by adjusting the applied gas pressure and the applied heat. An overview of the fibres produced by melt-PG can be seen in figure 4.78. As the melt temperature increased, the average diameter of the resulting fibres tended to decrease. This reduction in fibre diameter can be attributed to the reduction in viscosity observed at higher temperatures, which reduces the force opposing centrifugal force and the applied gas pressure. The thinnest fibres were achieved at a sample temperature of 200 °C (the maximum tested), the maximum rotational speed, and an applied gas pressure of 0.2 MPa (the maximum tested). The thinnest fibres had an average fibre diameter of 14 ± 8 μm, which is still considerably larger than those of PCL fibres produced using a solvent. Compared to fibres produced using a solvent, however, the fibre surface demonstrated an ultrasmooth topography that was suitable for applications in which surface features are unwanted.

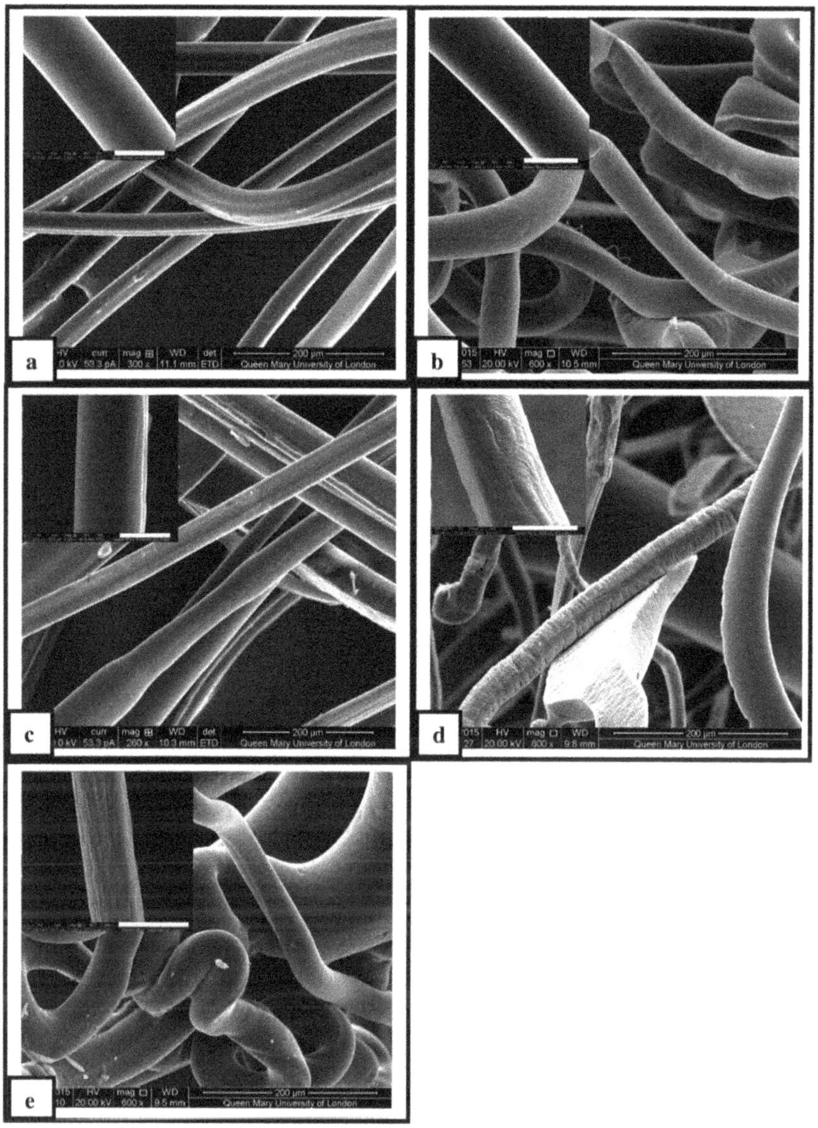

Figure 4.78. SEM images of PCL fibres obtained at 36 000 rpm and at a working pressure of 0.01 MP at the following temperatures: (a) 95 °C, (b) 105 °C, (c) 125 °C, (d) 155 °C, and (e) 200 °C. The scale bars in the inset images are 20 μm [150] John Wiley & Sons. [2016].

Silver-loaded PCL fibres were also produced using melt-PG and tested for their antimicrobial activity against Gram-negative *E. coli* and Gram-positive *P. aeruginosa.* All the tested fibres containing silver showed an antibacterial response rate of about 100% against *E. coli*, depicting a very potent bactericidal ability. At higher temperatures, the surfaces of the fibres attracted small defects that affected their smoothness. It was observed that at higher temperatures, the antibacterial effect against *P. aeruginosa* reduced, suggesting that surface topography may have an impact on the antibacterial properties of the fibres.

4.8.3 Core–sheath pressurised gyration

Although the production of nonwoven tubular fibres has proved to have excellent utility in many healthcare applications, there has been a recent uptick in the exploration of fibres consisting of more than a single component. Core–sheath fibres contain two distinct phases, namely a core structure, which in enclosed within the interior of the fibre strand and a sheath which surrounds the core and offers many benefits [151]. Electrospinning with a concentric needle setup can be used to produce such fibres, but the addition of further needles creates problems such as needle clogging and charge interference. PG has been explored as a possible means with which to produce core–sheath fibres which benefit from a high production rate and scalability. About six years after the introduction of PG, a setup capable of producing core–sheath fibres was demonstrated in 2019 [152].

The introductory PG device was constructed out of aluminium and housed two concentric reservoirs. The inner reservoir contained two nozzles on its exterior walls that had diameters of 80 mm; this inner reservoir was encased by a second reservoir which also had two outer nozzles with diameters of 100 mm. The larger nozzle was encased within the smaller nozzle so that the polymer containing the core could be inserted into the smaller reservoir whilst the sheath polymer was placed in the larger reservoir. The design features of the original core–sheath PG setup can be seen in figure 4.79. The core–sheath PG technique is also capable of operating at an applied gas pressure of up to 0.3 MPa and a rotational speed of up to 6000 rpm.

The first instance of core–sheath PG utilised PEO as the core polymer and PMMA as the sheath material to produce core–sheath fibres. Through the use of different dyes in the two components, fluorescent microscopy was used to highlight differences in shade between the sheath and core to confirm the presence of distinct core and sheath layers. In addition, focused ion beam techniques were used to dissect a section of the fibre in order to analyse its cross section using SEM. Images showing visualisations of the compartments can be seen in figure 4.80.

In another study, to demonstrate the capability of the core–sheath device, PEO and PVP fibres were used together to form core–sheath fibres using different operating parameters [153]. The effect of increasing rotational speeds on the fibre morphology can be seen in figure 4.81. We can see from the images that these fibres have good unidirectional alignment and a smooth topography. As typically seen, an increase in the rotational speed yields thinner fibres. At the highest tested speed of 6000 rpm in centrifugal spinning mode (no additional pressure), the core–sheath fibres had an average diameter of 625 nm, which was reduced to only 430 nm at an applied gas pressure of 0.1 MPa. The ability to combine both centrifugal spinning and solution blowing in this setup leads to superior control over the core–sheath morphology.

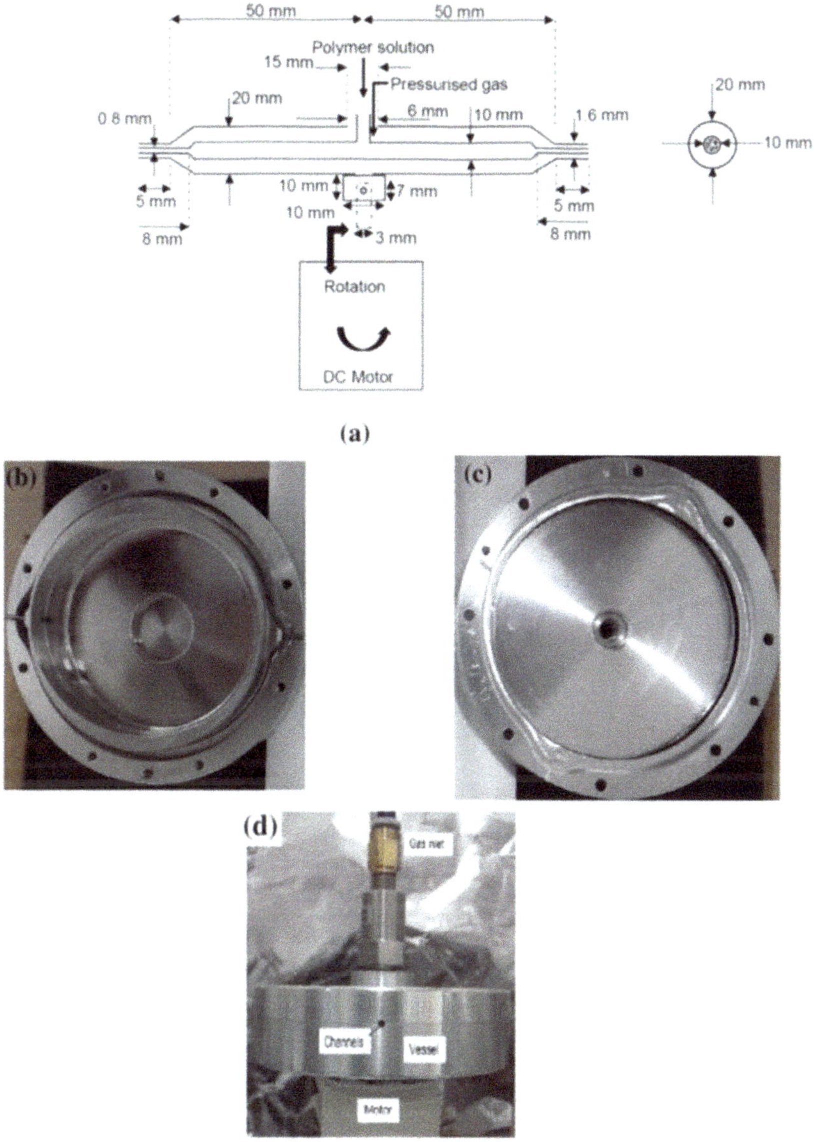

Figure 4.79. (a) Design features of the core–sheath PG device. Interior views: photographs of (b) the inner reservoir photograph, (c) the outer reservoir photograph, and (d) the experimental setup. Reprinted from [152], Copyright (2019), with permission from Elsevier.

The PEO-PVP fibres were also imaged using focused ion beam milling in order to visualise their cross sections. The resulting images can be seen in figure 4.82. It is clear from these micrographs that the core and sheath components within these fibres are separate. Within the interior of the core–sheath PG vessel, the two polymer solutions are separated by the concentric walls of the reservoirs and do not have the

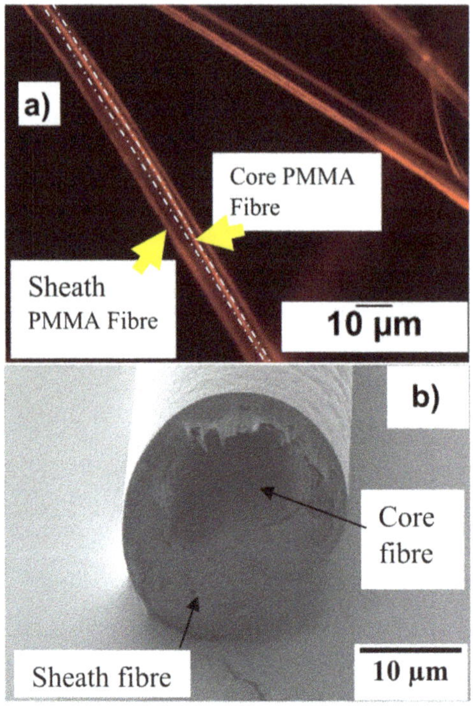

Figure 4.80. (a) Fluorescence micrograph showing the formation of a core–sheath fibre in a PMMA core–PEO sheath system. (b) Cross-sectional SEM image of a PMMA core–PEO sheath fibre depicting the distinct core compartment and sheath material. Reprinted from [152], Copyright (2019), with permission from Elsevier.

opportunity to mix; instead, as they leave the nozzles as a high-speed jet, the core is encased by the sheath material. It is possible that the polymer solution placed in the outer (sheath) reservoir experiences greater centrifugal force, as it has a larger radius, making this the first polymer solution to exit, followed shortly by the core solution. For this reason, the core encapsulation is less than 100%, which is also impossible using other such techniques such as electrospinning.

The core–sheath technology can be used to make fibrous scaffolds for bone tissue engineering applications. One study used this device to produce PCL and PVA core–sheath fibres with hydroxyapatite nanocrystals embedded into the sheath to improve bone regeneration [154]. The produced fibres contained a PCL core for mechanical rigidity and a PVA sheath which was able to release the hydroxyapatite particles. The average diameter of the PCL–PVA core–sheath fibres at a hydroxyapatite loading of 3% was 3.97 ± 1.31 μm. Cell culture and cytotoxicity analyses of the scaffolds showed that they were able to facilitate a high level of cell viability and that the hydroxyapatite nanocrystals embedded in the PVA sheath acted as cell binding sites. The osteogenic activity of these scaffolds was measured using alkaline phosphatase tests, which showed that this activity increased with higher loadings of hydroxyapatite.

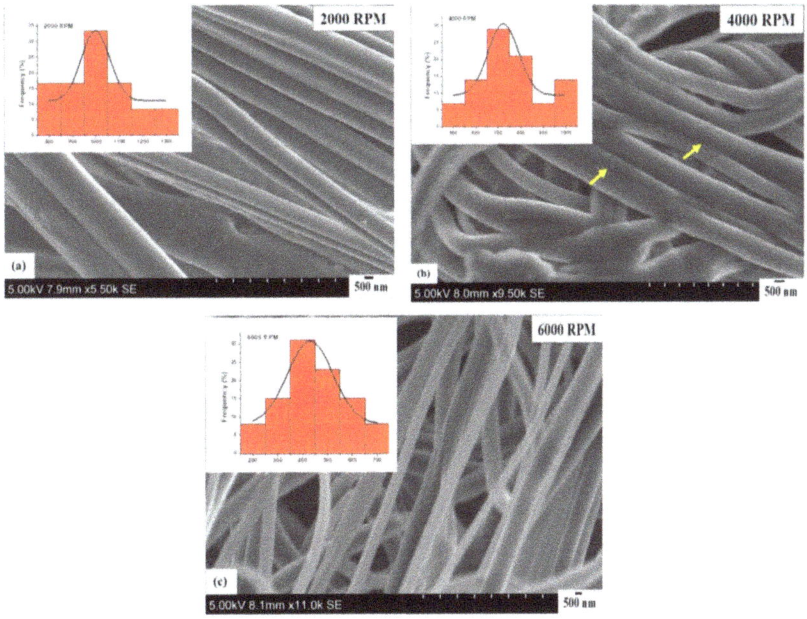

Figure 4.81. SEM images of core–sheath nanofibres obtained using a constant working pressure of 0.1 MPa at: (a) 2000 rpm, (b) 4000 rpm, and (c) 6000 rpm. The insets show the corresponding fibre size distributions of the core–sheath nanofibres for each case. Reproduced from [153]. CC BY 4.0.

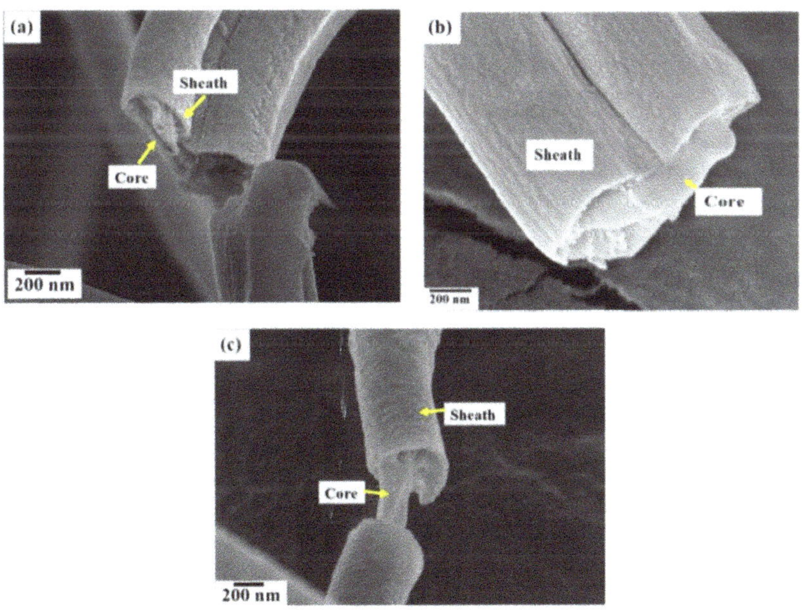

Figure 4.82. Cross-sectional micrographs of core–sheath nanofibres uncovered using focused ion beam milling. The nanofibres were produced at a rotational speed of 6000 rpm and at different working pressures of: (a) 0.1 MPa, (b) 0.2 MPa, and (c) 0.3 MPa. Reproduced from [153]. CC BY 4.0.

The manufacture of core–sheath also has great utility in drug delivery, especially in the context of engineering solubility enhancements for various drugs. Because of the distinct phases of the core–sheath fibres, new approaches can be taken when manufacturing drug release mechanisms. For example, it can be decided that the core and the sheath will contain different drugs loaded into different polymers. As the sheath dissolves, it releases a certain drug using a particular release profile; the fibre can then release another drug from the core on a different timescale. The possibilities of utilising multilayered polymeric fibres for drug release are nearly limitless.

Core–sheath PG has been used to provide an optimised release profile for tetracycline hydrochloride (TEHCL), an antibiotic used to treat a wide range of infections [155]. Utilising this approach to fibre manufacturing, a biphasic drug delivery system can be created which can release the drug via two modes (burst release and sustained release) at different time intervals. The core consisted of the drug dissolved in PVP, a rapidly dissolving hydrophilic polymer which is capable of burst release, and the sheath consisted of PCL, which contributed to a slowdown in release kinetics, thus allowing for sustained release. The fibres produced at maximum rotational speed at an applied gas pressure of 0.1 MPa had an average diameter of 5.0 ± 1.4 μm and showed an overall strong unidirectional alignment. When the applied gas pressure was increased to 0.2 MPa, the average fibre diameter reduced to 4.1 ± 1.1 μm. Because PCL was used as the sheath material and chloroform was used to dissolve it, the resulting core–sheath fibres had a topography which included many surface nanopores. Confocal microscopy was used to capture an image which shows the core–sheath PVP–PCL/TEHCL fibres and the distinctions between the core and the sheath material, this can be seen in figure 4.83.

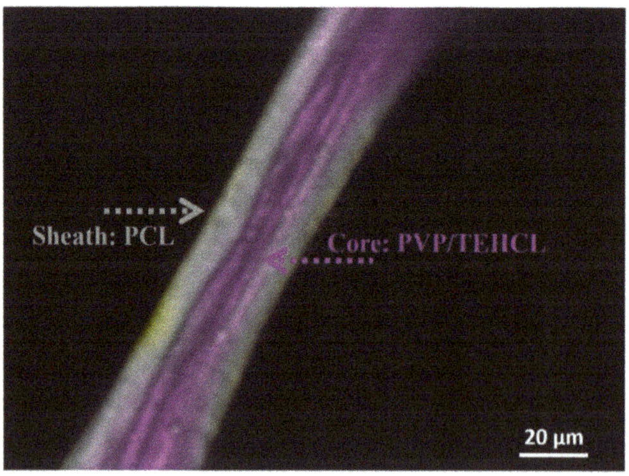

Figure 4.83. A confocal micrograph showing the distinction between the sheath and core regions. Purple dye was used to highlight the PVP core that contained TEHCL. Reprinted from [155], Copyright (2020), with permission from Elsevier.

The core–sheath fibres were then tested to determine their drug release kinetics and compared with single-layered PCL fibres loaded with TEHCL. In comparison to the PCL fibres, the core–sheath fibres showed a release profile only previously observed in hydrophobic polymers. The core–sheath fibres showed a more subdued sustained release than the PCL:TEHCL fibres, even though the drug was loaded onto the hydrophilic PVP core. This approach to drug delivery was the first to allow for the possibility of utilising hydrophilic drug carriers without the drawbacks of instant release. Due to the high frequency of the surface nanopores, the PCL sheath was able to facilitate the diffusion of the drug molecules into the aquatic environment. This work showcases the possibilities of exploiting core–sheath gyratory processes for novel drug delivery approaches.

The core–sheath gyratory technology continues to evolve to meet the ever-increasing demands of the biomedical field. This technology has seen many upgrades and iterations due to the complex nature of producing core–sheath polymeric structures. A second version of the core–sheath PG device was designed and manufactured to improve production quality and increase the potential of this approach for industrial scale-up [156]. The new device improves upon all aspects of the novel core–sheath PG device and provides greater control over the resulting morphology. The reservoirs have been redesigned to optimise polymer flow and a purpose-built collector houses the equipment to support a more optimised workflow. The schematics of this novel device can be seen in figure 4.84.

The novel device was used to spin core–sheath fibres using PLA and PEO, in which PLA was used in the sheath and PEO was used in the core. The resulting fibres

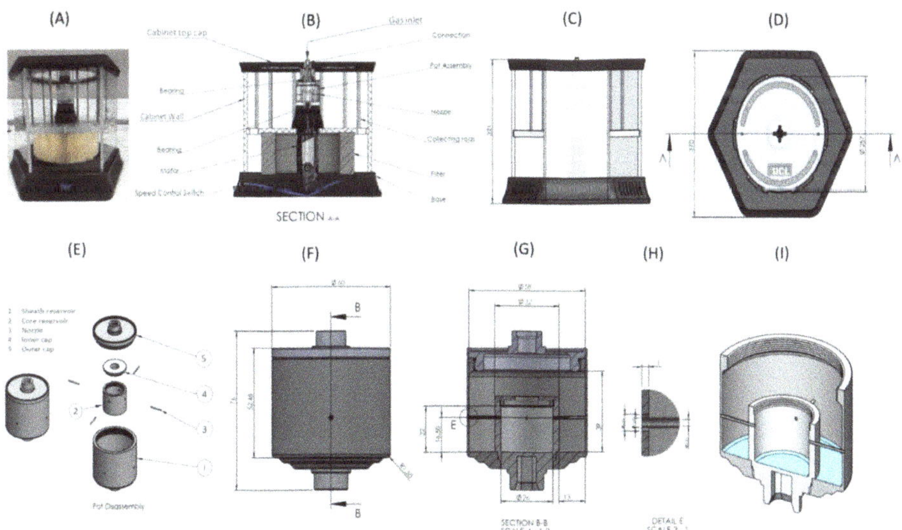

Figure 4.84. Schematics of the novel core–sheath vessel: (a) full view, (b) cross-sectional view of device parts, showing (c) height, (d) width, (e) disassembled core–sheath reservoir, (f) the reservoir's external dimensions, (g) the reservoir's internal dimensions, (h) orifice dimensions, and (i) the reservoir's cross-sectional side view. Reprinted with permission from [156]. Copyright (2021) AIP Publishing.

were analysed using focused ion beam electron microscopy in order to acquire cross-sectional images of the fibres. These images can be seen in figure 4.85. The thinnest fibres produced had an average diameter of less than 530 nm, demonstrating the excellent capability of newer devices to produce products with more desirable properties.

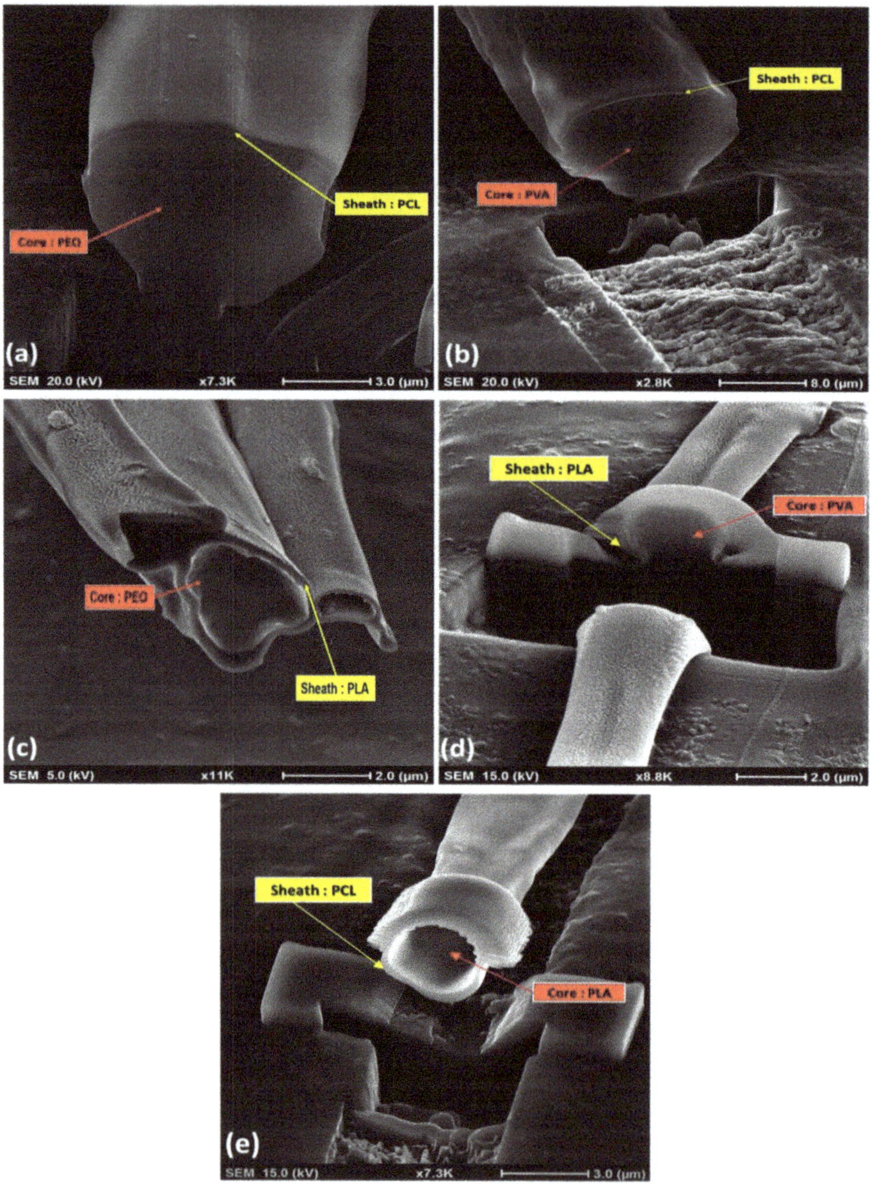

Figure 4.85. Focused ion beam–SEM cross-sectional images of core–sheath fibres: (a) PEO/PCL, (b) PVA/PCL, (c) PEO/PLA, (d) PVA/PLA, and (e) PLA/PCL. Reprinted with permission from [156]. Copyright (2021) AIP Publishing.

4.8.4 Nozzle pressurised gyration

PG is an excellent manufacturing method for the production of highly unidirectionally aligned fibres. Based on this premise, a newer modification to the PG setup has allowed for even greater control over the fibre alignment. This modified PG setup has been given the name nozzle-PG and involves the use of protruding nozzles instead of orifices to guide the exiting polymer solution [157]. Figure 4.86 shows the difference between the original PG design and nozzle-PG and shows how this affects the gas flow to produce a more directional polymer jet.

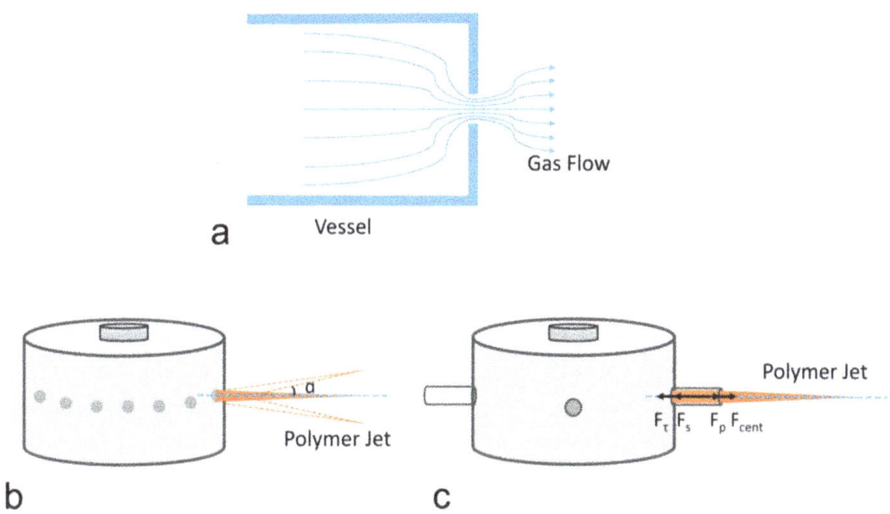

Figure 4.86. A diagrammatic representation of: (a) the gas flows through the orifice, (b) the liquid flow ejected from orifices in the original PG, (c) the liquid flow ejected from nozzles in the nozzle-PG process [157] John Wiley & Sons. [2022].

PCL fibres were spun under identical conditions (maximum speed and 0.2 MPa of applied gas pressure) using both the original PG setup and the nozzle-PG setup and then analysed. There were significant differences between their fibre morphologies, which can see seen in figure 4.87.

The original PG setup produced PCL fibres with an average diameter of 2.8 ± 2.8 μm. Under identical working conditions, the nozzle-PG setup yielded a fibre thickness that dropped to 2.1 ± 1.1 μm, producing significantly thinner and more uniform fibres. Furthermore, the nozzle-PG-produced fibres can be seen to be more unidirectionally aligned and to have much higher coherency when their alignment orientation is taken into consideration. This work further showed that the collection distance plays a crucial role in the alignment of fibres and that by allowing for an optimal distance, the unidirectional alignment can be enhanced. Together with the original PG setup and its derivative technologies, nozzle-PG adds value in the space of the mass production of polymeric fibres with a high degree of uniformity and alignment for specific biomedical applications, such as nerve tissue engineering, in which these properties could lead to increased bioactivity.

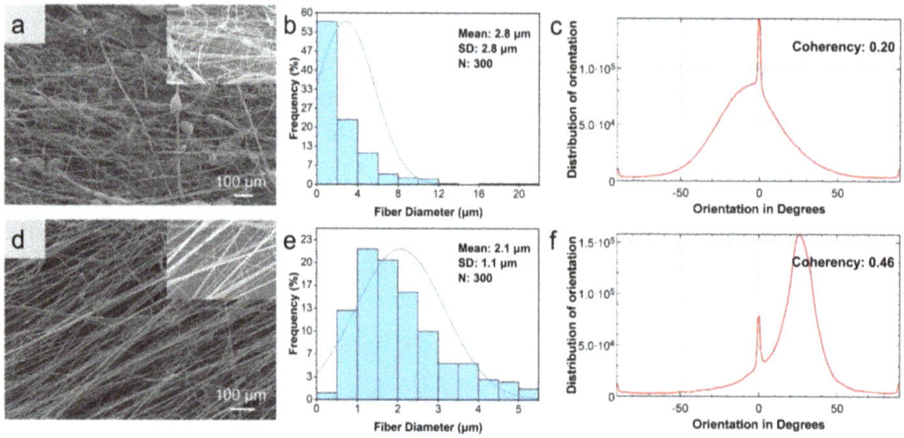

Figure 4.87. SEM images, fibre diameter distribution graphs, and orientation distribution graphs of PCL fibres produced by: (a–c) PG and (d–f) nozzle-PG at a working pressure of 0.2 MPa. The inset shows higher-magnification close-ups of the fibres [157] John Wiley & Sons. [2022].

4.9 The future scope of pressurised gyration

From all that has been shown in this chapter, we can see that centrifugal spinning and other gyratory techniques have worked to revolutionise the way in which fine fibres can be produced for use in a range of biomedical applications. These gyratory techniques benefit hugely from the rapid rotational speed and the ability to scale these units to meet the soaring demands of industry. We have seen how techniques such as PG and its derivates can be used to provide additional control over the fibre morphology and offer simplicity in the use of composite materials and additions. However, there is no such thing as a perfect system; therefore, going forward, we believe there are a number of key points of focus that should be attended to in order to make this technology more suitable for mass adoption.

First, although massive strides have been made to better scale the technology for industrial adoption, there are a number of obstacles which have to date prevented it. The technology needs to be completely automated to reduce dead time and increase production output. In order for this to occur, there must be an element of nonhuman automation and production assembly. For example, the use of robotic manufacturing and artificial intelligence systems can be incorporated to ensure that the production assembly can keep moving without distractions. Robotic arms can, for example, assist with the collection of the fibres and place them at the next stage of the production line where they can be sterilised and packaged. Utilising more modern technologies such as artificial intelligence and modelling, we can detect problems and reduce errors; for example, these technologies can be used to prevent polymer blockages and optimise working parameters and they can be used as a predictive tool to produce the most desirable products at the lowest possible costs to the consumer. For PG at least, work has already begun on using machine learning artificial intelligence and robotic elements in the production line to more efficiently optimise solution and operating parameters. Furthermore, the fully automated PG setup is currently being developed and investments made in a fully-automatic production machine.

As the biomedical landscape and its applications evolve, it is important to continue to innovate and continue to develop upon the current approaches to fields such as tissue engineering and drug delivery. For example, core–sheath and multi-layered fibres are becoming more popular due to their superior properties in tissue engineering applications. The development of gyratory techniques which can produce large amounts of these fibres is in the best interest of the field. Moving forward, tri-layered fibres with more than one sheath can be utilised for applications that require the release of different materials under different environmental conditions. PG-based technologies that can address this demand are being worked on currently; these include the ability to produce multilayered fibres made of distinct polymeric phases.

Although great work has been produced by gyratory processes in terms of the production of polymeric products, one concern which must be addressed is the environmental impact caused by the processing of these polymers. Even with the best intentions, many of these hydrophobic polymers take years to decades to degrade in compost; in addition, the use of harsh solvents creates a concern related to their long-term environmental residence. It is therefore crucial that the selection of polymers and solvents is aligned with continued support for sustainability and environmental longevity. Water-soluble polymers, for example, are increasingly adopted for gyratory-based manufacturing techniques due to their biodegradable nature and their ability to spin fibres without the use of environmentally unfriendly solvents.

All in all, gyratory techniques have contributed greatly to the current healthcare landscape, while leaving plenty of scope for more optimised techniques which would ensure the mass adoption of gyratory techniques in the field of biomaterials for healthcare.

References

[1] Zannini Luz H and Loureiro dos Santos L A 2022 Centrifugal spinning for biomedical use: a review *Crit. Rev. Solid State Mater. Sci.* **48** 1–16

[2] Kambic H E and Nosé Y 1997 Spin doctors: new innovations for centrifugal apheresis *Ther. Apher.* **1** 284–305

[3] Chen C, Dirican M and Zhang X 2019 Chapter 10—Centrifugal spinning—high rate production of nanofibers ed B Ding, X Wang and J Yu *Electrospinning: Nanofabrication and Applications* (William Andrew Publishing) 321–38

[4] Zhiming Z, Jun S, Yaoshuai D and Binbin L 2018 Research on modeling, simulation and experiment based on centrifugal spinning method *J. Brazil. Soc. Mech. Sci. Eng.* **40** 488

[5] Sarkar K, Gomez C, Zambrano S, Ramirez M, de Hoyos E, Vasquez H and Lozano K 2010 Electrospinning to forcespinning™ *Mater. Today* **13** 12–4

[6] Agubra V, Zuniga L, De la Garza D, Gallegos L, Pokhrel M and Alcoutlabi M 2016 ForceSpinning of polyacrylonitrile for mass production of lithium-ion battery separators *Mater. Today* **286** 72–82

[7] Bazrafshan V, Saeidi A and Mousavi A 2020 The effect of different process parameters on polyamide 66 nano fiber by force spinning method *AIP Conf. Proc.* **2205** 020–8

[8] Martín-Alonso M D, Salaris V, Leonés A, Hevilla V, Muñoz-Bonilla A, Echeverría C, Fernández-García M, Peponi L and López D 2023 Centrifugal force-spinning to obtain multifunctional fibers of PLA reinforced with functionalized silver nanoparticles *Polymers* **15** 1240

[9] Mahalingam S and Edirisinghe M 2013 Forming of polymer nanofibers by a pressurised gyration process *Macromol. Rapid Commun.* **34** 1134–9

[10] Zhang X and Lu Y 2014 Centrifugal spinning: an alternative approach to fabricate nanofibers at high speed and low cost *Polym. Rev.* **54** 677–701

[11] Daristotle J L, Behrens A M, Sandler A D and Kofinas P 2016 A review of the fundamental principles and applications of solution blow spinning *ACS Appl. Mater. Interfaces* **8** 34951–63

[12] Dai Y, Ahmed J and Edirisinghe M 2023 Pressurized gyration: fundamentals, advancements, and future *Macromol. Mater. Eng.* **308** 2300033

[13] Weitz R T, Harnau L, Rauschenbach S, Burghard M and Kern K 2008 Polymer nanofibers via nozzle-free centrifugal spinning *Nano Lett.* **8** 1187–91

[14] Mahalingam S, Raimi-Abraham B T, Craig D Q M and Edirisinghe M 2015 Solubility–spinnability map and model for the preparation of fibres of polyethylene (terephthalate) using gyration and pressure *Chem. Eng. J.* **280** 344–53

[15] Xu X and Luo J 2007 Marangoni flow in an evaporating water droplet *Appl. Phys. Lett.* **91** 124102–124102.

[16] Lu Y, Li Y, Zhang S, Xu G, Fu K, Lee H and Zhang X 2013 Parameter study and characterization for polyacrylonitrile nanofibers fabricated via centrifugal spinning process *Eur. Polym. J.* **49** 3834–45

[17] Raimi-Abraham B T, Mahalingam S, Davies P J, Edirisinghe M and Craig D Q 2015 Development and characterization of amorphous nanofiber drug dispersions prepared using pressurized gyration *Mol. Pharm.* **12** 3851–61

[18] Khan A H *et al* 2020 Effectiveness of oil-layered albumin microbubbles produced using microfluidic T-junctions in series for *in vitro* inhibition of tumor cells *Langmuir* **36** 11429–41

[19] Beachley V and Wen X 2009 Effect of electrospinning parameters on the nanofiber diameter and length *Mater. Sci. Eng. C: Mater. Biol. Appl.* **29** 663–8

[20] Heseltine P L, Ahmed J and Edirisinghe M 2018 Developments in pressurized gyration for the mass production of polymeric fibers *Macromol. Mater. Eng.* **303** 1800218

[21] Illangakoon E U, Mahalingam S, Matharu K R and Edirisinghe M 2017 Evolution of surface nanopores in pressurised gyrospun polymeric microfibers *Polymers* **9** 508

[22] Prabhakaran M P, Vatankhah E and Ramakrishna S 2013 Electrospun aligned PHBV/collagen nanofibers as substrates for nerve tissue engineering *Biotechnol. Bioeng.* **110** 2775–84

[23] Alenezi H, Cam M E and Edirisinghe M 2019 Experimental and theoretical investigation of the fluid behavior during polymeric fiber formation with and without pressure *Appl. Phys. Rev.* **6** 041401

[24] Truong Y B, Glattauer V, Lang G, Hands K, Kyratzis I L, Werkmeister J A and Ramshaw J A M 2010 A comparison of the effects of fibre alignment of smooth and textured fibres in electrospun membranes on fibroblast cell adhesion *Biomed. Mater.* **5** 025005

[25] Zhang Y Z, Feng Y, Huang Z M, Ramakrishna S and Lim C T 2006 Fabrication of porous electrospun nanofibres *Nanotechnology* **17** 901–8

[26] Serajuddin A T 1999 Solid dispersion of poorly water-soluble drugs: early promises, subsequent problems, and recent breakthroughs *J. Pharm. Sci.* **88** 1058–66

[27] Williams H D, Trevaskis N L, Charman S A, Shanker R M, Charman W N, Pouton C W and Porter C J H 2013 Strategies to address low drug solubility in discovery and development *Pharmacol. Rev.* **65** 315

[28] Ku M S 2008 Use of the biopharmaceutical classification system in early drug development, *AAPS J.* **10** 208–12

[29] Katti D S, Robinson K W, Ko F K and Laurencin C T 2004 Bioresorbable nanofiber-based systems for wound healing and drug delivery: optimization of fabrication parameters *J. Biomed. Mater. Res.* B **70B** 286–96

[30] Sun D D, Wen H and Taylor L S 2016 Non-sink dissolution conditions for predicting product quality and *in vivo* performance of supersaturating drug delivery systems *J. Pharm. Sci.* **105** 2477–88

[31] Ahmed J, Matharu R K, Shams T, Illangakoon U E and Edirisinghe M 2018 A comparison of electric-field-driven and pressure-driven fiber generation methods for drug delivery *Macromol. Mater. Eng.* 1700577

[32] Walani S R 2020 Global burden of preterm birth *I. J. Gynecol. Obstet.* **150** 31–3

[33] Romero R *et al* 2017 Vaginal progesterone decreases preterm birth and neonatal morbidity and mortality in women with a twin gestation and a short cervix: an updated meta-analysis of individual patient data *Ultrasound Obstet. Gynecol.* **49** 303–14

[34] de Araújo Pereira R R and Bruschi M L 2012 Vaginal mucoadhesive drug delivery systems *Drug Dev. Ind. Pharm.* **38** 643–52

[35] Neves J d, Palmeira-de-Oliveira R, Palmeira-de-Oliveira A, Rodrigues F and Sarmento B 2014 Vaginal mucosa and drug delivery *Mucoadhesive Materials and Drug Delivery Systems* (New York, NY: Wiley) 99–132 https://www.wiley.com/en-gb/Mucoadhesive+Materials+and+Drug+Delivery+Systems-p-9781119941439

[36] Brako F, Raimi-Abraham B, Mahalingam S, Craig D Q M and Edirisinghe M 2015 Making nanofibres of mucoadhesive polymer blends for vaginal therapies *Eur. Polym. J.* **70** 186–96

[37] Brako F, Raimi-Abraham B T, Mahalingam S, Craig D Q M and Edirisinghe M 2018 The development of progesterone-loaded nanofibers using pressurized gyration: a novel approach to vaginal delivery for the prevention of pre-term birth *Int. J. Pharm.* **540** 31–9

[38] Khosravi D, Taheripanah R, Taheripanah A, Tarighat Monfared V and Hosseini-Zijoud S M 2015 Comparison of oral dydrogesterone with vaginal progesteronefor luteal support in IUI cycles: a randomized clinical trial *Iran. J. Reprod. Med.* **13** 433–8

[39] Brako F, Thorogate R, Mahalingam S, Raimi-Abraham B, Craig D Q M and Edirisinghe M 2018 Mucoadhesion of progesterone-loaded drug delivery nanofiber constructs *ACS Appl. Mater. Interfaces* **10** 13381–9

[40] Smart J D 2005 The basics and underlying mechanisms of mucoadhesion *Adv. Drug Deliv. Rev.* **57** 1556–68

[41] Huang Y, Leobandung W, Foss A and Peppas N A 2000 Molecular aspects of muco- and bioadhesion: tethered structures and site-specific surfaces *J. Control. Release* **65** 63–71

[42] Khdair A, Hamad I, Al-Hussaini M, Albayati D, Alkhatib H and Alkhalidi B 2013 In vitro artificial membrane-natural mucosa correlation of carvedilol buccal delivery *J. Drug Deliv. Sci. Technol.* **23** 603–9

[43] Khutoryanskiy V V 2011 Advances in mucoadhesion and mucoadhesive polymers *Macromol. Biosci.* **11** 748–64

[44] Cam M E *et al* 2020 A novel treatment strategy for preterm birth: intra-vaginal progesterone-loaded fibrous patches *Int. J. Pharm.* **588** 119782

[45] Husain O, Lau W, Edirisinghe M and Parhizkar M 2016 Investigating the particle to fibre transition threshold during electrohydrodynamic atomization of a polymer solution *Mater. Sci. Eng.* C **65** 240–50

[46] Grela E, Kozłowska J and Grabowiecka A 2018 Current methodology of MTT assay in bacteria—a review *Acta Histochem.* **120** 303–11

[47] Neuberger T, Schöpf B, Hofmann H, Hofmann M and von Rechenberg B 2005 Superparamagnetic nanoparticles for biomedical applications: possibilities and limitations of a new drug delivery system *J. Magn. Magn. Mater.* **293** 483–96

[48] Perera A S, Zhang S, Homer-Vanniasinkam S, Coppens M-O and Edirisinghe M 2018 Polymer–magnetic composite fibers for remote-controlled drug release *ACS Appl. Mater. Interfaces* **10** 15524–31

[49] Han G and Ceilley R 2017 Chronic wound healing: a review of current management and treatments *Adv. Ther.* **34** 599–610

[50] Han L, Shen W-J, Bittner S, Kraemer F B and Azhar S 2017 PPARs: regulators of metabolism and as therapeutic targets in cardiovascular disease. Part II: PPAR-β/δ and PPAR-γ *Future Cardiol* **13** 279–96

[51] Yu T, Gao M, Yang P, Liu D, Wang D, Song F, Zhang X and Liu Y 2019 Insulin promotes macrophage phenotype transition through PI3K/Akt and PPAR-γ signaling during diabetic wound healing *J. Cell. Physiol.* **234** 4217–31

[52] Chen H, Shi R, Luo B, Yang X, Qiu L, Xiong J, Jiang M, Liu Y, Zhang Z and Wu Y 2015 Macrophage peroxisome proliferator-activated receptor γ deficiency delays skin wound healing through impairing apoptotic cell clearance in mice *Cell Death Dis* **6** e1597–7

[53] Richter B, Bandeira-Echtler E, Bergerhoff K, Clar C and Ebrahim S H 2006 Pioglitazone for type 2 diabetes mellitus *Cochrane Database Syst. Rev.* **4** CD006060

[54] Cam M E *et al* 2020 Evaluation of burst release and sustained release of pioglitazone-loaded fibrous mats on diabetic wound healing: an *in vitro* and *in vivo* comparison study *J. R. Soc. Interface* **17** 20190712

[55] Houchin M L and Topp E M 2008 Chemical degradation of peptides and proteins in PLGA: a review of reactions and mechanisms *J. Pharm. Sci.* **97** 2395–404

[56] Khan F, Dahman Y and Novel A 2012 Approach for the utilization of biocellulose nanofibres in polyurethane nanocomposites for potential applications in bone tissue implants *Des. Monomers Polym.* **15** 1–29

[57] Xie J, MacEwan M R, Schwartz A G and Xia Y 2010 Electrospun nanofibers for neural tissue engineering *Nanoscale* **2** 35–44

[58] Yang F, Murugan R, Wang S and Ramakrishna S 2005 Electrospinning of nano/micro scale poly(l-lactic acid) aligned fibers and their potential in neural tissue engineering *Biomaterials* **26** 2603–10

[59] Karimpoor M, Ilangakoon E, Reid A G, Claudiani S, Edirisinghe M and Khorashad J S 2018 Development of artificial bone marrow fibre scaffolds to study resistance to anti-leukaemia agents *Br. J. Haematol.* **182** 924–7

[60] Kapałczyńska M, Kolenda T, Przybyła W, Zajączkowska M, Teresiak A, Filas V, Ibbs M, Bliźniak R, Łuczewski Ł and Lamperska K 2018 2D and 3D cell cultures—a comparison of different types of cancer cell cultures *Arch. Med. Sci.* **14** 910–9

[61] Aljitawi O S, Li D, Xiao Y, Zhang D, Ramachandran K, Stehno-Bittel L, Van Veldhuizen P, Lin T L, Kambhampati S and Garimella R 2014 A novel three-dimensional stromal-based model for *in vitro* chemotherapy sensitivity testing of leukemia cells *Leuk. Lymphoma* **55** 378–91

[62] Broughton G, Janis J E and Attinger C E 2006 Wound healing: an overview *Plast. Reconstr. Surg.* **117** 1e-S–32e-S

[63] Ahmed J, Gultekinoglu M and Edirisinghe M 2020 Bacterial cellulose micro-nano fibres for wound healing applications *Biotechnol. Adv.* **41** 107549

[64] Naeem M A, Alfred M, Lv P, Zhou H and Wei Q 2018 Three-dimensional bacterial cellulose-electrospun membrane hybrid structures fabricated through *in situ* self-assembly *Cellulose* **25** 6823–30

[65] Altun E *et al* 2018 Novel making of bacterial cellulose blended polymeric fiber bandages *Macromol. Mater. Eng.* **303** 1700607

[66] Altun E *et al* 2018 Co-culture of keratinocyte-*Staphylococcus aureus* on Cu–Ag–Zn/CuO and Cu-Ag-W nanoparticle loaded bacterial cellulose:PMMA bandages *Macromol. Mater. Eng.* 1800537

[67] Heseltine P L, Hosken J, Agboh C, Farrar D, Homer-Vanniasinkam S and Edirisinghe M 2019 Fiber formation from silk fibroin using pressurized gyration *Macromol. Mater. Eng.* **304** 1800577

[68] Heseltine P L, Bayram C, Gultekinoglu M, Homer-Vanniasinkam S, Ulubayram K and Edirisinghe M 2022 Facile one-pot method for all aqueous green formation of biocompatible silk fibroin-poly(ethylene oxide) fibers for use in tissue engineering *ACS Biomater. Sci. Eng.* **8** 1290–300

[69] Rai R, Tallawi M, Grigore A and Boccaccini A R 2012 Synthesis, properties and biomedical applications of poly(glycerol sebacate) (PGS): a review *Prog. Polym. Sci.* **37** 1051–78

[70] Gultekinoglu M, Öztürk Ş, Chen B, Edirisinghe M and Ulubayram K 2019 Preparation of poly(glycerol sebacate) fibers for tissue engineering applications *Eur. Polym. J.* **121** 109297

[71] Broughton G I, Janis J E and Attinger C E 2006 The basic science of wound healing *Plast. Reconstr. Surg.* **117** 12S–34S

[72] Haque E, Chand R and Kapila S 2008 Biofunctional properties of bioactive peptides of milk origin *Food Rev. Int.* **25** 28–43

[73] Sato H and Feix J B 2006 Peptide–membrane interactions and mechanisms of membrane destruction by amphipathic α-helical antimicrobial peptides *Biochim. Biophys. Acta (BBA)—Biomembr.* **1758** 1245–56

[74] Afshar A, Yuca E, Wisdom C, Alenezi H, Ahmed J, Tamerler C and Edirisinghe M 2020 Next-generation antimicrobial peptides (AMPs) incorporated nanofibre wound dressings *Med. Devices Sensors* e10144

[75] Curtin John J and Donlan Rodney M 2006 Using bacteriophages to reduce formation of catheter-associated biofilms by *Staphylococcus epidermidis* *Antimicrob. Agents Chemother.* **50** 1268–75

[76] Weber B, Emmert M Y, Schoenauer R, Brokopp C, Baumgartner L and Hoerstrup S P 2011 Tissue engineering on matrix: future of autologous tissue replacement *Semin. Immunopathol.* **33** 307–15
[77] Basnett P *et al* 2021 Harnessing polyhydroxyalkanoates and pressurized gyration for hard and soft tissue engineering *ACS Appl. Mater. Interfaces* **13** 32624–39
[78] Behbehani M, Glen A, Taylor C S, Schuhmacher A, Claeyssens F and Haycock J W 2018 Pre-clinical evaluation of advanced nerve guide conduits using a novel 3D *in vitro* testing model *Int. J. Bioprint* **4** 123
[79] Daud M F, Pawar K C, Claeyssens F, Ryan A J and Haycock J W 2012 An aligned 3D neuronal-glial co-culture model for peripheral nerve studies *Biomaterials* **33** 5901–13
[80] Siemionow M, Bozkurt M and Zor F 2010 Regeneration and repair of peripheral nerves with different biomaterials: review *Microsurgery* **30** 574–88
[81] Radhakrishnan J, Kuppuswamy A A, Sethuraman S and Subramanian A 2015 Topographic cue from electrospun scaffolds regulate myelin-related gene expressions in schwann cells *J. Biomed. Nanotechnol.* **11** 512–21
[82] Chen Y, Yang Z, Zhao Z-A and Shen Z 2017 Direct reprogramming of fibroblasts into cardiomyocytes *Stem Cell Res. Ther.* **8** 118
[83] Conceição J, Adeoye O, Cabral-Marques H M and Lobo J M S 2018 Cyclodextrins as excipients in tablet formulations *Drug Discov. Today* **23** 1274–84
[84] Kelly A, Ahmed J and Edirisinghe M 2022 Manufacturing cyclodextrin fibers using water *Macromol. Mater. Eng.* **307** 2100891
[85] Xu Z, Mahalingam S, Rohn J L, Ren G and Edirisinghe M 2015 Physio-chemical and antibacterial characteristics of pressure spun nylon nanofibres embedded with functional silver nanoparticles *Mater. Sci. Eng.,* C **56** 195–204
[86] Shakiba M, Rezvani Ghomi E, Khosravi F, Jouybar S, Bigham A, Zare M, Abdouss M, Moaref R and Ramakrishna S 2021 Nylon—a material introduction and overview for biomedical applications *Polym. Adv. Technol.* **32** 3368–83
[87] Illangakoon U E, Mahalingam S, Wang K, Cheong Y K, Canales E, Ren G G, Cloutman-Green E, Edirisinghe M and Ciric L 2017 Gyrospun antimicrobial nanoparticle loaded fibrous polymeric filters *Mater. Sci. Eng.,* C **74** 315–24
[88] Ortolano G A, McAlister M B, Angelbeck J A, Schaffer J, Russell R L, Maynard E and Wenz B 2005 Hospital water point-of-use filtration: a complementary strategy to reduce the risk of nosocomial infection *Am. J. Infect. Control* **33** S1–S19
[89] Frankland S J V and Harik V M 2003 Analysis of carbon nanotube pull-out from a polymer matrix *Surf. Sci.* **525** L103–8
[90] Godoy-Gallardo M, Eckhard U, Delgado L M, de Roo Puente Y J D, Hoyos-Nogués M, Gil F J and Perez R A 2021 Antibacterial approaches in tissue engineering using metal ions and nanoparticles: from mechanisms to applications, *Bioact. Mater.* **6** 4470–90
[91] Pugin B, Cornejo F A, Muñoz-Díaz P, Muñoz-Villagrán C M, Vargas-Pérez J I, Arenas F A and Vásquez C C 2014 Glutathione reductase-mediated synthesis of tellurium-containing nanostructures exhibiting antibacterial properties *Appl. Environ. Microbiol.* **80** 7061–70
[92] Matharu R K, Charani Z, Ciric L, Illangakoon U E and Edirisinghe M 2018 Antimicrobial activity of tellurium-loaded polymeric fiber meshes *J. Appl. Polym. Sci.* **135** 46368
[93] Salgado C D, Sepkowitz K A, John J F, Cantey J R, Attaway H H, Freeman K D, Sharpe P A, Michels H T and Schmidt M G 2013 Copper surfaces reduce the rate of healthcare-acquired infections in the intensive care unit *Infect. Control Hosp. Epidemiol.* **34** 479–86

[94] L'Vov N P, Nosikov A N and Antipov A N 2002 Tungsten-containing enzymes *Biochemistry (Moscow)* **67** 196–200
[95] Matharu R K, Ciric L, Ren G and Edirisinghe M 2020 Comparative study of the antimicrobial effects of tungsten nanoparticles and tungsten nanocomposite fibres on hospital acquired bacterial and viral pathogens *Nanomaterials (Basel)* **10** 1017
[96] Doerrbecker J, Friesland M, Ciesek S, Erichsen T J, Mateu-Gelabert P, Steinmann J, Steinmann J, Pietschmann T and Steinmann E 2011 Inactivation and survival of Hepatitis C virus on inanimate surfaces, *J. Infect. Dis.* **204** 1830–8
[97] Matharu R K, Porwal H, Chen B, Ciric L and Edirisinghe M 2020 Viral filtration using carbon-based materials, *Med. Dev. Sensors* e10107
[98] Patial S, Kumar A, Raizada P, Le Q V, Nguyen V-H, Selvasembian R, Singh P, Thakur S and Hussain C M 2022 Potential of graphene based photocatalyst for antiviral activity with emphasis on COVID-19: a review *J. Environ. Chem. Eng.* **10** 107527
[99] Donskyi I S, Azab W, Cuellar-Camacho J L, Guday G, Lippitz A, Unger W E S, Osterrieder K, Adeli M and Haag R 2019 Functionalized nanographene sheets with high antiviral activity through synergistic electrostatic and hydrophobic interactions *Nanoscale* **11** 15804–9
[100] Meades G, Henken R L, Waldrop G L, Rahman M M, Gilman S D, Kamatou G P P, Viljoen A M and Gibbons S 2010 Constituents of cinnamon inhibit bacterial acetyl CoA carboxylase *Planta Med.* **76** 1570–5
[101] Toussaint-Samat M 2009 *A History of Food* (New York: Wiley)
[102] Sedighi M *et al* 2018 Protective effects of cinnamon bark extract against ischemia–reperfusion injury and arrhythmias in rat *Phytother. Res.* **32** 1983–91
[103] Ahmed J, Altun E, Aydogdu M O, Gunduz O, Kerai L, Ren G and Edirisinghe M 2019 Anti-fungal bandages containing cinnamon extract *Int. Wound* J **16** 730–6
[104] Ahmed J, Gultekinoglu M, Bayram C, Kart D, Ulubayram K and Edirisinghe M 2021 Alleviating the toxicity concerns of antibacterial cinnamon-polycaprolactone biomaterials for healthcare-related biomedical applications *MedComm* **2** 236–46
[105] Cooper R A, Molan P C and Harding K G 2002 The sensitivity to honey of Gram-positive cocci of clinical significance isolated from wounds *J. Appl. Microbiol.* **93** 857–63
[106] Visavadia B G, Honeysett J and Danford M H 2008 Manuka honey dressing: An effective treatment for chronic wound infections *Br. J. Oral Maxillofac. Surg.* **46** 55–6
[107] Matharu R K, Ahmed J, Seo J, Karu K, Golshan M A, Edirisinghe M and Ciric L 2022 Antibacterial properties of honey nanocomposite fibrous meshes *Polymers* **14** 5155
[108] Novoselov K S, Geim A K, Morozov S V, Jiang D, Zhang Y, Dubonos S V, Grigorieva I V and Firsov A A 2004 Electric field effect in atomically thin carbon films *Science* **306** 666
[109] Rao C N R, Sood A K, Subrahmanyam K S and Govindaraj A 2009 Graphene: the new two-dimensional nanomaterial *Angew. Chem. Int. Ed.* **48** 7752–77
[110] Sun X, Liu Z, Welsher K, Robinson J T, Goodwin A, Zaric S and Dai H 2008 Nano-graphene oxide for cellular imaging and drug delivery *Nano Res.* **1** 203–12
[111] Yang K, Zhang S, Zhang G, Sun X, Lee S-T and Liu Z 2010 Graphene in mice: ultrahigh *in vivo* tumor uptake and efficient photothermal therapy *Nano Lett.* **10** 3318–23
[112] Wan Y, Wang Y, Wu J and Zhang D 2011 Graphene oxide sheet-mediated silver enhancement for application to electrochemical biosensors *Anal. Chem.* **83** 648–53

[113] Sengupta R, Bhattacharya M, Bandyopadhyay S and Bhowmick A K 2011 A review on the mechanical and electrical properties of graphite and modified graphite reinforced polymer composites *Prog. Polym. Sci.* **36** 638–70
[114] Cataldi P, Athanassiou A and Bayer I S 2018 Graphene nanoplatelets-based advanced materials and recent progress in sustainable applications *Appl. Sci.* **8** 1438
[115] Amir A, Mahalingam S, Wu X, Porwal H, Colombo P, Reece M J and Edirisinghe M 2016 Graphene nanoplatelets loaded polyurethane and phenolic resin fibres by combination of pressure and gyration *Compos. Sci. Technol.* **129** 173–82
[116] Liu C-K, Lai K, Liu W, Yao M and Sun R-J 2009 Preparation of carbon nanofibres through electrospinning and thermal treatment *Polym. Int.* **58** 1341–9
[117] Feng L, Xie N and Zhong J 2014 Carbon nanofibers and their composites: a review of synthesizing, properties and applications *Materials* **7** 3919–45
[118] Chae H G, Choi Y H, Minus M L and Kumar S 2009 Carbon nanotube reinforced small diameter polyacrylonitrile based carbon fiber *Compos. Sci. Technol.* **69** 406–13
[119] Wu X, Mahalingam S, Amir A, Porwal H, Reece M J, Naglieri V, Colombo P and Edirisinghe M 2016 Novel preparation, microstructure, and properties of polyacrylonitrile-based carbon nanofiber-graphene nanoplatelet materials *ACS Omega* **1** 202–11
[120] Akhavan O and Ghaderi E 2010 Toxicity of graphene and graphene oxide nanowalls against bacteria *ACS Nano* **4** 5731–6
[121] Matharu R K, Porwal H, Ciric L and Edirisinghe M 2018 The effect of graphene–poly (methyl methacrylate) fibres on microbial growth *Interface Focus* **8** 20170058
[122] Frias J, Ribas F and Lucena F 2001 Effects of different nutrients on bacterial growth in a pilot distribution system *Anton. Leeuw.* **80** 129–38
[123] Amir A, Porwal H, Mahalingam S, Wu X, Wu T, Chen B, Tabish T A and Edirisinghe M 2020 Microstructure of fibres pressure-spun from polyacrylonitrile–graphene oxide composite mixtures *Compos. Sci. Technol.* **197** 108214
[124] Matharu R K *et al* 2020 Microstructure and antibacterial efficacy of graphene oxide nanocomposite fibres *J. Colloid Interface Sci.* **571** 239–52
[125] Aranda A, Sequedo L, Tolosa L, Quintas G, Burello E, Castell J V and Gombau L 2013 Dichloro-dihydro-fluorescein diacetate (DCFH-DA) assay: a quantitative method for oxidative stress assessment of nanoparticle-treated cells *Toxicol. In Vitro* **27** 954–63
[126] Paek S-M, Yoo E and Honma I 2009 Enhanced cyclic performance and lithium storage capacity of SnO_2/graphene nanoporous electrodes with three-dimensionally delaminated flexible structure *Nano Lett.* **9** 72–5
[127] Ahmed J, Tabish T A, Zhang S and Edirisinghe M 2021 Porous graphene composite polymer fibres *Polymers* **13** 76
[128] Gerratt A P, Michaud H O and Lacour S P 2015 Elastomeric electronic skin for prosthetic tactile sensation *Adv. Funct. Mater.* **25** 2287–95
[129] Xu J *et al* 2017 Highly stretchable polymer semiconductor films through the nanoconfinement effect *Science* **355** 59–64
[130] Kim Y, Yuk H, Zhao R, Chester S A and Zhao X 2018 Printing ferromagnetic domains for untethered fast-transforming soft materials *Nature* **558** 274–9
[131] Nurhamiyah Y, Amir A, Finnegan M, Themistou E, Edirisinghe M and Chen B 2021 Wholly biobased, highly stretchable, hydrophobic, and self-healing thermoplastic elastomer *ACS Appl. Mater. Interfaces* **13** 6720–30

[132] Mahalingam S, Ren G G and Edirisinghe M J 2014 Rheology and pressurised gyration of starch and starch-loaded poly(ethylene oxide) *Carbohydrate Polym.* **114** 279–87
[133] Aydogdu O M, Altun E, Ahmed J, Gunduz O and Edirisinghe M 2019 Fiber forming capability of binary and ternary compositions in the polymer system: bacterial cellulose–polycaprolactone–polylactic acid *Polymers* **11** 1148
[134] Altun E, Ahmed J, Onur Aydogdu M, Harker A and Edirisinghe M 2022 The effect of solvent and pressure on polycaprolactone solutions for particle and fibre formation *Eur. Polym. J.* 111300
[135] Vandenburg H J, Clifford A A, Bartle K D, Carlson R E, Carroll J and Newton I D 1999 A simple solvent selection method for accelerated solvent extraction of additives from polymers *Analyst* **124** 1707–10
[136] Li T, Ding X, Tian L and Ramakrishna S 2017 Engineering BSA-dextran particles encapsulated bead-on-string nanofiber scaffold for tissue engineering applications *J. Mater. Sci.* **52** 10661–72
[137] Hong X, Edirisinghe M and Mahalingam S 2016 Beads, beaded-fibres and fibres: Tailoring the morphology of poly(caprolactone) using pressurised gyration *Mater. Sci. Eng.* C **69** 1373–82
[138] Han P, Gomez G A, Duda G N, Ivanovski S and Poh P S P 2022 Scaffold geometry modulation of mechanotransduction and its influence on epigenetics *Acta Biomater.* **163** 259–74
[139] Hosseini F S and Laurencin C T 2022 Advanced electrospun nanofibrous stem cell niche for bone regenerative engineering *Regen. Eng. Transl. Med.* **9** 165–80
[140] Illangakoon U E, Mahalingam S, Colombo P and Edirisinghe M 2016 Tailoring the surface of polymeric nanofibres generated by pressurised gyration, *Surf. Innov.* **4** 167–78
[141] Curtis A and Wilkinson C 1997 Topographical control of cells *Biomaterials* **18** 1573–83
[142] Mahalingam S, Raimi-Abraham B T, Craig D Q M and Edirisinghe M 2015 Formation of protein and protein–gold nanoparticle stabilized microbubbles by pressurized gyration *Langmuir* **31** 659–66
[143] Rajesh S, Peddada S S, Thiévenaz V and Sauret A 2022 Pinch-off of bubbles in a polymer solution *J. Non-Newtonian Fluid Mech.* **310** 104921
[144] Mahalingam S, Xu Z and Edirisinghe M 2015 Antibacterial activity and biosensing of PVA-lysozyme microbubbles formed by pressurized gyration *Langmuir* **31** 9771–80
[145] Ibrahim H R, Higashiguchi S, Koketsu M, Juneja L R, Kim M, Yamamoto T, Sugimoto Y and Aoki T 1996 Partially unfolded lysozyme at neutral pH agglutinates and kills gram-negative and gram-positive bacteria through membrane damage mechanism *J. Agric. Food Chem.* **44** 3799–806
[146] Yağmuroğlu O and Diltemiz S E 2020 Development of QCM based biosensor for the selective and sensitive detection of paraoxon *Anal. Biochem.* **591** 113572
[147] Zhang S, Karaca B T, VanOosten S K, Yuca E, Mahalingam S, Edirisinghe M and Tamerler C 2015 Coupling infusion and gyration for the nanoscale assembly of functional polymer nanofibers integrated with genetically engineered proteins *Macromol. Rapid Commun.* **36** 1322–8
[148] Hong X, Mahalingam S and Edirisinghe M 2017 Simultaneous application of pressure-infusion-gyration to generate polymeric nanofibers *Macromol. Mater. Eng.* **302** 1600564

[149] Hong X, Harker A and Edirisinghe M 2019 Empirical modelling and optimization of pressure-coupled infusion gyration parameters for the nanofibre fabrication *Proc. R. Soc.* A **475** 0008

[150] Xu Z, Mahalingam S, Basnett P, Raimi-Abraham B, Roy I, Craig D and Edirisinghe M 2016 Making nonwoven fibrous poly(ε-caprolactone) constructs for antimicrobial and tissue engineering applications by pressurized melt gyration *Macromol. Mater. Eng.* **301** 922–34

[151] Mahalingam S, Matharu R, Homer-Vanniasinkam S and Edirisinghe M 2020 Current methodologies and approaches for the formation of core–sheath polymer fibers for biomedical applications *Appl. Phys. Rev.* **7** 041302

[152] Mahalingam S, Homer-Vanniasinkam S and Edirisinghe M 2019 Novel pressurised gyration device for making core–sheath polymer fibres *Mater. Des.* **178** 107846

[153] Mahalingam S, Huo S, Homer-Vanniasinkam S and Edirisinghe M 2020 Generation of core–sheath polymer nanofibers by pressurised gyration *Polymers* **12** 1709

[154] Mahalingam S, Bayram C, Gultekinoglu M, Ulubayram K, Homer-Vanniasinkam S and Edirisinghe M 2021 Co-axial gyro-spinning of PCL/PVA/HA core–sheath fibrous scaffolds for bone tissue engineering *Macromol. Biosci.* 2100177

[155] Majd H, Harker A, Edirisinghe M and Parhizkar M 2022 Optimised release of tetracycline hydrochloride from core–sheath fibres produced by pressurised gyration *J. Drug Deliv. Sci. Technol.* **72** 103359

[156] Alenezi H, Cam M E and Edirisinghe M 2021 Core–sheath polymer nanofiber formation by the simultaneous application of rotation and pressure in a novel purpose-designed vessel *Appl. Phys. Rev.* **8** 041412

[157] Dai Y, Ahmed J, Delbusso A and Edirisinghe M 2022 Nozzle-pressurized gyration: a novel fiber manufacturing process *Macromol. Mater. Eng.* **307** 2200268

Chapter 5

Future perspectives

This chapter brings together chapters 2–4 to highlight the positives of bubbles, particles, and different morphologies of particles and fibres. It also highlights shortcomings which prevail at present and illustrates how some of these can be overcome to make these processes truly amenable to mass production and manufacturing. This can also involve combining some of the processes described in chapters 2–4.

5.1 Biomaterials in healthcare

Great leaps and bounds have been made in the development of biomaterials for various biomedical applications, including all the topics discussed in this book. As is always the case, plenty more work can be done to further improve the suitability of these materials for the ever-growing landscape that is healthcare. In this chapter, we detail the key areas of focus that we believe will be vital in the future for the use of biomaterials in healthcare.

5.1.1 Industrial scale-up

Firstly, there will be a significant development in fabrication methods to meet the demands of industrial scale-up. Currently, electrospinning is being used to produce biomaterials for many industrial applications, but the real challenge is to increase yields and improve production rates. For example, it is well-known that the electrospinning technique is difficult to scale up due to factors such as charge interference between neighbouring nozzles and the clogging that inevitably occurs within these nozzles due to stagnation. These techniques must therefore focus on ramping up the production output so that the increasing demands for these materials can be met. Utilising the state-of-the-art methodologies available can help to maximise the production output by increasing the efficiency of material consumption and reducing the overall costs of production.

doi:10.1088/978-0-7503-5187-4ch5

5.1.2 Energy usage

As the importance of energy is becoming increasingly apparent in a world where major economies have an undeniable fuel reliance on other nations, we have learnt how essential it is to reduce energy consumption and work with more efficient processes. Therefore, ambient technologies such as pressurised gyration (PG), which does not require the energy-intensive application of an altered working environment, become increasingly attractive as energy costs become more volatile due to the changing tensions between countries. Increasing the power efficiency of biomaterial manufacturing techniques leads to greater stability in times of economic austerity and ensures that the production of vital materials can continue undisturbed. A similar situation was witnessed during the 2019 COVID outbreak, when many production lines of important materials were halted, affecting worldwide supplies of urgent medical equipment. Lower energy consumption is also a global focus, as countries unite to reduce their emissions, a necessary evil which is caused by the majority of global power generation.

5.1.3 Environmental considerations

This push towards improving the energy efficiency of current technologies is also aligned with the common goal of improving the environment, as a result of which, all major governments are committed to environmental initiatives in the coming decades. The use of materials and solvents which cause less environmental harm has led to an ongoing effort in the biomaterials field to incorporate more materials which are biodegradable and non-polluting. Currently, the term biodegradable can be seen to be attributed to a wide range of materials with vastly different degradation rates under numerous differing conditions. For example, many polymers classified as 'biodegradable' still require years to degrade; they are not naturally found in the environment and require additional treatment. Going forward, there could be a better classification of biodegradability that would allow both researchers and healthcare professionals to better understand how a given material will behave under the specific conditions of their applications. Another important component of biodegradability is whether a specific material is also bioresorbable; while some polymers may be biodegradable, the degradation products of biomaterials may also pose a risk of cytotoxicity. PLA is a fascinating example of a polymer which is both biodegradable and bioresorbable; its degradation product is lactic acid, naturally found in small quantities inside the body, which can be safely metabolised. Polymers can also degrade via widely different techniques inside the body such as via 'bulk erosion', 'surface erosion', 'bioabsorption', and 'bioerosion', so these must be given detailed consideration when biomaterials are used in healthcare.

5.1.4 Drug delivery

Biomaterials have been used to revolutionise drug delivery by enabling the targeted and sustained release of active pharmaceutical ingredients (APIs), which can improve their therapeutic efficacy and reduce side-effects. One of the main advantages of using biomaterials is their ability to target specific cells or tissues. For example, more work will go into biomaterials which can release drugs directly into cancer cells, while, for example, sparing healthy tissue. These approaches can increase the effectiveness of treatments while reducing their side-effects.

Biomaterials have also been designed to release APIs in a sustained profile, which can improve the efficacy of treatments by maintaining therapeutic levels of drugs over an extended period. This is particularly important for drugs that have a rapid degradation rate or require frequent dosing. Biomaterials can also be used for drug delivery, as they have the ability to protect drugs from degradation or clearance by the body. Some drugs may otherwise be rapidly cleared from the body, limiting their effectiveness. By encapsulating the drug within a biomaterial, the drug can be protected and released over a longer period. There are several different types of biomaterials that can be used for drug delivery, including polymers, liposomes, and nanoparticles. Each biomaterial has its unique properties and advantages, and the choice of biomaterial is extremely important for each application. In the future, we can expect to see more natural polymers and an increased use of highly hydrophilic drug carriers such as cyclodextrin. Core–sheath and multilayered fibre production will also contribute to polypharmacy administration, in which more than one drug can be given to a patient in a single package.

5.1.5 Biosensors

Another area in which there is an expectation of increased growth in biomaterials is the fabrication of biosensor components. The development of novel approaches to medical diagnostics is essential to eradicate disease and increase global living standards. Cancers can have many variations, and they can be difficult to culture in two-dimensional cell lines. The development of microfluidics and its many technologies has made it possible to miniaturise many biochemical tests, which has the benefit of improving sensitivity and reducing the costs associated with higher reagent volumes. Although this book has discussed microfluidics in relation to creating microbubbles for healthcare applications, it can also be used to make organ-on-chip platforms and components for advanced biosensors. We believe that future work will look into incorporating cell cultured models into microfluidic devices that can offer superior analysis and diagnosis compared to their two-dimensional petri-dish counterparts. For these three-dimensional organs-on-chips to succeed, however, there will need to be material-based biosensor detection systems which can be used to monitor the microenvironment of the cell culture. This book has shown how fabrication techniques such as electrospinning and PG can be used to produce some of these biosensor parts. The novel use of materials can help to improve the sensitivity of these biosensors; for example, highly precise oxygen concentration measurements can be made within these microfluidic environments by phosphorescence-based oxygen biosensors and functional porous materials such as PMMA can used to improve the analyte detection levels. Through the use of core–sheath fibre manufacturing techniques, fibres with more than one material constituent can be used to provide more reliable detection. Real-time monitoring is becoming more popular, as up-to-date metrics are desired, which can then provide the patient with more relevant data and the clinician with superior diagnostic abilities.

We have recently seen a substantial development in technology in the field of wearable devices, with the result that smart watches and health monitoring have become incredibly popular. As a result of innovations in the use of biomaterials in biosensors, we will see the further development of wearable technologies, which will empower their users with more data and statistics to allow them to live healthier and more productive lives. These wearable devices can provide continuous monitoring of various health parameters, allowing for the early detection and treatment of medical conditions.

5.1.6 Regenerative medicine and tissue engineering

One of the best arguments for the advancement of biomaterials is the hope that one day it will provide a means for the easy replacement of damaged tissues and other anatomical structures. Therefore, tissue engineering and regenerative medicine are at the forefront of potential biomaterials breakthroughs. The field of tissue engineering scaffolds made from polymeric materials has seen many attempts to create structures that can mimic the *in vivo* environment of the body. The development of polymers based on natural materials such as cellulose and milk proteins provide a strong basis for *in vivo* biocompatibility, an essential consideration for any biomaterial that is considered for use in tissue engineering. Furthermore, these naturally derived materials often lead to less environmental harm and raise fewer concerns related to cytotoxicity. The development of further novel polymeric structures such as porous fibres, core–sheath fibres incorporating many layers, and other concentric fibre shapes will help to provide a greater choice of tissue engineering structures that can better facilitate mechano-transduction cues such as surface stiffness and other topological features.

One of the biggest obstacles which prevents the success of tissue engineered structures is the role of the immune system, which often leads to loss of implant function. Recently, the term 'immune engineering' was coined to describe the use of engineering tools to target different cell types of the immune system. This approach can be applied to tissue engineering to create constructs that can evade the host's defence system and create their intended long-term effects. Much future work must therefore go into immune engineering and tissue engineering; by combining these two disciplines, we can learn more about the specifics of the innate and adaptive immune systems and approach a future in which engineered tissue replacements will become an integral part of general surgery. This endeavour will make essential healthcare available to more patients, allowing the reliance on human donors to be significantly reduced or even eradicated.

5.1.7 Cell encapsulation

The encapsulation of cells within polymeric materials such as bubbles, particles, and fibres has become increasingly popular in the development of biomaterials which target healthcare applications. The idea is that biocompatible structures that can accept seeded cells can be fabricated using techniques such as electrospinning; such structures have a superior bioactive effect on the target tissue. These cell-encapsulated biomaterials have the ability to allow metabolic transport but are isolated from the host's immune system; an example is the treatment of diabetes in humans, in which porcine islet cells are used in an encapsulated form. However, the use of technologies such as electrospinning has raised concerns about the viability of these cells; an open question remains as to whether or not the use of a high-voltage electric field reduces cell viability. In addition, gyration technologies can produce encapsulated cells, but this raises a concern that the high shear forces involved contribute to a reduction in cell viability. Further work needs be carried out on the viability of cells under such manufacturing and mass production conditions.

5.1.8 Graphene and its derivatives

Following the recent discovery of single-atom-thick graphene, there has been an enormous push to utilise this material in nearly every conceivable application. Graphene, including its derivatives such as graphene oxide and graphene nanopores mentioned in this book, has remarkable properties such as excellent mechanical strength and electrical conductivity. However, it has proven a difficult material to produce and scale up, and its uses in secondary structures such as fibres have been limited to date. Still, this material possesses properties which would be a tragedy to waste, and further work to support the current research by producing further fibrous materials using techniques such an electrospinning will only promote the widespread use of this fascinating material.

Graphene oxide can also be used to provide a long-lasting physical antibacterial effect. At specific concentrations of graphene oxide, a bactericidal effect has been noticed, which arises from the sharp protrusions of the graphene flakes. Physical antimicrobial features are very difficult for evolution to compensate for; therefore, the likelihood that bacterial cells will adapt to it are very slim. It thereby combats a high degree of antimicrobial resistance. Graphene oxide and other graphene-based materials can also be used as surface coatings, for example, in hospitals where infection is a very common issue. The use of physical antimicrobial attacks is also preferred, as it reduces the need for antibiotics, which ultimately create the selection pressure that leads to microbial resistance. We believe that a lot more effort will be input to introduce graphene as a common biomaterial in the future, and its use in healthcare will subsequently become ubiquitous.

5.1.9 Artificial intelligence and machine learning

Artificial intelligence (AI) and machine learning (ML) are new technologies based on the use of computer algorithms to generate intelligence that is equal to or superior to human intelligence. Although this technology has seen commercial success and is touted as the next big evolutionary step for mankind, its use in biomaterials and healthcare has been less discussed. AI and ML can be used to better optimise production assemblies and operating parameters and give researchers more time to spend on other ventures. For example, AI can be used to simulate or predict the optimal solution parameters and working parameters for fibre manufacture, a process that has thousands to millions of possible variations. AI can also be used to augment experimental data and make models based on fewer data points, increasing the accuracy of many procedures whilst also saving time and expensive resources. In cases in which human trials are required, AI and ML can use limited data and extrapolate the required outcomes, saving lives as a result.

Furthermore, ML can be used for corrective scenarios and can help to complete the automation of production assemblies. For example, a fully automated electrospinning setup still requires continuous monitoring and adjustments; the lack of these could lead to a loss of production yield due to factors such as needle clogging. Many data points can be gathered using sensors; when fed into an ML system, this data can be translated directly into the adjustments that need to be executed.

5.1.10 Soft robotics

We have discussed the necessity for fully automated fabrication techniques, which are required for full industrial scale-up. In order to complete a chain that has advanced sensory equipment and AI, there needs to be a robotic element at the end of it. Soft robotics is an excelling field of robotics which focusses on robots that have precise control over the pressure and handling of delicate materials. An example of this can be seen in surgical robotics, in which the pressure applied to an open wound must be precise in order to prevent severe injury. Soft robotics can also be applied to an assembly line where fibres are produced and collected. The collection of nanofibres is a very delicate process which is often handled manually. However, human interactions create bottlenecks, as these interactions lack accuracy and have high associated costs. In order to facilitate widespread adoption, the costs associated with production must come down. Consequently, there would be a huge benefit to the biomaterial and healthcare world if soft robotic technologies could be applied to the production routes of biomaterials.

5.2 The future of microfluidic technologies

Microfluidic technology offers precision, accuracy, and repeatability for screening and fabrication in biomedical applications. Lab-on-a-chip applications developed to function as miniaturised total chemical analysis systems have demonstrated the ability to perform high-yield fabrication and high-sensitivity analysis using small quantities of reactants and analytes, respectively. In the last few decades, the development of microfluidics has undoubtedly contributed to the development of modern biology. Biological studies developed using microfluidic and nanofluid systems were limited to proof-of-concept studies in their very first years. Further growth in microfluidic technologies was then experienced as a result of an increase in the variety of materials used in microfluidic chip production. Parameters such as the organic or inorganic material used, optical permeability, resistance to flow, solvents, and conductivity have a significant impact on the development of microfluidic platforms. In addition, the desirability of the material used is also affected by features such as its ease of processing, economic cost, and reusability.

The importance of microchips can be exemplified by the revolution in the use of microfluidic technologies in the biomedical field that followed the discovery of polydimethylsiloxane. The increase in versatility in terms of material choice and production techniques has made it convenient to produce microfluidic chips easily and quickly in an application-specific manner. The development and rapid prototyping of microfluidics has allowed for the development of rapid diagnostic kits, the increase in sensor application areas, improved drug delivery systems, and tissue-cell culture platforms that enable the needs of target-specific applications to be readily met.

Microfluidic technologies have been at the forefront of the COVID-19 pandemic, which has deeply affected the whole world in recent years. The diagnosis, prevention, and treatment possibilities offered by microfluidic platforms have been used during the pandemic and will continue to be used as needed. Loop-mediated isothermal amplification, polymerase chain reactions, clustered regularly interspaced short palindromic repeats, and recombinase polymerase amplification techniques were adapted to microfluidic devices for virus detection and particularly the detection of COVID-19. In addition, aptamer- and immunoassay-based techniques contributed to virus detection analysis techniques in the field of microfluidic technology. The detection apparatus has been simplified to cell phones and paper-based colorimetric methods to save time and money.

Microfluidics has also gained a pivotal role in drug and vaccine studies. Microfluidics, which offers low-cost, reproducible, and high-efficiency production techniques, has made a significant contribution to the development of COVID-19 vaccines and has taken its place on the market. In addition to the production step of vaccine and drug studies, microfluidics provides significant advantages compared to the traditional methods used for *in vitro* test studies. Cellular toxicity tests performed under dynamic microfluidic culture conditions and organ-on-a-chip models are replacing static cell culture tests and animal experiments on a daily basis. Their low cost, low toxicity, and high reproducibility and verifiability have allowed FDA-approved drug and vaccine studies to accelerate and increase. The replacement of animal experiments by microfluidic platforms based on dynamic culture environments has also contributed to reducing the amount of global carbon emissions.

The future perspective on microfluidic technology is that it will provide simple and fast solutions to complex biological systems. By supporting human-on-a-chip applications with artificial intelligence (AI) in future studies, it is expected to offer widespread, personalised diagnosis and treatment opportunities for biological systems that are today limited by our understanding and our ability to provide solutions.

5.3 The future of electrohydrodynamic technologies

Electrohydrodynamic systems are superior among biofabrication techniques because they allow a wide range of production types using a single method. EHD, which is a bottom-up production technique, has many biomedical applications due to its nanoscale production capability. It offers varied production capabilities from nanoparticle production to microbubbles and from nano- to microfibres. Precision control over the design and manufacture of these products can be achieved via the electrical voltage applied, depending on the solution properties and the distance between the nozzle and the collector.

The control ability and increased precision in nanoparticle and microbubble production offer advantages that can overcome the disadvantages, such as resolution and loading capacity, experienced in conventional systems. In addition, it is possible to produce particles with a porous surface by utilising the volatility of the selected solvent. In this way, the diffusion rate can be differentiated. It is also possible to produce multilayered particles by modifying the nozzle design. The production of multilayer structures from polymers with different degradation rates or hydrophilic/hydrophobic characteristics enables the creation of carriers that can provide multiple therapeutic effects as well as sequential and sustained release. In addition, particulate systems obtained using EHD, which is a direct production method, also offer a more environmentally friendly approach than conventional methods. The nanoprecipitation or emulsion systems used in traditional methods create organic waste and need more energy and time, as they require a purification step.

On the other hand, fibre production via EHD is quick, easy, and economical compared to traditional methods. Decreased fibre sizes which easily encompass the nanoscale allow fibre membranes or surface modification layers to be prepared with increased surface areas. The increased surface area of these fibres also helps to increase drug loading capacity and effectiveness.

The EHD technique, which offers diverse solutions from drug delivery systems to imaging agents, from tissue scaffolds to wound dressings, and from implant surface modifications to wearable sensor applications in biomedical applications, is expected to evolve over the next few years to offer faster, portable, and more complex solutions to health problems in a single step. Aspects that will continue to be developed in the near future include offering solutions to the complex health problems encountered in the human body, designing multilayered structures with different features, and gaining increased capabilities using multilayered particle and fibre applications alone or in combination. In addition, it is predicted that studies in which cells are loaded onto the tissue scaffold during EHD production, especially in tissue engineering applications, and studies that increase cell penetration and viability will gain momentum. In this way, these studies have the potential to succeed at developing solutions for larger tissue regeneration areas, such as full-thickness wound treatment, by increasing the layer thickness of the scaffold. One of the most important factors in this development is to increase the number of design studies in the field of industrial-scale production and to continue to attach importance to the gun assemblies developed for use in portable bedside applications. Portable EHD guns with direct application features in first aid applications are particularly useful to counter military injuries, where they can be used to stop bleeding and prevent infection. Since they do not need expert users, they have the potential to meet very important and widespread use today and in the rapidly evolving future.

5.4 The future of gyration-based manufacturing techniques

In this book, we have seen that centrifugal spinning and other gyratory techniques have worked to revolutionise the way in which fine fibres can be produced for use in a range of biomedical applications. These gyratory techniques benefit hugely from rapid rotational speeds and the ability to scale these units to meet the soaring demands of industry. We have seen how techniques such as PG and its derivatives can be used to provide additional control over the fibre morphology and enable the simple use of composite materials and additives. However, there is no such thing as a perfect system; therefore, going forward, we believe there are a number of key focal points that should be attended to in order to make this technology more suitable for mass adoption.

First, although massive strides have been made to better scale this technology for industrial adoption, until now, a number of obstacles have prevented it. This technology needs to be completely automated to reduce downtime and increase production output. In order for this to occur, there must be an element of nonhuman intervention and production management. For example, the use of robotic manufacturing and artificial intelligence systems can be incorporated to make sure that the production assembly can keep moving without distractions; robotic arms, for example, can assist with the collection of the fibres and move them to the next stage of the production line where they can be sterilised and packaged. Utilising more modern technologies, such as artificial intelligence and modelling, we can detect problems and reduce errors. For example, these technologies can be used to prevent polymer blockages, optimise working parameters, and function as predictive tools to generate the most desirable products at the lowest possible cost to the consumer. In the domain of PG, work has already begun on the use of machine learning/artificial intelligence and robotic elements in the production line to create more efficiently optimised solutions and operating parameters. Furthermore, a fully automated PG setup is currently being developed and investments made in a fully-automatic production machine.

As the biomedical landscape and its applications evolve, it is important to continue to innovate and to develop upon the current approaches in fields such as tissue engineering and drug delivery. For example, core–sheath and multilayered fibres are becoming more popular due to their superior properties in tissue engineering applications, and the development of gyratory techniques which can produce large quantities of these fibres is of significant interest for specific applications, such as healthcare, in which the active biomaterial can be contained in the sheath, e.g. in antimicrobial filters. The experience gained during the COVID-19 pandemic and the need to deliver effective antiviral masks in very large quantities has accelerated the need for such core–sheath strategies. Moving forward, tri-layered fibres with more than one core can be utilised for applications that require the release of different materials under different environmental conditions. PG-based technologies are currently being developed to address this demand; these include the ability to produce multilayered fibres made of distinct polymeric phases.

Although very significant effort has been expended on the production of polymeric products using gyratory processes, one concern which must be addressed is the environmental impact of such polymer processing. Even with the best intentions, many of these hydrophilic polymers take years to decades to degrade in compost. In addition, the use of harsh solvents creates concerns related to their long-term environmental persistence. It is therefore crucial that the selection of polymers and solvents considers sustainability. Water-soluble polymers, for example, are increasingly being adopted for gyratory-based manufacturing techniques due to their biodegradable nature and their ability to form fibres without the use of environmentally unfriendly solvents.

Overall, gyratory techniques have contributed immensely to the current healthcare landscape, but there is vast scope for improved techniques which would enable the mass adoption of gyratory techniques for the production of healthcare biomaterials discussed in this book and beyond.

www.ingramcontent.com/pod-product-compliance
Ingram Content Group UK Ltd.
Pitfield, Milton Keynes, MK11 3LW, UK
UKHW051307130926
8556IPUK00048B/733

9 780750 351850